"Finally, a book that does more than skim the surface of accountable care, and explains why it is the likely lynchpin of the coming transformation of our healthcare payment and delivery systems. Bard and Nugent provide a comprehensive and comprehensible analysis of the essential values, capabilities, and collaborative dynamics that define all viable variants of the accountable care organization. A trenchant and rich exposition that inspires as it illuminates the path to a truly patient-centered healthcare system that is rational, effective, and affordable."

–Alan D. Aviles, Chief Executive, New York City Health and Hospitals Corp.

"[This book] provides valuable information to anyone involved in accountable care development. It is an excellent resource as we transition from volume to value. The compelling point is that an ACO is not an entity, but rather a set of competencies and relationships that are foundational for transformation of care delivery."

–Joseph R. Swedish, FACHE
President and Chief Executive Officer
Trinity Health

"The last 40 years has shown that more money, more technology, and more facilities alone will not improve the health of the community and we now face the reality that reliance on money alone has lead to an economically unsustainable cost for a model of care that yields progressively poorer health outcomes for a growing number of Americans. We in the medical profession need to learn how to become more responsible stewards of the resources already in the system through better organization and delivering care that provides the best value for the patient. Accountable care organizations represent a pathway toward sustainability, and getting there starts by sharing best practices from progressive provider organizations that are already working as ACOs. Dr. Bard's years of experience with organizations like ours enable him to offer critical insights about what it takes to form a successful ACO."

–H. Eugene Lindsey, MD, President and Chief Executive Officer, Atrius Health, Newton Massachusetts

Accountable Care Organizations

Accountable Care Organizations

*Your Guide to Strategy,
Design, and Implementation*

Marc Bard and Mike Nugent

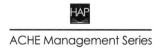

ACHE Management Series

Your board, staff, or clients may also benefit from this book's insight. For more information on quantity discounts, contact the Health Administration Press Marketing Manager at (312) 424-9470.

This publication is intended to provide accurate and authoritative information in regard to the subject matter covered. It is sold, or otherwise provided, with the understanding that the publisher is not engaged in rendering professional services. If professional advice or other expert assistance is required, the services of a competent professional should be sought.

The statements and opinions contained in this book are strictly those of the authors and do not represent the official positions of the American College of Healthcare Executives or the Foundation of the American College of Healthcare Executives.

Library of Congress Cataloging-in-Publication Data

Bard, Marc.
   Accountable care organizations : your guide to design, strategy, and implementation / Marc Bard, Michael Nugent.
      p. ; cm.
   Includes bibliographical references and index.
   ISBN 978-1-56793-415-1
   1. Medical care--United States. 2. Health care reform--United States. I. Nugent, Michael (Michael Edward) II. Title.
   [DNLM: 1. Delivery of Health Care--organization & administration--United States. 2. Health Care Reform--United States. W 84 AA1]
   RA395.A3B269 2011
   362.1'0425--dc22
                                        2010051673

The paper used in this publication meets the minimum requirements of American National Standard for Information Sciences—Permanence of Paper for Printed Library Materials, ANSI Z39.48-1984. ∞ ™

Acquisitions editor: Janet Davis; Project manager: Eduard Avis; Typesetting: Putman Productions Cover and chapter-opener illustrations: Craig Frazier. Copyright © 2011 by Craig Frazier. Exhibits: Joyce Mihran Turley.

Found an error or a typo? We want to know! Please e-mail it to hap1@ache.org, and put "Book Error" in the subject line.

For photocopying and copyright information, please contact Copyright Clearance Center at www.copyright.com or at (978) 750-8400.

Health Administration Press
A division of the Foundation of the American
   College of Healthcare Executives
One North Franklin Street, Suite 1700
Chicago, IL 60606-3529
(312) 424-2800

I would like to dedicate my share of the book to the brilliant clients whose trust and confidence have enabled me to learn and grow over the past 30 years as a consultant and whose personal friendship and good spirit have sustained me through the effort it takes to bring us together.

—*M.B.*

I would like to dedicate my portion of the book to those on the front lines of care delivery and financing—that this book can shed light on where accountability is needed most, so we can each take part in changing how the system is organized and financed to achieve the quality, access, and affordability improvements we all know exist.

—*M.N.*

Contents

Foreword

Long before provisions in the Patient Protection and Affordable Care Act of 2010 focused attention on accountable care organizations as a new model for providing care, Geisinger Health System was working to change the healthcare delivery and payment system. By capitalizing on our unique anatomy as a fully integrated and connected health services organization, we have been able to assume accountability for coordinating and organizing care to reduce variability, align incentives, decrease costs, and improve patient outcomes.

More than three million people in Pennsylvania already benefit from our efforts, but we are committed to working with healthcare leaders from across the country to find out if what we do at Geisinger can be scaled and generalized for use in other environments.

That goal is one of the reasons I am excited about Marc Bard and Mike Nugent's book, *Accountable Care Organizations: Your Guide to Strategy, Design, and Implementation.* Bard and Nugent provide functional definitions, prescriptive steps, processes, and best practices that can be adopted by almost any healthcare provider seeking to reengineer care, regardless of the organization's practice milieu.

The authors share a wealth of experience and breakthrough insights that will enable physician leaders and professional healthcare managers to improve care and lower the presently unsustainable cost trajectory. They also provide guidance on how to tap the profession-alism, creativity, and energy of our nation's doctors. This practical approach and tangible advice will be useful to every healthcare execu-tive contemplating change, because transformation is only possible with providers leading the charge.

At Geisinger, we have been blessed with a unique set of circumstances that have helped us move to the forefront of care redesign in the United States. But you don't have to be as far along the organizational or cultural curve as Geisinger to start applying the lessons of better-integrated and more accountable care. As this book shows, any provider can take steps—clinically, organizationally, and culturally—to transform care delivery, with substantial benefits for patients, payers, and the community.

Clearly, the move to accountable care will create winners and losers in the market. Healthcare providers that generate the most value—both better outcomes and cost savings—will thrive. Leaders of healthcare organizations that want to become marketplace winners in the emerging world of accountable care will get a head start by reading and learning from this book.

Glenn D. Steele Jr., MD, PhD
President and Chief Executive Officer
Geisinger Health System

Preface

Some might think it more than a little presumptuous to write a book describing how to build something that has never been built before. Indeed, to some extent, we include ourselves among those critics. The accountable care organization (ACO) today is more a *concept* than a *construct*, and as such there is no blueprint, road map, instruction manual, or recipe. What is clear at this time is that the ACO is a healthcare delivery system that will be capable of providing consistently high-quality care and service to a population of patients, satisfying them so that they prefer to obtain care from their "system," reducing the resources required to provide the care and achieve those outcomes, and operating within different delivery and reimbursement models to achieve the outcomes.

And that seems like a pretty good idea.

Those outcomes represent, in engineering terms, performance specifications. More important, they are the very sets of outcomes that the authors of this book have devoted their clinical practice and consulting careers helping organizations achieve through more effective organizational design and improved delivery. So while an ACO has technically never been designed and built before, many departments, programs, clinical service lines, organizations, and systems have been designed and built to achieve the *outcomes* intended within the accountable care organization. That experience and knowledge along with rational and bounded optimism compelled the authors to write this book.

A great deal is written about ACOs every week. Most of what has been written to date has focused on definitions, descriptions, predictions, and policy. Those are logical starting points. The goal of this book is to turn policy into pragmatics, answering the following set of crucial questions:

- What will it take to produce the outcomes necessary for success within an ACO model?
- What trade-offs must be evaluated by a healthcare provider considering an ACO strategy?
- What are the potential benefits to the stakeholders, most importantly the patients?
- What steps and actions should an organization take, and how should it accomplish them?
- What should leaders be doing to make all this happen?

Answering these questions will enable healthcare executives to bring the debate into their own organization and replaces "its" with "our."

Our primary goal, then, is to help healthcare executives consider whether the pursuit of this strategy is right for them, their organizations, and their patients. Our secondary goal is to help leaders start or advance the necessary conversations with others in their organizations and their communities: Do we have the capabilities, capacity, and commitment to make the trade-offs necessary in an ACO delivery and reimbursement system? What will it take to build the capabilities necessary for *our* success? To be sure, the ACO is *not* for every organization, every healthcare executive, every physician, or every patient. For those who believe in this model, there is reason to believe that it can work. It will be a more rational model for healthcare delivery, and represent one of many noble experiments designed to improve America's irrational healthcare ecosystem, in which organisms and entities fight for survival in a hostile environment. It is that singular hope and belief of improving healthcare delivery and outcomes that drove the authors to manage their hubris and write this book.

The book is divided into three broad sections. The first focuses on the external environmental forces that have set the stage for accountable care. The first section also describes how the ACO is currently envisioned by those setting policy and initiating design. The second section describes the design features required for success in this model, using a medical analogy of "anatomy" (structures, systems, programs, and relationships), "physiology," (functionality and processes), "sociology" (leadership and culture), economy (the economics associated with payment reform and the restructuring of the delivery of care), and information technology. Finally, the third section is devoted to an assessment process and a road map that will enable delivery system leaders to decide whether the destination is worth the journey, and for those who consider themselves ready, to begin the journey.

How to Use This Book

Starting with Chapter 2, each chapter of this book ends the same way. First is a set of questions the chapter should have provoked in the reader and that can be used to facilitate critical conversations within the organization. Second is a table organized according to the three categories of readers: (1) those *interested* in exploring ACOs, (2) those *engaged* in planning their journey, and (3) those already *committed* and on their way. For each category of readers, we supply a brief summary of the points within the chapter that are germane to that group's perspectives, along with a set of recommended actions that can be considered to advance the chapter's concepts within their own organizations.

Most important, we—and all our fellow citizens—wish you great success on that journey.

Squam Lake, New Hampshire, October 2010

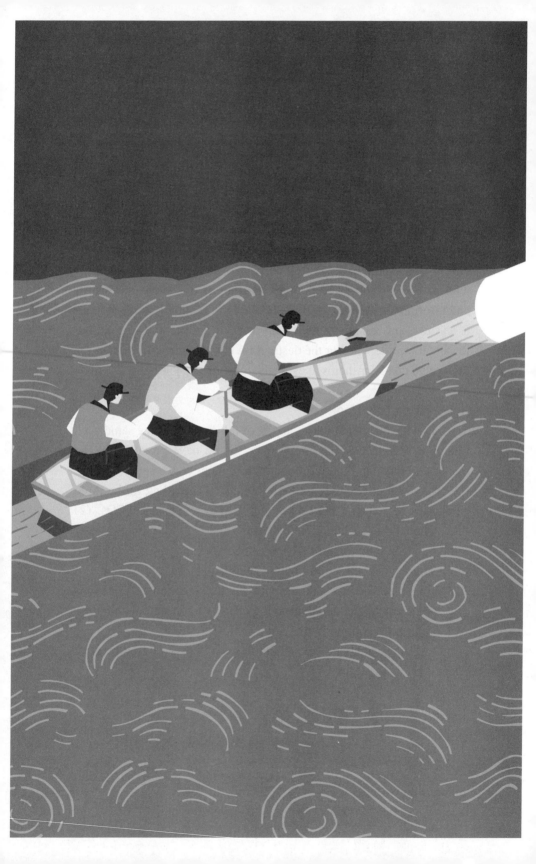

1

Setting the Stage for the ACO Strategy

We may have problems in our healthcare system, but we do have the best healthcare system in the world by far.

—Representative John Boehner (R-OH)

The Longest Day Ever

At 11:05 a.m., the emergency department (ED) at a Massachusetts hospital is starting to heat up. Only 13 of the department's 23 beds are occupied, but many of the patients are especially demanding.

"It's a very, very busy day," says the chief of emergency medicine (CEM). "We have many high-acuity psychiatric patients. The number of actual patients is quite deceptive." Since 7 a.m., the CEM has been the only physician in the unit. He is joined by two physician's assistants (PAs) and six nurses. Another physician won't arrive until after noon.

The ED feels cramped. The ceilings are low. The beds are arranged along two walls, and there isn't a good flow to the department. The CEM and his PAs are stuck in a small alcove that is barely 10 feet across. A sign on the wall says "The Batcave." Even with 10 empty beds, the ED feels crowded, in part because each of the psychiatric patients is overseen by a hospital public safety officer in a blue uniform.

Fifteen minutes later, shouts break out. A man brought in that morning for psychiatric evaluation decides he's ready to go. In his hospital gown, he dashes out of his exam room, grabs a handful of medication off a nearby cart, and sprints for one of the exits. Safety officers give chase. Making a turn for the exit, the patient grabs a wheelchair and flings it to the nearest officer. The chair smashes the officer's left hand, but she tackles the patient and sits on top of him until other officers arrive.

An hour later, she reflects on the experience: "I've been bit, kicked, punched, spit on, and scratched—and that's on a good day. But I've never had a wheelchair thrown at me before."

The incident gives the CEM a new patient to care for. He x-rays the officer's left hand and scans the images.

"I don't want to miss any work," the officer tells him. "I like my job."

But the CEM spots a tight break in the proximal phalanx of her pinky. "It's fractured," he says.

"Oh, no." The officer is upset, knowing that this injury will mean mandatory time off, even if she's only wearing a finger splint.

From the standpoint of the hospital and its parent system, the real drama is taking place down the hall in exam room 18. There, a 29-year-old Brazilian immigrant is in the middle of his second visit to the ED in four days.

The previous Friday, the man came in with an eye infection. It turned out to be mild conjunctivitis, a common childhood affliction. He was sent home with a topical antibiotic. But over the weekend, he was cleaning the eye directly with his bare fingers, inadvertently making the irritation worse. So he's wearing wraparound shades in the exam room because he is embarrassed about how his left eye looks.

This morning, the man, who works for a company that delivers home appliances, woke up with abdominal pain. He endures palpations and throat swabs as the CEM tries to determine if he has a strep infection or appendicitis.

The problem isn't the man's symptoms, which are less complex than many they see. It's that he's going to the ED for episodes that should be treated in a primary care physician's (PCP's) office. The patient says he has a PCP, but he's forgotten her name. "I don't like doctors," he says. He says he doesn't have health insurance, but that's not really the case: His chart says he's covered by the Massachusetts Health Safety Net, a mechanism put into place by the state's landmark healthcare reform law of 2006. This law has extended coverage to about 97 percent of the state's residents.

Patients who show up in the ED when they don't belong there cost the hospital money. Had the man gone to a PCP or one of the hospital's numerous clinics, his conjunctivitis could have been treated at minimal cost. The Health Safety Net reimburses the same as MassHealth, the state Medicaid program. That means the hospital is getting about 70 cents on the dollar for treating this patient.

As it turns out, the patient did the right thing this morning. A computed tomography (CT) scan shows acute appendicitis, and he is admitted for emergency surgery. But still, the hospital suffers financially: For this entire $4,700 episode, the hospital will be reimbursed only about $3,300. Other reimbursement rules also hurt the hospital.

"From the moment the patient comes into the ED to the moment he is discharged from the inpatient hospital, that is considered a single episode," explains the hospital's chief financial officer. "Whatever care he gets in the ED doesn't generate any incremental revenues for the hospital. It gets bundled into one inpatient episode of care." The hospital's parent system lost nearly $12 million in fiscal 2009 because of underpayment, as compared to costs, by the state's Health Safety Fund.

Another hour goes by in the ED. A 37-year-old man who works at the nearby college comes in with severe abdominal pain. The pain is so intense that he retches into a plastic container as he is wheeled into an examination room. A kidney stone is initially suspected. On the bed, he curls into a fetal position, writhing in pain. A CT scan shows an obstruction of the small bowel. The man is admitted for surgery.

In an adjacent bed, a 49-year-old man is waiting to be seen. He awoke the previous night with shortness of breath and pain radiating down his left arm. Because of his history of heart disease, he thinks he might be suffering another heart attack. His medical background is extraordinarily complex: cardiac disease, bouts of non-Hodgkin's lymphoma, and he is missing all his teeth due to complications from cancer treatments. The man, who previously worked at a dry cleaning shop, now lives on disability payments and was recently kicked out of his apartment.

Still, his mood is upbeat. "I have perfect blood pressure," he says. "The rest of me is falling apart, but my blood pressure is perfect." He came to the ED, which is close to his temporary home, because his primary care physician left Massachusetts two years ago, and he hasn't been able to get a new one. He's on a waiting list. "I came here because it's so close by," he says.

At 2 p.m., the CEM's physician's assistant, who has worked in the hospital ED for six years, announces to no one in particular: "This is the longest day ever. We got in here a long, long time ago."

Healthcare in America Is Not a System–It's an Ecosystem

In 2009, the battle over healthcare reform generated a seemingly endless debate on the US healthcare system. But does such a *system* even exist?

Consider, for example, a major city's municipal water system. On the supply side, the system typically consists of the following:

- a reservoir;
- a treatment plant to ensure that the supply is clean, free of contaminants, and treated with fluoride and other chemicals; and
- a network of mains, pipes, and pump stations to deliver the water under pressure into every house, business, and facility within the city.

On the waste side, there is a network of pipes and sewers to carry waste water away from millions of users; a treatment plant to eliminate or mitigate harmful and noxious elements of human waste; and a dispersal system to return treated water to the environment.

Every element in the water system is planned by the government, designed by engineers, and built to exacting standards. The average house has hundreds of connections between pipe sections that carry water under pressure. How often does one of them fail? Rarely, although the emergency call to the plumber always seems to happen frequently. Older houses often have original brass plumbing that is more than 100 years old but is still functioning.

No such system exists in US healthcare. If anything, our healthcare resembles an *ecosystem*—a defined community of living and nonliving things that work together to sustain themselves. Most natural ecosystems contain entities that play unique roles: producers, or plants, create energy from sunlight. Consumers, most of them animals, make use of that energy. And decomposers break down dead plants and animals into materials that can be reused.

Each player in the ecosystem is only concerned about its own survival. It responds to environmental changes to gain advantage for itself. In the Darwinian world of the ecosystem, each player competes with the others, seeking to expand its niche.

The US healthcare system is just such an ecosystem. Individual providers and payers all operate independently, looking out for their own success. The environment is crowded: There are many players trying to survive, and new ones constantly enter. It is also marked by scarcity: There aren't enough dollars for each player to thrive.

Consumers are another class of player in the healthcare ecosystem. For them, survival means obtaining adequate, high-quality healthcare services at a reasonable cost. They are faced with multiple, confusing choices. And the environment is also marked by scarcity: The demand for healthcare services almost always exceeds supply.

Finally, there is the government, which can effect sweeping changes in the overall environment and upset the balance between the many players.

In this ecosystem, the constant struggle for dominance and survival often perverts the real purpose for which healthcare exists. Incentives get twisted, and unintended consequences abound.

Atul Gawande (2009), a surgeon at Boston's Brigham and Women's Hospital and a staff writer for *The New Yorker*, illustrated the unintended consequences of the healthcare ecosystem in a widely discussed article published in June 2009. He looked at McAllen, Texas, a low-income community that has among the highest healthcare costs in the country. In McAllen, Medicare spending in 2006 was around $15,000 per enrollee, or around twice the national average.

After speaking with doctors, hospital executives, local businessmen, and academics, Gawande arrived at a shockingly simple conclusion: Too many doctors in McAllen had become entrepreneurs with financial stakes in how they practiced medicine. These doctors purchased diagnostic equipment so that they could profit from high reimbursements, or they became partners in for-profit institutions. Some doctors outright asked for kickbacks in exchange for referrals. As a result, patients in McAllen were getting too much medicine—too many tests, too many operations, too many days in the hospital—that showed little or no beneficial impact on health outcomes.

In one of the article's devastating quotes, a surgeon told Gawande: "There is overutilization here, pure and simple. [In the past 15 years] the way to practice medicine has changed completely. Before it was about how to do a good job. Now it is about 'How much will you benefit?'"

Is this bad behavior? Not for an ecosystem; each player in the ecosystem looks to exploit opportunities to grow and thrive at the expense of the others. But it's definitely bad medicine.

Gawande concludes, "The lesson of the high-quality, low-cost communities is that someone has to be accountable for the totality of care. Otherwise, you get a system that has no brakes. You get McAllen."

Birth of the US Healthcare System

Schoolboys were once taught that baseball, the national pastime, was invented by Abner Doubleday in 1839 in Cooperstown, New York. That tale has since been dismissed as myth; Doubleday may never have set foot in Cooperstown. The actual origins of the game are much more complex and less romantic. One unattractive fact is that baseball probably descended from popular British folk games such as stool ball, cricket, and rounders.

The origins of the US healthcare system are similarly shrouded in myth, with the actual truth being a little less appealing. On its website, Blue Cross Blue Shield of Massachusetts (2010) says it was originally created in 1937 "by a group of community-minded business leaders" to "spread the cost of hospital treatment among a large group of employed persons." The actual origins of group health insurance in the United States are a little less quaint.

In the nineteenth century, many hospitals were essentially shelters where the sick or dying poor were cared for; these shelters were often supported by churches or other religious organizations. In the early twentieth century, medical science advanced, and hospital care became more expensive. In what has become a common refrain 100 years later, hospital administrators searched for ways to pay for the resource-intensive innovations that were revolutionizing care.

Baylor University Hospital in Dallas, Texas, was one of those institutions struggling to pay for care. A university official—Justin Ford Kimball—devised a scheme in which a group could make affordable monthly payments (50 cents to start with) in exchange for 21 days of free care at the hospital. The plan was marketed to teachers, and they signed up in droves.

The American Hospital Association (AHA) popularized the idea in other parts of the country. By 1935, there were 15 similar hospital insurance plans. The AHA created the Hospital Service Association, which became a trade group for the nascent health insurance industry, codifying rules, setting standards, and lobbying state and federal regulators.

But where did the Blue Cross come from? An official at an early insurance plan in St. Paul, Minnesota, put a blue cross on his stationery and later used it on a poster. The symbol was powerful, and the name caught on. In 1939, the Hospital Service Association officially adopted the Blue Cross name for its plans.

However, the most important events that shaped the development of the United States's unique system of employer-based healthcare were the result of a series of historical accidents, rather than any government or industry plan.

In the middle of World War II, much of the US labor force had joined the military. That left private companies scrambling for fewer job applicants. Left unchecked, supply and demand would ensure that salaries rose, as those companies competed for scarce labor. Rather than risk unchecked inflation, the Roosevelt administration put national wage controls in place.

But there was a loophole. Fringe benefits, such as healthcare coverage, were exempt from the wage controls. So companies began offering health plans as a way of enticing workers. In 1943, the Internal Revenue Service ruled that healthcare benefits should be exempt from income taxes. A later ruling strengthened the tax advantages. Ever since, the US healthcare system has tied healthcare coverage for those of working age to one's job. South Africa was one of the few other countries that adopted a similar system. Among industrialized nations, the United States became an outlier in this regard.

The history of the US healthcare system was a source of significant irony in the national debate on healthcare reform in 2009 and 2010. Opponents of reform frequently declared that the United States has the best healthcare system in the world, and any effort to change it would be tantamount to socializing medicine and would lead to a government takeover. Those positions ignored the fact that it was a socially minded president—Franklin D. Roosevelt—and a series of socially focused rulings during World War II that created the current system that is deemed to be "the best." Few politicians who espoused the superiority of the US system would support the wage controls that led to that system.

The Long, Slow Rise and Rapid Decline of Managed Care Plans

Blue Cross plans became a sort of gold standard for healthcare coverage. As traditional insurance indemnity plans, they paid for everything; there were few exclusions. If you had Blue Cross or another managed care plan, your healthcare costs were fixed. You just had to pay the premiums or premium contributions that were not covered by your employer.

Little surprise, then, that healthcare turned out to be expensive. A major response to the rising costs in the 1980s and 1990s was the growth of managed care plans. Payers found that shortening hospital stays, moving patients from hospitals to ambulatory settings, and limiting access to specialists saved money.

Employers, eager to control rising health insurance expenses for workers, embraced the new approach. Between 1984 and 1993, the percentage of employees in large firms enrolled in managed care plans increased from 5 percent to 50 percent (Lagoe, Aspling, and Westert 2005). State and local governments also jumped on the bandwagon.

The intention of managed care plans was to control costs by managing utilization, the mix of services provided, and unit reimbursement. In retrospect, it more-or-less worked, at least for a time. The annual increase in per capita healthcare spending in the United States fell to about 2 percent from 1994 to 1996, which was less than the rate of inflation. Growth in healthcare premiums also slowed, but at the cost of increasing tension, divisiveness, and dispirit among providers at every level of healthcare delivery.

But managed care plans were perhaps too successful for their own good. It turns out that healthcare consumers didn't like being told where they could and could not go and what procedures would and would not be covered. Horror stories arose of patients dying because specialized care was denied by pencil-pushing insurers. There were also tales of insurance companies using red tape and delay tactics to avoid paying patient claims. Lawsuits proliferated, many of which attained class-action status that represented thousands of plaintiffs. "Managed care" became a dirty word among consumers. Doctors also rebelled, angered because they believed accountants and actuaries were telling them how to practice medicine. In fact, there would have been a great deal that each party could have learned from the other if the system had been managed differently. But, unfortunately, there was no system to manage.

The inevitable backlash came in the late 1990s. Health plans loosened their grip on utilization, and patients used more healthcare services. In an ironic throwback to the 1940s, companies offered richer benefit plans to attract employees. The economy was in the midst of the longest post-war expansion ever, and firms could afford to spend more on healthcare. Consumers also enjoyed a period of prosperity, with a steady increase in income for middle-class families. They could handle premiums that began to rise more each year.

By the early 2000s, medical inflation had rebounded, and the media reported each year on double-digit premium increases for consumers. Soon, politicians and policymakers started calling the annual increases "unsustainable." (The claim was somewhat weakened by the fact that the same script replayed each summer, as health plans set their premiums for upcoming open-enrollment periods.)

There were renewed efforts to control costs. "Consumer-driven healthcare" was an Orwellian euphemism for shifting costs to patients through increased out-of-pocket costs such as co-pays and deductibles. The basic thought behind the movement was that patients consumed too much healthcare because insurance shielded them from the true costs of their healthcare purchases. With more "skin in the game," the thinking went, patients would make more careful decisions. In essence, they would begin to behave more like shoppers in a clothing store, buying lots of high-value items and carefully evaluating special or designer purchases.

The Bush administration promoted the consumer-driven approach with proposals for health savings accounts and other mechanisms for patients to accumulate money to pay for out-of-pocket healthcare expenses. They never really caught on. In retrospect, it seems unreasonable to assume that Americans, who have nearly the lowest savings rate among citizens of industrialized nations, would suddenly start putting money away for unexpected medical expenses. Moreover, the Bush economic recovery wasn't long or sustained, and the income gap between the upper class and the middle and lower classes expanded to record levels. Middle-class families never achieved a feeling of prosperity that might have promoted greater savings. Many people binged on credit and depended on the real-estate bubble to support spending beyond their means.

The lack of a unified approach, let alone a successful technique for controlling healthcare costs in the first decade of the 2000s, set the stage for a new idea that might achieve the seemingly contradictory goals of controlling costs while improving patient outcomes.

That idea seems to be accountable care organizations. This idea is discussed fully in the chapters that follow.

Inconvenient Truths

All hospitals are unique. Each provides a different mix of clinical care, teaching, and research. Each has a different relationship with doctors and other caregivers. Cambridge Health Alliance (CHA) is unique among hospital systems in Massachusetts. It is nominally an instrument of the Cambridge Public Health Commission, making it the only public acute care health system in the state. At the same time, CHA's hospitals are a few of a handful of true "safety net" hospitals in the state. Safety net hospitals serve concentrations of urban poor who have nowhere else to go for care. These patient populations lead to poor payer mixes, with a predominance of Medicare, Medicaid, and state-subsidized care; relatively few of these patients have private insurance. Thirty percent of the people in CHA's primary service areas have incomes of less than 200 percent of the federal poverty level (about $20,000 a year) and are not native English speakers. The system spends $6 million a year just on interpreters, with Portuguese, Spanish, and Haitian Creole being the predominant foreign languages.

Several circumstances make CHA's difficult mission tougher than that of other safety net providers in Massachusetts. After being formed in 1996, CHA was asked by the state to take over two troubled safety net hospitals. The system took over Somerville Hospital, located in a densely populated, relatively poor city that neighbors Cambridge, in 1996 and took over Whidden Memorial Hospital in blue-collar Everett in 2001. The takeovers saved the two institutions from being closed. CHA also acquired numerous neighborhood health clinics and school-based health centers as well as four facilities with a significant number of psychiatric beds.

But now the system contains three safety net hospitals, each an underperformer in terms of reimbursement. The uninsured made up 23 percent of the system's patients in 2006, prior to the state's health reform law. Medicaid accounted for another 25 percent. Both percentages were the highest among the state's community hospitals.

In addition, CHA contains the state's top two acute care providers of psychiatric care, which devote nearly 200 beds to behavioral health. Psychiatric care is among the worst paying specialties in the United States. So CHA is saddled with additional revenue shortfalls, even as it is tasked with providing almost the entire psychiatric safety net for metropolitan Boston. Before the Massachusetts healthcare reform, CHA provided one-third of the mental health inpatient care for the uninsured in the state.

The Perfect Storm

All that was before the financial storm hit. When Dennis Keefe, the chief executive officer of CHA, looks back over the past three years, his naturally serious demeanor softens somewhat and a look of resignation comes over his face.

"It was the perfect storm," he says of the forces that converged and pushed his hospital system from a nearly $14 million surplus in fiscal 2006 to a $25 million loss in fiscal 2009. "The perfect storm" is an overused expression, but it isn't mere hyperbole in this case. A set of unexpected forces came together in a way that no one could have foreseen, creating a fiscal maelstrom that came close to capsizing CHA.

In 2006, it looked as if CHA was about to turn the corner financially and enter an unusually prosperous period. In April of that year, then-Governor Mitt Romney signed the Massachusetts healthcare reform bill into law. Despite his efforts later as a presidential candidate to distance himself from the law, Romney played a lead role in crafting what was a progressive and ultimately successful effort to extend health coverage to nearly all Massachusetts residents.

"We actually felt we had things under control and headed in the right direction," recalls Keefe. "We were optimistic that the new administration of Governor Deval Patrick was coming in."

Before the reform effort, hospitals treated patients who walked in their doors regardless of whether they had insurance. Hospitals that incurred unpaid medical debt were reimbursed from the Uncompensated

Care Pool, essentially a fund created by the state in 1985 to ensure that all residents received care regardless of their ability to pay. It is funded by insurers, who contribute to the pool each year. (And how did the insurers meet this obligation? Essentially by raising rates on those who purchased insurance, creating another cross-subsidization within the ecosystem.)

Under the health reform law, previously uninsured Massachusetts residents were expected to buy low-cost commercial insurance or subsidized government-insurance plans. Hospitals and health systems, like CHA, would no longer be burdened by a huge number of uninsured patients. Moreover, as residents became covered, they might move to other caregivers, secure in the knowledge that they would be treated. Fewer patients would show up in the emergency department seeking routine treatment. That could ultimately give CHA, which relied on government payment for 73 percent of its revenues, a better payer mix.

It didn't work out that way. The world credit markets froze in the fall of 2007. Some of Wall Street's largest financial institutions failed. The stock market plunged, and home prices began their inevitable fall back to Earth. The Massachusetts economy was in crisis. A year later, with tax revenues falling and deficits looming, Governor Deval Patrick did the only thing he could: He imposed Draconian cuts.

Under state rules, the governor is allowed to make discretionary cuts in the state budget that has already been implemented. CHA was allotted $94 million for fiscal year 2008, which began on July 1. But in October of that year, under Governor Patrick's prerogative to impose the so-called 9C cuts, he cut $40 million of the allotment. CHA struggled to cope with the loss of nearly 10 percent of its annual operating budget of $450 million.

Keefe recalls that the bad news was delivered in a phone call from Dr. Judy Ann Bigby, the secretary of Massachusetts Executive Office of Health and Human Services. Forty million of the more than $90 million promised by the state, she told Keefe, "would not be forthcoming." Keefe recalls, "I told everyone at the time, 'We're four months into our fiscal year. There's no way we can deal with this!'"

It got worse. Under the new Health Safety Net payment system, Medicare outpatient rates for the system dropped precipitously, from $376.73 per visit in fiscal year 2008 to $311.31 per visit in fiscal 2010. CHA, with 300 beds, has about 17,000 annual discharges. But between its ambulatory care, primary care, and neighborhood health clinics, CHA sees about 660,000 ambulatory visits a year. So the Medicare cuts were especially hurtful to the system.

"A significant portion of the free care we give is through our neighborhood clinics," says Gordon Boudrow, CHA's chief financial officer. "Medicare pays poorly, and 70 percent of our uncompensated care is through the ambulatory setting. It reduces our aggregate rate." The total hit was about $12 million a year in unreimbursed costs because of the rate cuts. It didn't stop there. Medicaid inpatient reimbursement per case also dropped dramatically, from $5,541.53 in fiscal 2008 to $4,726.92 in fiscal 2010, which are lower than the rates from 10 years earlier, in fiscal 1998, before any adjustment for inflation.

Finally, none of the anticipated benefits from Massachusetts's healthcare reform materialized. Even when they had insurance and the ability to choose any provider, CHA patients proved remarkably loyal to the system. Between the implementation of the healthcare reform law in 2006 and June 2009, the proportion of the system's low-income patients and government-paid payer mix actually increased, which was the opposite of what was expected.

Allison Bayer, the system's chief operating officer, sums up what happened this way: "Under health reform, the state made a commitment to improve access and cover as many people as possible. Dollars that used to be allocated to the Uncompensated Care Pool (now known as the Health Safety Net Trust Fund) were redistributed; many of those dollars now go towards premium payments to enable more residents to have coverage. The underlying assumption around healthcare reform was that if you provide access and coverage for many more people, then there's no more need for safety net institutions like ours."

As for the newly insured patients who could now go anywhere they wanted? "In the past, they didn't have much choice," says Bayer. "Now, they could go anywhere. But that didn't happen. People stayed with us.

It's great for continuity of care. But those patients didn't disappear, so we continue to have a large proportion of care that reimburses below cost." The loyalty of patients was a great endorsement of the quality of care CHA delivered. But it also devastated the system's bottom line.

The final part of the financial storm was the recession itself. Like many hospital systems, CHA saw a drop in volume. Was it because of the patients who had lost jobs and could no longer afford co-pays and deductibles? Or was it because of the patients who were afraid of losing their jobs so they put off elective procedures in order to not lose time from work? For whatever reason, Cambridge Health Alliance hospitals had more empty beds. The choices were grim.

The Healthcare Ecosystem Weakens

Despite double-digit premium increases, millions of uninsured, and endless complaints from businesses that couldn't compete globally because of high healthcare costs, the healthcare ecosystem managed to muddle through. But there were increasing warning signs that the healthcare system was changing for the worse. Some called the situation a death spiral.

Decrease in Employer-Based Insurance Coverage

The most notable sign was the breakdown of the employer-based system. Companies increasingly found ways to avoid the costs of providing healthcare for their employees. Some shifted costs to employees, who had to pick up ever larger portions of premiums. Others found ways to categorize more workers as independent contractors, who weren't entitled to health coverage and other benefits. Finally, an increasing number just got out of the healthcare-providing business altogether, leaving employees to find coverage elsewhere.

The percentage of workers under age 65 (when citizens become eligible for Medicare coverage) has declined steadily for years. Among younger workers, the percentage has dropped even more quickly: In 2000, 67.7 percent of nonelderly Americans had employment-based health insurance. By 2009, the percentage had dropped to 55.8 percent, according to the US Census Bureau (2010).

This decline has been exacerbated by the process of adverse selection. All things being equal, older or sicker workers are more likely to purchase health insurance because they know they need it. Younger or healthier workers, on the other hand, are more likely to put off the expense because they think they don't need it. So insurance companies typically get a self-selecting group of ratepayers who are sicker than the overall population. That means healthcare costs cannot be spread across a healthier group, and premiums must rise to provide the extra care for the sicker population, which in turn drives more healthy people away.

Paul Krugman and Robin Wells (2006) reported that a form of adverse selection was under way in the workplace. Workers with health problems specifically sought jobs that provided generous health benefits. In the process, they made it more expensive for those firms to continue to provide health coverage.

The Medicare Part D Doughnut Hole

At the same time, the federal government passed the Medicare Prescription Drug Improvement and Modernization Act of 2003 (called Medicare Part D). This act highlighted the growing disarray within the ecosystem. Most everyone agreed that providing coverage for drugs for seniors was a huge step forward and would prevent the tragic situations where the poor elderly had to choose between buying food and buying medication. But as designed, Medicare Part D turned into a wasteful, complex mess.

The actual drug coverage was provided by insurance companies and not by the government, which added to administrative costs. The act specifically prohibited the government from negotiating drug prices with the pharmaceutical companies. So the potential savings of buying in bulk for millions was eliminated. And seniors were faced with literally dozens of plans to compare, an onerous task even for younger, computer-savvy caregivers. The federal government touted this plethora of choices as a benefit. But as economists have noted, consumers faced with too many choices often find themselves unable to make a decision.

Meantime, the benefit itself was flawed because of the infamous "doughnut hole." After paying a $310 deductible, seniors were given 75 percent coverage of all their prescription drug costs until they had reached $2,830 in costs. Then, after the $2,830 limit, they had to pay all costs out of their own pocket until costs reached $6,440. At that point, "catastrophic coverage" from the government kicked in, paying 95 percent of drug costs.

The system was and still is confusing, and it has angered many seniors who rightly thought that "prescription drug coverage" meant prescription drug coverage, yet found themselves paying full cost for their drugs when they fell into the payment gap.

It became harder and harder for the government, insurance company executives, or providers to pretend that the ecosystem was providing healthcare efficiently or yielding optimal medical outcomes. The destructive forces within the ecosystem were becoming clear to everyone.

The Long and Winding Road to Healthcare Reform

The fight for universal coverage and healthcare market reform didn't begin in 1994, when Bill and Hillary Clinton launched an effort to pass the Health Security Act. The plan ultimately failed because of its own shortcomings and political miscalculations on the part of the White House. The drama of that vicious battle weakened the Clinton administration for years.

Today's health reform is largely a case of déjà vu all over again, so to speak.

An early effort in the 1920s failed. In 1945, shortly after Harry Truman became president, he sought to pass a universal health plan "to assure the right to adequate medical care and protection from the economic fears of sickness" (Harry S. Truman Presidential Library n.d.). It was opposed by the American Medical Association and the drug industry. Inevitably, it was labeled "socialistic." Truman tried again after his reelection in 1948 but was again blocked by Congress.

In 1965, Lyndon Johnson passed Medicare and Medicaid as part of his Great Society program. But medical coverage for the elderly and indigent still left millions of Americans without insurance.

The next attempt was an effort of two Republican presidents: Richard Nixon and Gerald Ford. Nixon announced a plan for universal coverage in his 1974 State of the Union address. It was quickly forgotten when the Watergate scandal enveloped the administration. Gerald Ford, upon succeeding Nixon, championed national health insurance. It was blocked by insurance lobbyists and by labor leaders. (The unions were miffed by Senator Ted Kennedy [D-MA] because Kennedy introduced his own universal coverage plan in 1974 but didn't consult with organized labor.)

President Obama's Attempts at Reform

The debate over comprehensive healthcare reform in the United States gave politicians and pundits of all stripes an opportunity to promote all sorts of half-truths and mischaracterizations about American healthcare and the government's efforts. Perhaps the most ludicrous example of how this dialogue was hijacked was the pernicious misrepresentation that President Obama's healthcare plan would create "death panels" who would meet and vote on whom should be given or denied care. This story was started by Obama's opponents and repeated endlessly by the right-wing media establishment, giving it the semblance of reality. The mainstream media perpetuated this misrepresentation by including references in their reports about these alleged death panels, sowing fear among the public that healthcare reform would reduce access to care.

The incident illustrates the difficulty of having an informed discussion about such a fraught policy area. It completely eliminated the possibility of a meaningful discussion about current, let alone future, healthcare rationing in America. Members of both political parties were unwilling to talk about the reality of rationing out of fear that doing so might be misconstrued as support for rationing. But any physician or hospital official could easily describe how healthcare is already rationed because it is unattainable for many without government-sponsored or employer-based insurance.

From June 2009 through March 2010, as the White House and then the Democrats lost control of the healthcare debates, reform opponents clung to perhaps the most insidious falsehood about the US healthcare system: that it is the best in the world.

The Quality of US Healthcare

By any rational measure, US healthcare isn't the best in the world. It often ranks as the worst system of any major industrial nation. The Commonwealth Fund, the New York–based nonpartisan foundation that promotes better healthcare in the United States, issues an annual survey that compares the US healthcare system with those of other developed nations. The results are predictably miserable.

In its latest report, The Commonwealth Fund (2010a) states that despite spending the most per capita on healthcare—$7,290 in 2007, or 16 percent of the country's gross domestic product—the nation lagged behind Germany, Canada, the Netherlands, New Zealand, Australia, and the United Kingdom in almost all measures of medical outcome: "The US is last on dimensions of access, patient safety, coordination, efficiency and equity." It is apparent that the United States is slow in adopting national policies that promote primary care, quality improvement, and information technology.

These results, which show up in a slew of studies, should be familiar to all healthcare executives. Among 30 countries that belong to the Organisation for Economic Co-operation and Development (OECD) (2010), the United States was second worst in premature female mortality (with Hungary being first) and was fourth worst in measures of premature male mortality. Life expectancy rates were lower in the United States than in most industrialized nations, and the country also lags in measures of infant mortality (Commonwealth Fund 2010b).

Moreover, US patients experienced more safety problems than patients in other OECD countries. The United States came in last in a study of chronically or intensively ill patients in eight countries, with more than one in three American patients reporting errors in drug choice or dosage, medical errors, or delays in getting abnormal test results (OECD 2010).

Finally, 46 million American residents, or 16 percent of the population, are uninsured, making the United States one of only three

OECD countries (along with Mexico and Turkey) that have a large proportion of their population with no medical coverage. That will change under the Patient Protection and Affordable Care Act of 2010 (PPACA), but it will take years to reach its target. Even after full implementation of the PPACA in 2019, an estimated 23 million US residents will still lack healthcare coverage.

"The measures of US health, including life expectancy, infant mortality, and deaths preventable by medical care, remain mediocre compared to other rich nations," note Jonathan Oberlander and Theodore Marmor (2010) in the *New York Review of Books*. "At the same time, American medical care is notoriously the most expensive in the world. Premiums for family coverage under employer-sponsored insurance now average over $13,000 a year. Expenditures on health care in the United States amount to more than $2.5 trillion, or about 17 percent of national income, while Western European democracies average about 10 percent."

Despite these glaring deficiencies, reform opponents stuck to their script. "We may have problems in our healthcare system, but we do have the best healthcare system in the world by far," said Senator John Boehner, the Ohio Republican and Senate minority leader. "Having a government takeover of healthcare is a dangerous experiment that I don't think we should do with the best healthcare system in the world."

Emerging from the Jaws of Defeat

President Obama accomplished through a parliamentary maneuver what former presidents had tried to do for 60 years. The House adopted a version of the Senate bill, and then both chambers passed a reconciliation act that provides the final passage. (This only required 51 votes in the Senate, denying the chance for a filibuster.)

An immediate attack on the PPACA's constitutionality was launched, and vows to repeal the bill were made. But by mid-summer, the repeal effort had lost steam. Many think the theory that the federal government had somehow infringed states' rights in the PPACA was flawed to begin with. As the dust settled, many began to look again at what the health reform law actually contained. And what it contained didn't seem worth all the fuss.

The PPACA is moderate, is limited in scope, and builds substantially on the existing US healthcare system. The ecosystem isn't in immediate danger, although some changes in the environment will certainly, over time, favor some species and provide challenges for others.

More than anything, the PPACA looks a lot like Massachusetts's 2006 healthcare reform bill. The PPACA extends coverage to about 30 million people. It does not threaten private insurance companies with a government-sponsored health plan—the so-called "public option" that Democrats deemed unwinnable. And it contains a lot of small but significant measures that help the average American consumer obtain and pay for health coverage.

Exhibit 1.1 shows some of the details of the PPACA, several of which have already been enacted in late September 2010.

From Financial Catastrophe to Market Leader: CHA Looks to the Accountable Care Organization

When the shock from the Massachusetts governor's 9C cuts faded in late 2008, CHA tried to find a way forward after 22 percent of its future operating revenues had been swept away. The system hired an outside consultant to perform a sweeping assessment and to recommend cost-cutting measures that wouldn't endanger its long-term survival.

The cuts went deep, and they included the following:

- Shutting all inpatient services at the Somerville Hospital campus, one of the system's three main facilities
- Reducing headcount by 447 FTEs (full-time equivalents) out of 3,200
- Shedding 35 adult mental health beds and 26 addictions beds
- Reducing outpatient mental health services by 20 percent
- Consolidating six primary care sites, four specialty clinics, and a dental clinic with other facilities

Employees who remained also took a hit. Executives and physician leaders gave back 9 percent in compensation, and all managers reduced annual time off by five days, saving $1 million annually.

Employees' share of health insurance premiums also increased, and salaries were frozen for fiscal 2010.

But the more CEO Keefe and his team worked at keeping the system afloat, the more obvious the shortcomings of the existing business model became. Cost cutting, consolidation, or revenue cycle improvement did not change the fundamental problem that faced CHA: Reimbursements didn't cover costs for most services, and there were no high-profit service lines that could cross-subsidize the system's money-losing operations. All the usual steps to enhance revenues made Keefe feel more and more like a hamster running on a spinning wheel, working hard but not getting anywhere. His doctors felt the same way.

"When you talk to physicians about this, you find out they are so tired of the current treadmill of increasing productivity, making their targeted numbers of office visits, and generating income," says Keefe. "They've completely lost the whole context of why they're in medicine in the first place."

Another state effort moved CHA in another direction, however. A commission established by Therese Murray, president of the State Senate, undertook a study of healthcare payments in Massachusetts. In early 2010, the commission recommended a course of action that was as bold as Governor Romney's healthcare reform had been four years earlier. The commission said the state should move from a fee-for-service payment scheme to one of global payments. Capitation was coming back. Keefe participated in focus groups for the payment reform commission. He told people he was ready for change.

"Right now," Keefe says, "we're at the bottom of the food chain. We're severely handicapped by fee-for-service. Global payments? Bring it on. If you greatly benefit from the current system, you don't want it to change. The gap between the haves and the have-nots has become greater. The whole payment system needs to be fixed."

The solution, Keefe concludes, was not just to change the medical payments but also to move his entire healthcare system to an accountable care organization (ACO) built around a medical home model.

CHA, he says, has most of the pieces to become a functioning ACO, including the following:

- Two secondary care hospitals
- A salaried physician organization
- Neighborhood clinics that function as feeders to the hospitals
- A relatively advanced electronic medical record system that is fully implemented for ambulatory care
- An in-house health insurer—Network Health—that already serves as a capitated payer for a significant portion of CHA's patients

"We're rethinking what a hospital really is," says Keefe. "We want to become a virtual high-performing ACO and then adopt more of an ACO structure."

Despite having so many pieces of the puzzle, COO Bayer says turning CHA into a real ACO won't be easy: "Physicians and other care providers don't have historical experience working as a care team to focus on managing the patient. In the current fee-for-service system, it's all about making the appointment, getting the patient in, getting the charge out, and getting the money back. We, as a system, are still paid per click. That hasn't changed yet. But we're trying to restructure the system before the payment system changes. We're moving forward.

"We've got smart, talented, creative people who work here, but they're limited by the transactional environment that exists in healthcare," Bayer adds. "They're stifled and trapped in the current system. They know how to design care that works, but the system doesn't allow it. They're demoralized. They're laboring under perverse incentives that deny needed care and encourage care that isn't needed. The ACO is our opportunity to deliver a rational system of healthcare."

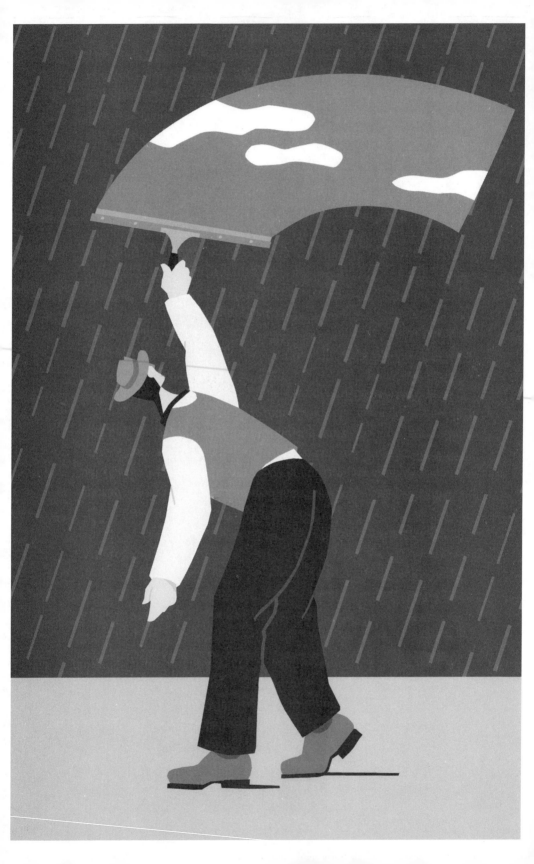

2

The Accountable Care Organization

This has been a journey that has required an "all-in" leadership commitment. No dabbling in an ACO.... This model fundamentally changes the way we do business. This journey is not for the timid; it is full of risk and potential obstacles, but it is the necessary path for us to fulfill our core mission of providing exemplary healthcare with access for all in our community. It puts us into a full partnership with our medical staff.

—Judy Rich
President and Chief Executive Officer
Tucson Medical Center/TMC Healthcare, ACO Pilot Site

Only a few pages—four to be precise—of the Patient Protection and Affordable Care Act of 2010 (PPACA) are devoted to the development and deployment of the accountable care organization (ACO). Other than Medicare rate regulation, no other issue within the PPACA has stirred more interest, passion, and imagination among healthcare providers than the ACO.

But what exactly is an ACO? It's hard to say. There are three ACO pilot projects in development, but none is fully operational at this time. Many feel that describing an ACO is like the familiar parable about the three blind people and the elephant. One touches the trunk and says the elephant is a snake. Another touches a leg and says the elephant is a pillar. And another touches the ear and says it is a fan. Of course, they are all right. And they are also all wrong.

It's much easier to say what an ACO is not.

Contrary to common perception, an ACO is not an entity. Calling it an *organization* is, in many respects, a misnomer. It is really a *system*. The actual entity is the integrated delivery system (IDS), whether it is traditional or a new model. The IDS enters into an agreement with the Centers for Medicare & Medicaid Services (CMS) and, presumably in the future, with other nongovernment payers to deliver care to a population of patients. Then, as long as the IDS achieves predetermined quality outcomes, it shares in any savings generated by its clinical effectiveness and operating efficiencies. So the ACO is really an umbrella financial and clinical care delivery redesign *strategy* that uses fee-for-service, pay-for-performance, bundled payments, and partial or full-risk capitation tactics to improve quality and efficiency.

Various ACO Perspectives and Interpretations

Those looking at the ACO today can only see part of the whole, because many of the requirements, regulations, and policies that govern the ACO have not yet been established. And many project what they want to see onto the four ambiguous pages of the PPACA (2010):

- Those passionate about clinical quality improvement see the ACO as a means to achieve their goals.
- Those driven by the need for greater efficiency and cost management see the ACO as a potential pathway to that end.
- Those seeking improvements in population management see the ACO as a potential step in the right direction.
- Those focused on physician development and alignment see the ACO as an opportunity to achieve those goals.

The ACO lives at the complicated intersection of all four of these perspectives. The ACO will eventually succeed through the successful integration of all four.

Three different strategies to adopt the ACO are emerging for provider organizations interested in learning more about ACO opportunities or already committed to the new approach. Each strategy is based on an interpretation of the ACO.

1. The first interpretation places the emphasis on *accountable* and sees the ACO as a movement or way of being, just as the environmentally minded do in trying to reduce their carbon footprints. For these interpreters—either healthcare organizations or their leaders—accountability is imminently supportable and far superior to the current healthcare system, which fails to link payment to performance in any meaningful way. For many of these interpreters, there is enough clarity about what the ACO will be that they support it emotionally. But there is not enough clarity to make the investment and take meaningful action. In short, these interpreters are *interested* but far from committed.

2. The second interpretation places the emphasis on *care* and uses the ACO to set the organization's compass. The ACO sets a direction for a journey without a clear end. While still not completely tangible, the current understanding on the part of these interpreters is that accountable care focuses primarily on clinical integration and coordination. For them, the linkages to value-based purchasing of care are clear enough to be able to set a general direction and start the journey. If the first category of interpretation describes those who are interested, this second category describes those who are *engaged* in making the ACO a reality. Those who support this interpretation appreciate the value proposition of care integration across all dimensions. Ultimately, the laboratory for innovation will be in the overall integration and coordination of care and how that integration gets translated into new reimbursement strategies. For those who set their compasses, the driving motivation appears to be a desire to be in the pole position when the initial ACO implementation rules and regulations are finally promulgated by the federal government. This could happen anytime before 2012. For many of these

interpreters, the designated CMS Center for Innovation will be the real pot of innovative "gold" at the end of the ACO rainbow.

3. The third interpretation places the emphasis on *organization*. Those who interpret the ACO in this way see the new care delivery and financing model as a life raft amid a rising tide of real and immediate financial, competitive, and operational threats. For these interpreters, the ACO is a true competitive destination and one to which they are *committed* before the system takes on any more water. Many of our nation's safety net and public hospitals, particularly those that provide relatively lower acuity care, face financial and operational challenges that cannot be solved operating in the current healthcare ecosystem, where reimbursement depends almost exclusively on independent, disconnected transactions. Like Cambridge Health Alliance (discussed in Chapter 1), they cannot survive under the current fee-for-service reimbursement system.

The CMS Strategy

Despite the fact that the entirety of the ACO description is limited to pages 277–281 of the PPACA, CMS has adopted a relatively clear strategy for creating the first ACO. CMS is promoting a series of noble experiments by well-intentioned and thoughtful people and organizations. Transforming the "nonsystem" into a system of care is fraught with complexity, resistance, trade-offs, and likely missteps along the way. But CMS understands that to accomplish this through the establishment of policy is like trying to perform delicate vascular surgery using a carving knife. By sponsoring pilots and promoting experiments, CMS will tease out the elements of success as the ACO strategy is adopted more widely.

To date, CMS has specified a limited number of design principles for the ACO. It appears as if CMS's intention is to rely on the innovative potential present in local, regional, and national healthcare delivery systems to design organized systems of care around those principles. At the present time, CMS is debating whether to establish regulations that will make only those with a high likelihood of success eligible to play or regulations that will enable many others to enter the fray as well. In similar fashion, CMS is debating the merits and liabilities of regulations to ensure that all those who participate "win," none of those who participate "lose," or some balance between the two.

We believe that the strategy is best served by ensuring that all the emerging ACO systems be based on a common set of principles, a common DNA. If designed around common core principles, emerging ACOs will have enough similarities to better evaluate what it takes to make an organized system of care work. There will also be enough differences to learn what elements offer greater or lesser benefit. In brief, it appears that CMS is supporting an experimental process in which the elements that make an ACO succeed are derived from creative but bounded experimentation. Over time, systems should gravitate toward common successful elements of a system of care without any one party (governments, health plans, or others) being forced to take full ownership of the process.

Transforming the Current Healthcare Nonsystem

T. R. Reid's (2009) examination of alternative national healthcare systems reinforces the observation that there is no perfect or best national healthcare model. Each system is an imperfect work in progress based on a rational and supportable set of principles, trade-offs, and choices. The challenge is in transforming an existing system to another. Still, the fact remains that several industrialized nations have successfully achieved that transformation. The most striking point in Reid's book is that what *most* differentiates the US healthcare system from those in other industrialized nations is the complete absence of anything resembling an organized system. The other striking point is that the United States is the only industrialized nation that does not recognize access to healthcare as a right of citizenship but rather sees it as a privilege of wealth.

Similarly, Atul Gawande (2009), in his recent article in *The New Yorker*, shows how Great Britain, France, Switzerland, and the United States all developed their unique healthcare systems by building on the circumstances at hand—something that social scientists call *path dependence*. The ACO is an attempt to free the US healthcare nonsystem from some of the burdens it carries because it took shape largely as a result of historical accidents. The ACO is intended to create an organized system of care that can, over time, evolve to provide a high level of care to every American as a right rather than as a privilege. The challenge is that it is much harder to modify a system that is already treating a population than to start from scratch. Unlike a restaurant that can close overnight for renovations, American healthcare cannot temporarily shut its doors during its renovation process.

What Is an ACO?

The term *ACO* is attributed to Glenn Hackbarth, chair of MedPAC, and Elliott Fisher, director of The Center for Health Policy Research at Dartmouth College. One of the first descriptions of the ACO appeared in the *New England Journal of Medicine* in 2009. In that article, the ACO was described as "a provider-led organization whose mission is to manage the full continuum of care and be accountable for the overall costs and quality of care for a defined population" (Rittenhouse, Shortell, and Fisher 2009).

Expanding on that definition, an ACO is a high-performing, organized system of care and financing that can provide the full continuum of care to a specific population over an event, an episode, or a lifetime while assuming accountability for clinical and financial outcomes.

For CMS, the emphasis is on a system of care that can hold itself accountable not only for the resources used and the cost of delivery but also for the outcomes produced. For healthcare delivery systems, the emphasis shifts from looking at one patient at a time to being accountable for a defined population of patients through all of their healthcare needs.

There is a common misconception about how the first ACOs will be reimbursed. Many of those who envision the ACO today are equating payment reform with capitation or a global payment mechanism. The reality is that only highly developed models will be using capitation as the payment model. CMS's initial programs are currently designed around Medicare fee-for-service reimbursement rather than partial or complete capitation. This will challenge the delivery system because it will need to provide a strong enough culture and set of incentives for teamwork to overcome the economic self-interests of those who provide care within the ACO.

In brief, the ACO is not really an entity as much as it is a contractual relationship that consists of delivery and financing tactics between an organized healthcare delivery system and CMS or another payer to provide measurably high quality care efficiently and to share the benefits of efficient delivery with CMS (and possibly with patients).

The Early Stages of ACO Implementation: An Overview

Currently, healthcare leaders and consultants assume that CMS will be sanctioning or designating delivery systems as "ACO approved." This will mean those systems are authorized to accept ACO payment strategies, at least from CMS. As with any assessment criteria, the requirements and standards can be expected to be refined and become increasingly rigorous over time. The PPACA specifies only a small number of requirements. Those requirements will certainly be expanded on the basis of experience from the initial pilots under way in 2010 and from the programs slated to begin in January 2012. Even with the evolving requirements, PPACA is never expected to be one size fits all. There will be a natural maturing process in which developing or evolving systems will be authorized to participate in low-risk, low-reward, shared-savings reimbursement strategies while fully integrated delivery systems will be authorized to participate in higher-risk, higher-reward savings models.

In the meantime, those organizations that choose to participate in the program will be able to choose at what level they wish to compete—novice, intermediate, or expert, each of which will have its own level of risk and reward. CMS and some delivery systems are concerned that the low-risk/low-reward model will not be attractive enough to encourage participation. For some, "the juice may not be worth the squeeze." We predict that, over time, if the experiment appears promising, the risk/reward systems will get richer, offering better paybacks for those with the most advanced ACO strategies.

It is not clear whether ACOs will be ranked for the purposes of determining which economic model will be used by CMS for contracting purposes. For example, delivery systems with a history of success managing risk contracts could be considered for a higher risk/reward model, while delivery systems without a history of successful risk management could be considered for a more modest shared savings model. But regardless of the economic model, common elements will likely be present in all ACO models.

Medicare is currently debating a number of different methodologies for enrolling patients in ACOs. We discuss these later in this chapter. Primary care, in turn, will be linked to a core group of clinical specialists and subspecialists, hospitals, and other institutions and programs that provide specific services. They will span the full spectrum of care, including urgent care, emergency care, acute inpatient care, rehabilitation, psychiatric treatment, subacute and long-term care, specialty care, ambulatory surgical care, home care, diagnostic evaluation, alternative therapy, and nutritional services, to name but a few. They could also include pharmacy networks, pharmacy benefits managers, and durable medical equipment suppliers. All of these institutions, programs, and caregivers will be linked to one another and their patients through an electronic health platform, medical record, and information exchange.

The question of ACO stratification will ultimately be determined by how tightly integrated the system is. There will be different formulas for assumption of risk and distribution of shared savings depending on the systems' level of integration and other capabilities. This will be further explored in the upcoming chapters on ACO anatomy, physiology, and sociology and economics, as the linkages are structural, operational, cultural, and financial.

ACO Requirements

In those four pages in the PPACA (2010), CMS manages to spell out a lot of details about what these local "microsystems" of care will look like. Under the requirements, the ACO must operate under the joint leadership of clinicians and professional managers working collaboratively. They must design and deliver a system of care based on the fundamental principles of efficiency and effectiveness. Efficiency targets resource utilization. Effectiveness targets clinical outcomes. Section 3022 of the PPACA, titled "Shared Savings Program," directs the US secretary of health and human services to establish a "shared savings program that promotes accountability for a patient population and coordinates items and services under [Medicare] parts A and B, and encourages investment in infrastructure and redesigned care processes for high quality and efficient service delivery." These stated PPACA requirements apply only to CMS's initial 2012 ACO programs. Exhibit 2.1 details the basic requirements.

Ultimately, the requirements that are spelled out seem to have been determined by political realities. Noncontroversial, politically safe attributes are spelled out in great detail. Politically charged areas have been deliberately left vague. (For more details on the requirements in the law, see the sidebar.) For example, the requirement that ACOs cover only 5,000 beneficiaries is unrealistic with regard to the required infrastructure investment. Moreover, 5,000 lives is too small a number for a healthcare provider to accept actuarial risk or be able to determine whether measured outcomes are causal or simply accidental.

Must an ACO Contain a Hospital?

At first glance, a highly integrated, 400-physician group practice that generates excellent clinical outcomes would be a logical choice for an ACO. Unfortunately, such a physician practice may well be one of the higher-cost delivery systems in its market, and it may have only middle-of-the-road performance in its risk contracts, partly because of its relationship with a very high-cost/highly reimbursed hospital for inpatient services. Is this "system" well suited for ACO contracting? Until this practice has a full hospital partner with real skin in the game—one that will win or lose on the basis of the shared savings all

Exhibit 2.1 PPACA's Basic Requirements for ACO Programs

- ACOs must have a mechanism for shared governance; governance here is broadly defined as governance, management, and contracts that link the participants to one another.
- The following providers are eligible:
    - ACO professionals in group practice arrangements,
    - Networks of individual practices of ACO professionals,
    - Partnerships or joint-venture arrangements between hospitals and ACO professionals,
    - Hospitals that employ ACO professionals, and
    - Other groups of service providers and suppliers as the US secretary of health and human services determines appropriate.
- The ACO must be willing to become accountable for the quality, cost, and overall care of the Medicare fee-for-service beneficiaries assigned to it.
- The ACO must have a formal legal structure, including clinical and administrative leadership, that allows the organization to receive and distribute payments and shared savings to participating service providers and suppliers. (Though, surprisingly, in a recent confidential conversation, a MedPac official indicated that a contractual arrangement would meet the criteria of a "formal legal structure.")
- The ACO must have a minimum of 5,000 beneficiaries assigned to it for at least three years.
- The ACO must provide full transparency with regard to quality.

Source: PPACA (2010).

partners can achieve—it is unlikely to drive enough savings to thrive under a shared savings ACO model.

The more vexing question is whether a physician group practice can operate independently as an ACO. The answer must be considered within three planes. At a regulatory level, the answer is unequivocally "yes"; there is nothing in the statute that prevents it

ACO Provisions in the PPACA

The anatomy of organizations that contract for Medicare accountable care reimbursement is described more in Chapter 3, but here is a brief list of the required elements:

- A shared program governance (not necessarily organizational governance) that includes, at a minimum, hospital leadership and physician leadership* and may also include the payer
- A collection of physicians who operate with sufficient integrity to pass, as a minimum standard, the Federal Trade Commission definition of "clinical integration"
- Agreement to cover 5,000 patients for a minimum of three years
- Enough integration with at least one hospital and other care facilities to operate as a system; such facilities may include skilled nursing facilities, long-term acute care hospitals, nursing homes, or ambulatory surgical centers (Practically speaking, we believe that the hospital or healthcare system needs to be a full partner in the endeavor, as described in Chapter 3.)
- An advanced medical home model for primary care
- Innovative payer strategies, beginning with CMS
- Comprehensive information technology framework, fully linked across the system
- Comprehensive medical management system, including patient registries
- Internal systemwide education
- Patient education for those who elect to receive care within the ACO (assuming a formal enrollment rather than an attribution process)
- Committed leadership
- Supportive culture

Each of these elements is described in the forthcoming chapters. At present, what is abundantly clear is that inclusion of only 5,000 members is grossly insufficient to adequately serve the goals of the program.

*While Section 3022 of the PPACA suggests that a large multispecialty group practice can operate as an ACO, the practice will require a tightly integrated relationship with a hospital to operate as an ACO.

from doing so. At a theoretical level, the answer is "occasionally." This might be possible where a large, mature, and high-performing multispecialty group has enough market presence to effectively manage care along the continuum and has a well-developed infrastructure that requires little capital investment. At a practical level, however, the answer is "unlikely." Only a few group practices have the management expertise, strategic insights, span of influence, or capital to develop an ACO without a hospital partner. Therefore, in Chapter 3 we focus on the more common circumstances where a physician organization partners with a hospital as the two "anchor tenants" for the ACO "mall."

An even larger unanswered question at this time is whether the system can be created in such a way that the anticipated payoff is worth the effort. As noted earlier, will the "formula" for shared savings—where the first dollar goes back to the US Treasury and "above-threshold" savings are shared between CMS and the delivery system—create a large enough incentive for high-performing delivery systems to participate? Because the formulas are just now being considered, it is possible that the system will fail to create sufficient incentives to attract delivery systems to participate. We will all have to wait for the answer to this looming question.

The Six Goals of the ACO

The ACO, with its roots among academics and policy leaders, emerged out of growing frustration with the lack of "systemness" and organization in American healthcare delivery. This lack of systemness certainly contributes significantly to disappointing US healthcare outcomes, as noted in Chapter 1. While the United States ranked highest in overall per capita spending ($7,290 in 2007 compared with an estimated $3,387 in the Netherlands) (OECD 2010), it came in seventh out of seven in the outcomes ranking. World Health Organization rankings demonstrate similar relative performance, despite the fact that the United States spends more than $2.1 trillion a year on healthcare, or more than the entire gross domestic product of all but seven industrialized nations (Anderson et al. 2005).

The ACO model has six underlying principles and goals. These six goals are efficiency, quality, effectiveness, timeliness, patient-centeredness, and equitability.

1. The first goal is based on the belief that improved alignment of the structures, organizations, professionals, and functional systems will improve the *efficiency* of care, including reductions in avoidable costs. The rationale for this assumption comes from the demonstrated efficiencies produced by IDSs such as Kaiser Permanente, Intermountain Health Care, and Geisinger Health System.

2. The second goal is based on mounting data that support the positive correlation between integration and *quality*. Integration refers to an unspecified but commonly accepted standard of systemness across delivery settings, providers, specialties, disciplines, programs, delivery systems, and time. It was based largely on this growing body of data that the Federal Trade Commission created the standard of "clinical integration" to enable more closely integrated physician associations and health systems to negotiate as clinical delivery systems without running afoul of federal restrictions on collective bargaining. Common sense and experience support the notion that better clinical outcomes, greater employee and patient satisfaction, and improved efficiency result from better-integrated care.

3. The third goal is intended to address *effectiveness*—delivering the appropriate care in the safest and least resource-intense setting. The critical step in improving effectiveness is reducing treatment variations that simply don't add value. It is well known that orthopedic surgeons who standardize total hip-replacement processes can perform more surgeries in a given day than those who do not. The point was strongly underscored in Atul Gawande's (2007) *New Yorker* article that shows how standardized procedures for inserting central intravenous lines resulted in sharp drops in avoidable infections. He followed

up that article with the best-selling book *Checklist Manifesto*, which argues for standardization across a variety of clinical practices.

Loosely coupled systems (discussed further in Chapter 4) lack the capacity to reduce unnecessary variation; therefore, one of the core qualifications for becoming an ACO is demonstrating a level of structural integrity and a commitment and capacity for standardizing practices that will benefit from reductions in variation. This principle is the driving force behind Geisinger Health System's ProvenCare model, an approach to care in which standardization enables greater predictability of outcomes for patients, providers, and payers.

4. The fourth goal is access to healthcare. The Massachusetts healthcare reform law, enacted in 2006, shows that access to health insurance should not be confused with access to healthcare. Access to insurance may be a necessary prerequisite, but it is not a guarantor of access to care. For instance, in Massachusetts a severe shortage of primary care physicians meant that even residents with new subsidized or free healthcare policies still frequently showed up in the emergency department for routine treatment. Nevertheless, the ACO, along with the health insurance reform specified in the PPACA, is an attempt to address the problem of *timeliness*, an area in which American healthcare falls far short of that in other industrialized nations.

5. The fifth goal is envisioned to address the growing need for patient-centeredness in all clinical process design. David Hanna of RBL Group famously stated in 1988 that "All organizations are perfectly designed to get the results they get" (Hanna 1988). In American healthcare, most processes are designed around the needs and interests of those who deliver and finance care. Few follow the guiding principle of *patient-centeredness*. Doctors and other caregivers need to create proactive patient care plans and work with patients in a cooperative way to improve their overall health. This is considerably more than a marketing gimmick or an advertising slogan.

6. The sixth goal, with its emphasis on standardization and provision of the full continuum of care for a designated population, is envisioned as one response to the challenge of *equitability*—that is, turning healthcare into a right of citizenship rather than a privilege of status or wealth.

The shocking realization is that these are the same exact goals outlined by the Institute of Medicine's (IOM's) 2001 report *Crossing the Quality Chasm*. Though more than a decade separates the IOM report and the healthcare reform statute, the shortcomings of US healthcare haven't changed. The mere fact that it has taken more than a decade to meaningfully respond to the initial IOM report is testimony to the flagrant absence of a national system of care. While the problems are the same, the ACO strategy outlined in the PPACA at least provides a new way to try to address these long-standing problems.

The ACO model is also an attempt to integrate the many schools of thought regarding how to fix healthcare in the United States. One school believes in the power of markets and that the answer lies in increasing consumerism—that is, making patients pay more for healthcare so that they respond to price signals and treat healthcare like other services they purchase. Another school believes that the answer lies in technology, and another believes that the solution rests in quality. Another school believes strongly that payment reform is the ultimate answer, and yet another believes that management and organizational design can lead healthcare out of the morass. The ACO strategy is an attempt to combine all these approaches into a single, comprehensive solution.

Moreover, the concept of the ACO seems to be filling an unmet professional and psychological need for a large number of physicians and hospital leaders. It reminds them why they went into medicine or healthcare in the first place. It wipes away the cynicism that develops from being exposed to the corrupting and perverse financial incentives prevalent in today's ecosystem. The ACO has hit a nerve. It's no surprise that there is more interest in developing this new delivery strategy than in almost anything in healthcare today.

Definitely Not a Slam Dunk

ACOs will face many challenges. Here are just a few:

- Will enough providers want to integrate sufficiently to participate in this program?
- Will enough patients participate?
- How will participants pay for the massive infrastructure required to become functioning ACOs?
- If patients are not locked into ACO delivery systems, can costs really be managed over time?
- Will provider systems lose interest and drop out of the program?
- What quality measures and standards will ultimately be used to determine eligibility for shared-savings distribution?

Unless these questions are effectively addressed, there is (and should be) much concern over the viability of the approach. In late October 2010 the National Committee for Quality Assurance (NCQA) released its first set of quality-measure recommendations for public commentary. These initial measures provide some insight into the answer to the last question listed above. The NCQA's initial recommendations include measures directed at the following specific areas:

- Structure
- Resource stewardship
- Health services contracting
- Access availability
- Practice capabilities
- Data collection
- Initial health assessment
- Population management
- Practice support
- Information exchange
- Patient rights and responsibilities
- Performance reporting

Further details of the initial measures and standards and the assessment methodology can be found on NCQA's website at www.ncqa.org.

What is clear to everyone, however, is that setting too lofty a bar for eligibility, such that only highly evolved IDSs qualify, won't really advance the dial of healthcare improvement needed across America.

ACO's Roots in History

The ACO is neither radical nor entirely innovative. As a system of healthcare delivery, the ACO will bear many similarities to the more advanced health maintenance organization (HMO) of the 1970s, 1980s, and 1990s. The HMO was a system that successfully achieved care integration but was severely limited by a lack of information technology and evidence-based medical standards. Today's ACO will be supported by contemporary information and technology systems and exchanges along with quality metrics that were unavailable during the HMO heyday.

A number of programs have served as early pilots for ACOs. One pilot is the Physician Group Practice Demonstration, a project that was established at many different locations, including the Billings Clinic, Dartmouth-Hitchcock Clinic, Everett Clinic, Forsyth Medical Group, Geisinger Health System, Marshfield Clinic, Middlesex Health System, Park Nicollet Health Services, St. John's Health System, and University of Michigan Faculty Group Practice. Another pilot is the Brookings-Dartmouth ACO Collaborative, which includes, among others, private-sector groups in Irvine and Torrance, California. Others are the ACO pilot sites in Roanoke, Virginia; Louisville, Kentucky; and Tucson, Arizona. These pilot sites were selected to experiment with large and small group practices, different competitive environments, and different practice models that range from fully integrated systems to multiple independent provider groups. A pilot under way is the Medicare "646" Demonstration in Indianapolis, Indiana, and North Carolina.

The Physician Group Practice Demonstration, initiated by Medicare in 2005 to test the impact of efficiency and quality performance payment incentives and rewards within 10 selected provider organizations, has reported extensively on its results. McClellan and colleagues (2010) report that through the third year of the program, all 10 participating sites achieved success on most quality measures. The groups demonstrated cost reductions of $32 million, more than $25 million of which was distributed by CMS to the groups as incentives (McClellan et al. 2010).

The data from the Physician Group Practice Demonstration and the ACO pilot programs support the fundamental thesis that improved systemness demonstrably increases the efficiency and effectiveness of clinical care. Further support is provided by numerous other reports of pilot or demonstration programs that show a positive correlation between improved systemness of care and rational economic incentives, lowered costs of care, and better clinical outcomes.

A Disputable Assumption About Systems of Care

One of the core assumptions underlying the conceptualization of the ACO is that while IDSs in America are relatively rare, "virtual" delivery systems composed of community hospitals and their medical staffs are ubiquitous. But this is flawed thinking. To call a community hospital with its medical staff a system of care is akin to referring to US healthcare as a system. Having all the components of a system does not make a system or does not make it spontaneously generate the benefits of integrated care.

Measuring Effectiveness and Efficiency: The Core ACO Tenets

The first cornerstone of the ACO is the belief that optimal clinical outcomes and resource utilization are achievable only within an organized system of care. The second cornerstone is the observation that there is no single best model for that system of care. A growing body of quality standards enables CMS to feel reasonably secure in establishing clinical outcome standards, and increasingly sophisticated technology enables accurate reporting of results. Efficiency, however, is more elusive, and does not easily fit into a set of national standards. For this reason, CMS has set the benchmark for measuring efficiency as *showing improvement over current performance*.

Here's how it will work: Based on analysis of historic resource utilization, mix, and costs, CMS is able to extrapolate costs over the next period of time for defined populations. Currently available systems and controls will enable CMS to recalibrate those projections, thereby "bending the trend" downward. This recalibrated projection will become the benchmark for the shared-savings calculations. The difference between total cost of care to a defined population and the recalibrated benchmark represents the shared-savings pool, some of which will be shared between CMS and the delivery system using yet-to-be-determined formulas.

What is known at this time is that first dollars will go to CMS. Once a performance threshold is reached, additional shared savings will be distributed between CMS and the ACO. Those formulas will ultimately be adjusted on the basis of the ACO's appetite for risk: The greater the potential loss the ACO is willing to assume, the greater the reward within the shared-savings program. See Exhibit 2.2 for an illustration.

It is unlikely that any two systems will be satisfied with the same distribution formula, so it is expected that each ACO governing body will take on the responsibility of establishing and managing its own redistribution/funds flow formula. Clearly, internal checks and balances will need to be established and approved by CMS or the authorizing agency to ensure appropriate avoidance of underutilization and avoidance of adverse patient selection.

Underutilization—often because of rejection of physicians' and patients' requests—was one of the unforgiveable sins of the HMOs of the 1980s. It gave managed care a bad name. So there must be checks and balances to prevent underutilization in the ACO. To a certain extent, clinical quality standards ensure that adequate care will be provided. Moreover, underutilization becomes a self-defeating strategy when it prevents providers from meeting stated quality thresholds. The need to achieve excellent clinical outcomes will be a powerful balance against the impulse to single-mindedly pursue cost reductions.

Overutilization has its own internal implications and has to be managed internally through peer accountability. If a particular physician is ordering too many tests or performing too many procedures, the

Exhibit 2.2 Bending the Trend

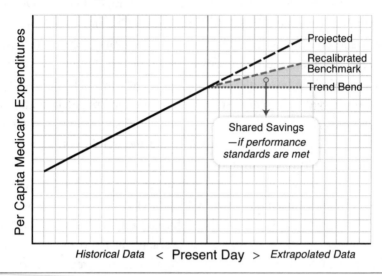

transparency of reporting using electronic health records will bring that behavior to light. The more sinister issue is the avoidance of adverse patient selection. Here the answer is not as clear. At first pass the assignment of "healthy" 65-year-olds to the ACO would seem advantageous. But if CMS risk- or cost-stratifies patients, older patients with multisystem diseases and higher projected costs that can be managed through better integration might prove strategically advantageous to the ACO.

The Five and One-Half Core Competencies of the ACO
We fully acknowledge that no single approach or organizational model will achieve the outcomes necessary for success in the ACO. But, it is clear that success will require the demonstration of five and one-half core competencies, as shown in Exhibit 2.3.

1. *Leadership and culture*. Leadership commitment is clearly critical for success. The laws of physics tell us that objects in motion will stay in motion while objects at rest will stay at rest unless energy is applied to change the present state. Organizational behavior

Exhibit 2.3 Core Competencies of an ACO

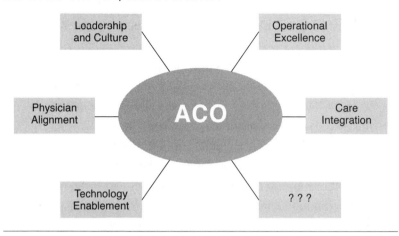

is based largely on the results of a complex set of organizational habits that developed over years as a result of direct and indirect reinforcement. Without that internal reinforcement, the habits would be extinguished. Declaration of an intention for change will initially produce resistance, because most in the system have learned to adapt to and therefore enjoyed success in the current system. Often, the *most* resistant are those who have "risen" highest within the current system. If these leaders do not support this strategy, it is doomed to failure. The real test of leadership commitment is whether leaders can acknowledge and respond rationally to the resistance while remaining true to their change goals.

Because culture ultimately trumps strategy, the most effective strategy implementation requires a supportive culture. This, in turn, requires clarification of values and consistency in adhering to those values as manifested in expectations, incentives, rewards, performance management, and group behavioral norms. Any dissonance between what the organization espouses and what is observed will ultimately lead to the staff's cynicism and deep resignation—the two powerful toxins to organizational performance and change. Taking the bold leap of redesigning incentives and rewards is often the most difficult transition for executive leadership to make, because it requires letting go of something that has been working long before there is any proof that the new strategy will work better. A culture of trust, optimism, and confidence is ultimately the only tool available for overcoming the lack of evidentiary basis for the proposed changes. This requires an investment in building social capital throughout all elements of the enterprise.

2. *Operational excellence*. Healthcare waste—resources consumed without added value—in America has been estimated at 30 percent or more of total spending (Skinner and Fisher 2010). Reduction in that number will challenge many core assumptions and will threaten sacred cows. Some sacred cows need to be fed; others ignored; and still others slaughtered, particularly if top line growth slows. Organizations need to become intolerant of steps, resources, and habits that add no measurable value—those that are based on beliefs, assumptions, former realities, habits, or rumors. Excellence must extend beyond the clinic to the strategic management suite. Operational expertise in managing the economics of the ACO must be developed, including revenue and expense management tactics, capital investment, managed care contracting, risk management, and funds flow/incentive design activities (see Chapter 7).

3. *Care integration*. This critical competency extends across the system and across key partnerships with providers and organizations, such as subacute or long-term-care settings that may be only contractually related to the ACO. This requires a patient-centered focus and vigilance in the adherence to evidence-based care. It also requires incorporation of some core design principles commonly ascribed to "concierge medicine" within everyday practice. The principles associated with concierge medicine will vastly improve information transfer, direct communication, and coordination of care. It will require a high degree of physician–physician and

physician–organization teamwork in design and delivery, which is explained in more detail in Chapter 4.

To balance performance with innovation, the entire system has to operate using simultaneous loose–tight properties, in which the system as a whole is tightly managed while the local components of the system operate with great flexibility. If the system is too loose, it threatens organizational integrity. If it's too tight, caregivers and patients will feel constricted and innovation will be stifled.

What are needed are well-defined systems and processes that can be customized according to the unique needs of the caregivers and an individual patient or patient's family. Care providers are always quick to demand the ability to invoke exceptions to rules, but remember that there cannot be exceptions to rules unless there are rules first.

4. *Physician alignment*. Physician alignment is difficult to describe and also difficult to achieve. Simply put, alignment represents the degree to which physicians, acting out of enlightened self-interest, operate with a common vision, mutual goals, balanced accountability and authority, and the acceptance of a shared destiny. Physician–physician alignment is often more difficult to achieve than alignment between the physicians and the hospital. While over the past 25 years hospitals and physicians have competed vigorously, more recent advances in science and technology have significantly intensified competition among procedural-based physicians. Those tensions require appropriate forums and processes for resolution; they cannot be addressed one conflict at a time. Care integration requires strong physician–physician alignment in order to assess, design, implement, and adhere to standardized care processes. Population management, in which the ACO uses information technology and standardized care to improve outcomes for the entire population covered by the organization, raises the bar and makes this even more important. (Governance and management

The Edge of Chaos Concept Applied to ACOs

There is no single or best model for organizing the components of an ACO. Whatever model is selected must include a legal structure that defines how the ACO relates to its external environment and an organizational structure that defines how the ACO's components relate to one another. More important, both external and internal elements of structure must enable the entity to operate according to the description of "the edge of chaos," a concept created and defined by author Michael Crichton (1995) in *The Lost World*:

> a zone of conflict and upheaval, where the old and the new are constantly at war. Finding the balance point must be a delicate matter—if a living system drifts too close, it risks falling over into incoherence and dissolution; but if the system moves too far away from the edge, it becomes rigid, frozen, totalitarian. Both conditions lead to extinction. Too much change is as destructive as too little. Only at the edge of chaos can complex systems flourish. And, by implication, extinction is the inevitable result of one or the other strategy—too much change, or too little.

Successful ACOs will need to operate in a zone of constructive tension between the forces of local control that support innovation and the systemwide standardization that supports efficiency, efficacy, and predictability. Both forces are vital to the success of the ACO. At times the forces of innovation must prevail; at other times, the forces of stability must prevail. Either way, the ACO structure must be designed to enable the healthy tension between the forces to be exposed, debated, analyzed, and managed. Too much innovation will be as destructive as too much standardization. Each of the structural elements can be designed in a way that either enables or limits the ability of the organization to manage the tension in a healthy and constructive way within the ACO's "edges of chaos."

structures for achieving and managing this integration are described in greater detail in Chapter 3.)

5. *Technology enablement.* A robust electronic health record system is the central nervous system that links together care processes and resource utilization to engineer care. Information technology (IT) must be substantial and sophisticated enough to integrate clinical effectiveness with operational efficiency. The growing belief is that common IT platforms are not the only option; IT "exoskeletons" or "umbrellas" are currently being piloted that can be superimposed to integrate disparate platforms and enable them to operate as a virtual common platform. In addition, information exchanges are also being developed to allow information to be shared across institutions and practices. That option makes the investment in electronic medical records more manageable for many health systems. Technology needs are discussed in greater detail in Chapter 6.

And the final one-half core competency? We will reveal it at the end of this chapter.

Organization of the ACO

Many hospitals and healthcare systems are looking for an ACO template. It does not yet exist. Washington policymakers are steeped in efforts to craft policy to produce intended outcomes and, as noted, are recognizing that trying to achieve a set of outcomes using policy as the only tool is a bit like trying to sculpt a delicate piece of alabaster with a dull chisel and a 10-pound mallet. Policy is powerful and potentially destructive. If it is too restrictive, innovation is stifled. If it is too broad, gamesmanship and chaos ensue. This delicate balance is yet another "edge of chaos" (see sidebar) for healthcare reform.

While this ambiguity is unsettling and paralyzing to some organizations, it is conversely energizing to others for whom it represents opportunity. These empowered organizations are reassured that the successful formula will be built around their own strengths, their culture, and their leadership. Despite the looseness of the current requirements, a limited set of elements and attributes will be common to most ACOs. They include the following:

1. Effective, collaborative, and enlightened leadership made up of both physicians and professional administrators
2. A culture that supports clinical and operational integration, care redesign, operating efficiency, innovation, and systemness
3. A medical home model for primary care providers able to provide care management, coordination, integration, and patient navigation
4. Comprehensive patient registries to identify high-risk patients and offer services to mitigate risk
5. A broad array of clinical specialists within or in relationship with the ACO (see Chapter 3)
6. One or more acute care hospitals, including associated ambulatory care sites, even though this is not required in the legislation
7. Affiliations, partnerships, joint ventures, or joint operating agreements with subacute care facilities with well-developed management that links and coordinates care across settings
8. Medical risk-management functions that have previously been the purview of the payers
9. Supportive compensation, incentive, and reward systems that align with what the market values and is willing to pay for
10. Systems and processes to encourage, manage, and reward patient "stickiness"—the propensity of patients to choose to stay within the system for all their care. (This point is further discussed in the next section.)

Which Patients Join and Which Stay?

A key factor for ACO success will be patient "stickiness," also referred to as customer loyalty. In the initial Medicare pilot programs, beneficiaries have been attributed retroactively to ACOs using evaluation and management codes. At present, CMS is debating whether to formally enroll members, rely on physicians to enroll members, or continue with the "double blind" methodology to minimize the potential for elimination of high-risk or high-cost patients. We believe strongly that patients should be full partners in the program, and that can only be achieved by a formal up-front enrollment process. Additionally, basing results on annual retroactive analysis limits organizational learning and the ability to influence real-time results. Few students would find acceptable a system that provided little or no feedback during the course of studies and awarded grades only at the time of graduation.

There is another issue with enrollment methodology. Systems could seek to avoid high-cost patients who will need a lot of care—called "high utilizers." Providers would be skeptical of patients assigned to them by Medicare, fearing a large number of high utilizers. If providers enroll the patients, the risk is at the other end. However, as noted, to the degree possible that Medicare could risk-adjust or calculate predicted expenses based on previous expenses for the patients enrolled, the ACO would desire to receive a "balanced portfolio" of patients. Having a certain number of heavy utilizers within the ACO leaves room for improvement. If an organization only enrolls healthy, low utilizers, there is very little room for improvement and shared savings. There's mutual incentive to have a mixed portfolio of members.

As the policy is currently crafted, however, patients will not be captive to the ACO program and will be free to receive care wherever they want. This is a clear reaction to the restrictions imposed by managed care in the 1990s, which consumers soundly rejected. It will be up to the ACO program to create "stickiness" for patients so that they voluntarily choose to stay within the system of care. There will be no formal agreements that bind patients to that system or its partners.

Many who study the HMOs of the 1970s and 1980s think that patient and employer demands for greater choice ultimately led to the HMOs' demise. Employees who felt forced by their employers to join restrictive HMO networks and had no other coverage options demanded more choice. They felt the restrictive networks disrupted relationships they had with existing physicians and hospitals. For these reasons, we believe voluntary enrollment is the preferred attribution option. We have already learned that patients don't like being forced into care relationships that they may not know or trust. Still, keep in mind that some patients were happier with the HMO provider networks. Those who valued "systemness" over "choice" were often highly satisfied, while those who favored choice over systemness often were not.

Physician Employment and Physician Alignment Are Not Synonyms

Many healthcare organizations equate "alignment" with employment, assuming that as long as physicians are employed by the system, their interests are aligned with the system or the hospital. This is a common and often costly error. For some workers, employment is the straightest path to alignment, but there are no guarantees that employment will lead to alignment. Many system leaders, for example, observe significant out-of-system "leakage" from employed physicians. This raises clear questions about how closely aligned the employed physicians actually are with their system. Why are they sending patients elsewhere? The inverse is often also true: Many healthcare systems enjoy high degrees of alignment with private physicians who are not employed and receive little or no direct compensation from the system.

At the most basic level, physician–hospital alignment represents the degree to which physicians and hospitals, each acting out of enlightened self-interest, operate with a shared vision, mutual goals, balanced accountability and authority, and the recognition of a common destiny. Employment is not a precondition for alignment.

In many hospital-based systems, the hospital's relationship with physician "employees" mirrors the relationship it has with other employed caregivers, such as respiratory therapists, radiology technicians, or dieticians—these are the individuals under employment agreements with the hospital or system. But unlike what it gives to other skilled workers, the hospital often does not provide the physicians with leadership, performance management, or support systems necessary to ensure their success as employees in a traditional sense. Hospitals often rely on the physicians to provide that for themselves. Aggregating a collection of independent specialists without common context or shared vision and then assuming that self-governance and management will occur is an optimistic delusion. This is a developmental need for many system-employed practices. The physicians will need to develop those supports before they can function fully in an ACO partnership.

To further accentuate the problem, many of the employment agreements represent past deals developed between individual physicians or small group practices and for potentially rational reasons. Often the affiliation was part of the hospital's larger defensive strategy, which is no longer relevant to the ACO going forward. Employment agreements are often created without the benefit of a strategic framework, common design principles, or shared values. Any sense of teamwork engendered by this kind of relationship is purely accidental. The members of these employed practices resemble a track team rather than a soccer team: Each member of the track team competes individually rather than as part of an organized group. But the nature of healthcare requires that the delivery team operate more like a World Cup soccer team, with each player simultaneously supporting the common goal (pun fully intended) of care integration and efficiency optimization.

These physician groups with "leftover" agreements typically fall short of the level of alignment and integration required for success in an ACO. Therefore, the first step toward more effective physician–hospital alignment must focus on physician–physician alignment: Design and help the physicians build the level of professional relationships required for optimal efficiency and clinical care outcomes.

Payment Models Within the ACO

Many health systems have concluded that CMS's preferred or intended payment methodology for the ACO is global capitation. This is a widespread belief, and it is incorrect. Both CMS and commercial payers fully acknowledge that capitation is only supportable for those systems with more advanced clinical and operational integration.

As already noted, simply designing a payment system in which the Geisingers, Mayo Clinics, and Kaiser Permanentes operate as ACOs will not advance healthcare in America one iota. These advanced healthcare systems are already integrated, and their patients are already reaping the benefits of that model. Rewarding these organizations doesn't help change the larger healthcare crisis in the United States. It's the other 99 percent of healthcare in America that needs to be influenced by the PPACA.

The Medicare programs are initially intended to operate using a fee-for-service model and organized around shared savings within an asymmetric risk model that provides potential upside for the delivery system and with little or no downside risk for the providers. CMS understands that no interests are served by encouraging health systems to assume any risk until they have demonstrated the capacity to generate intended clinical and economic outcomes. Rather than help to improve the US healthcare system, this model would only put it in even greater jeopardy. Consequently, the payment model will likely evolve over time from traditional fee for service to selective capitation, bundling, and other arrangements.

Fully integrated delivery systems, such as those mentioned, can accept risk because they have demonstrated the capacity to manage it and achieve predictable quality outcomes without falling into the traps of overutilization or underutilization of services. But most delivery systems will use alternative integrative models, such as co-management agreements, independent practice associations, physician organizations, physician hospital organizations, or foundations as the functional physician alignment vehicle (these are described in Chapter 3). In general, the more integrated and experienced the medical organization, the higher the level of risk it can safely assume, as shown in Exhibit 2.4a. The same two parameters—risk tolerance and level of integration—can be used to profile reimbursement strategies that might be considered by organizations with different levels of integration, as shown in Exhibit 2.4b.

Pay-for-performance (P4P) strategies yield mixed quality and efficiency improvements in systems with relatively low levels of integration. Where P4P metrics have focused on process improvements, process has arguably improved although costs have not. Consequently, ACOs need to think hard about linking P4P bonuses, specific cost-savings opportunities, and shared savings *together* with the "bundling" approach that is used.

Exhibit 2.4a Practice Type and Risk Tolerance

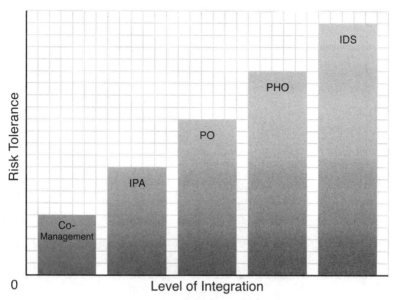

The higher the level of integration, the higher the level
of risk that can safely be assumed

NOTE: IPA = independent practice assoc.; PO = physician organization; PHO = physician hospital organ.;
IDS = integrated delivery system

Here's how it works (see Exhibit 2.5). Payers and providers start by distinguishing between core, evidence-based, and avoidable costs within the hospital (e.g., heart bypass surgery) or even across the care continuum "bundle" (e.g., diabetes). They subsequently agree to reduce avoidable costs (e.g., infection, emergency department visit rate) over time. To hold providers whole, both sides agree to share in the savings, as calculated by the actual versus expected performance on prior period's cost savings. That way, new P4P bonus or shared-savings payments (black) are partly funded by actual avoidable cost savings. In this way, P4P bonuses and shared-savings arrangements are evolving from a "no-risk" model to one in which providers have at least some skin in the game.

Bundled and episodic payment methods are essentially different ways to aggregate resources into packages/products that patients buy.

Exhibit 2.4b Reimbursement Strategy and Risk Tolerance

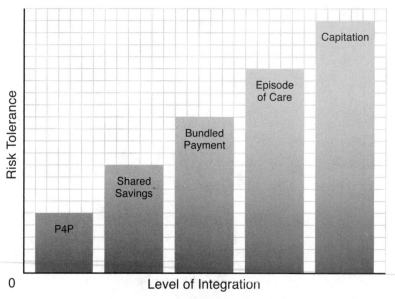

The higher the level of integration, the higher the level
of risk that can safely be assumed

The resources and actors that are bundled together influence the cost and quality improvement potential. Emerging examples include a 30-day hospital and physician bundle that pays for the initial admission and associated readmissions within 30 days. In this model, hospitals and physicians could retain any variable or fixed cost savings associated with avoidable readmissions, similar to the cost savings hospitals achieved from reduced length of stay when prospective DRG (diagnosis-related group) payments were implemented in the early 1980s. Furthermore, providers could even get an additional P4P bonus for satisfying additional quality and efficiency standards. These additional payments could be manifested as a P4P "value-based multiplier" on top of a negotiated, 30-day DRG case rate-based fee schedule.

Finally, capitation (PM/PM or PM/PY) assumes full risk for a "covered life" over a defined period of time (one year) and, for all

Exhibit 2.5 Bending the Cost Curve and the Integration of P4P, Shared
Savings, and Bundles

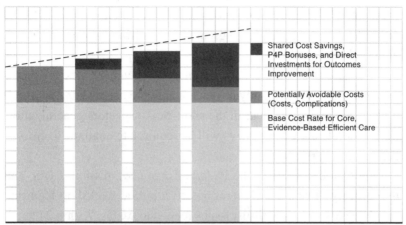

Keys to Success
1. Agree to fair, evidence-based costs
2. Tie bonus payment to actual versus expected avoidable costs
3. Share cost savings for better outcomes
The result: lower yearly cost increases than in the past

practical purposes, assumes full financial risk for the Medicare benefi-
ciary. Payments would certainly need to be risk adjusted, as is the case
with some of the bundling approaches profiled earlier.

Capitation, of course, also carries potential reward: Innovation, pre-
ventive care, and coordination can all contribute significantly to potential
cost savings and improved outcomes. The level of clinical and systems
integration required for full capitation reimbursement is typically greater
than that required for bundled payment because bundled payments can be
limited to a select group of services, physicians, and staff. Consequently,
global capitation requires the full commitment of the system, but it is not
necessarily the end game for all ACOs.

Potential Legal Impediments
The perverse incentives in the US healthcare system have led, over
time, to a number of outrages: self-referrals, kickbacks, and other

forms of self-serving and financial abuse. Many responses have been implemented over the past 25 years, including the Stark law, antikickback regulations, and other consumer protections. But do these legal and regulatory rules now threaten the nascent ACO movement, which requires greater integration among disparate economic entities?

It is safe to assume that, over time, enforcement of the legal protections will remain roughly proportional to the perceived need. But it is also safe to assume that, in the short run, inspectors general, attorneys general, and US attorneys will be required to continue to enforce the existing legislation.

On October 5, 2010, the Federal Trade Commission, CMS, and the Office of Inspector General hosted a public workshop featuring panel discussions on antitrust issues related to ACOs. Within 24 hours of that meeting, the Federal Trade Commission issued an announcement that it will develop antitrust safe harbors for ACOs as well as an expedited review process for ACOs that do not qualify for those safe harbors. At the conference, CMS administrator Donald M. Berwick sought to reassure participants that his agency was not looking to trip up well-intentioned ACO innovators: "We have underlying statutory requirements. For example, CMS will have to enforce Stark provisions. But, we can interpret those statutes wisely and in a manner that, while still consistent with the plain language and intent of the applicable statutes, does not unnecessarily impede the development of ACOs" (Berwick 2010).

Fundamental antitrust principles will continue to apply to the formation and operation of ACOs. More specifically, ACOs developed and operated to improve quality and reduce healthcare costs that do not create undue market concentration will be considered "pro-competitive," while ACOs formed by independent, competing providers solely to raise prices will not be considered favorably.

Long-Term Versus Short-Term Solution
Albert Einstein is often quoted as having said, "The significant problems we face today cannot be solved at the same level of thinking we

were at when we created them." This applies to the current healthcare system. Today's system is a highly developed transactional framework designed to favor the interests of those who deliver and finance care over those who receive it. Reversal of that highly evolved system will take time and patience. Success will be marked by a series of rational, bounded, and responsible experiments that, over time, will coalesce into a new system of care. The ultimate goal of the ACO strategy is to organize care rather than to create a true national system of care, or to create microsystems of care rather than a national health system. Promotion of a national health system would be folly in today's divisive and politically charged environment.

CMS recognizes that a Big Bang approach is doomed to failure. Healthcare systems in every developed nation have supporters and critics. The American healthcare system will continue to have both as it transforms itself, though the ACO strategy is clearly intended to create a little more balance between the supporters and the critics. No one expects to achieve universal satisfaction. More achievable will be a set of healthcare outcomes that demonstrates improvement in the health of our population, access to reasonable care for every American as a right of citizenship, and the provision of care at a cost that is affordable and sustainable.

Even in its most optimistic form, the ACO strategy is imperfect, making trade-offs that will be hailed by some and lambasted by others. That is the nature of democracy and the natural history of change. The ACO represents a rational system of care delivery and financing that unites purchasers, payers, and providers (and, here's hoping, patients as well) in a system that can, over time, evolve and improve. Therefore, the ACO must be seen as a long-term solution rather than as a short-term fix. It will certainly emerge as the result of countless experiments and approximations based on a limited common set of principles set forth in the PPACA. It is not for everyone—not for all purchasers, payers, providers, or patients. As such, it is not *the* solution but rather one of many solutions to the crisis of America's fractured health system. And like any change process, it will be adopted by the innovators first, the early adopters next, and the late adopters last.

ACO Pilot Site: Tucson Medical Center

Describing the innovative process is best left to the voice of one innovator—Judy Rich, president and CEO of Tucson Medical Center/TMC Healthcare, which was selected as an ACO pilot site by the Engelberg Center for Health Care Reform at the Brookings Institution and the Dartmouth Institute for Health Policy and Clinical Practice. Here is Rich (2010) discussing the project in her own words:

> At Tucson Medical Center (TMC) we have created the TMC Accountable Care Organization, LLC. The ACO earns a bonus pool from payors that is based on lowered costs and improved quality. The ACO Steering Committee, composed of both hospital and physician representation, is responsible for setting the quality measures to be used in determining the distribution of the bonus pool. TMC's ACO is unique in that the overwhelming number of participants are community, non-hospital-employed physicians. Physicians have been invited into the ACO based on the value that their respective practices bring to the goal. We have settled upon a patient attribution model that will assign the practice's patients to the ACO, and the data collection will track improvement over time. Physician willingness to participate in the ACO has far exceeded our initial expectations. The next step in the process will be to develop an MSO (management services organization) that will sell services to the ACO. These services will improve the primary care of patients through case management and data throughout the continuum of care. This requires a robust electronic medical record with the ability to share data.
>
> At TMC we have embraced the ACO as an alignment strategy with our physicians and as a means to improve the health of our community through coordinated care. Unlike models in the past this one is not designed to produce volume for the hospital. This model keeps patients out of the hospital. We have learned that our physicians value a partnership that is focused on the patient and "doing the right thing." It has been a journey that has required an "all in" leadership commitment. No dabbling in an ACO...this model fundamentally changes

the way we do business. It put us into a partnership with our medical staff that is supporting their autonomy and expertise as managers of patient care. It lowers the costs of care by reducing repetitive, unnecessary care, lowering length of stay and utilization of expensive resources. TMC's ACO is a model for the future of healthcare in Southern Arizona, which I am sure will evolve in its appearance and makeup over the next few years. This journey is not for the timid. It is full of risk and potential obstacles, but it is the necessary path for us at TMC to fulfill our core mission of providing exemplary healthcare with access for all in our community.

Building ACO Readiness

Because there is no ACO template, there is no right formula for building ACO readiness. Chapter 9 focuses on a reasonable set of steps to consider in building an ACO. Exhibit 2.6 outlines the five steps that are serving a number of organizations well today as they prepare to apply for ACO status in 2012.

1. *Envision and educate.* Step 1 is envisioning the overall ACO delivery model that will work best within the primary organization and educating those within the organization, including their governing bodies, about the intention, rationale, vision, and requirements and competencies. Some providers also use this step to educate and engage external organizations that are likely to become partners within the ACO system.
2. *Assess and analyze.* Step 2 concentrates on assessment and analysis to determine which resources and programs currently exist within the organization and whether they are configured in a manner that improves quality and efficiency. This step underscores the Stockdale Paradox discussed in Jim Collins's book *Good to Great*: Organizational leaders must remain confident in their vision but at the same time face the brutal

Exhibit 2.6 Five Steps to an ACO

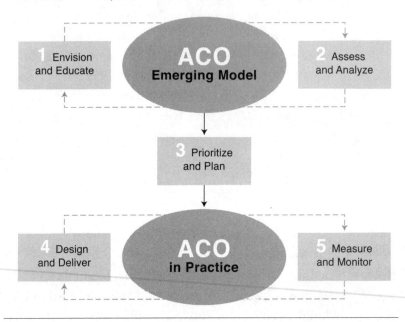

facts of their current reality. As we visit more health systems, we find that many seem to want to believe they are more advanced than they really are. The Stockdale Paradox posits than an organization won't truly advance until it recognizes the reality of where it is, regardless of how brutal those facts are.

3. *Prioritize and plan.* Step 3 is used for establishing priorities and developing a plan. Given finite tangible and intangible resources, especially capital and leadership, each organization must determine which areas to concentrate on first. The important outcome of this step is momentum. Many organizations may not have made the decision to contract as an ACO. But they have already determined that clinical integration and improved operating efficiency are crucial competencies. They are actively engaged in initiatives to improve clinical effectiveness, care integration, and operating efficiencies, which can only be beneficial regardless of their ultimate ACO strategy.

4. *Design and deliver.* Step 4 is detailed design and delivery. While some design elements can be borrowed from other systems, many must be crafted around the particular strengths and weaknesses of the current delivery system. That process, by definition, will generate a series of repetitive experiments. It is wise to remember that today's Mayo Clinic is Version 10.0 of the Mayo brothers' initial vision, just as Geisinger is Version 10.0 of Abigail Geisinger's vision. Few organizations can design and deliver Version 10.0 in the first round. This leads us to our final step.

5. *Measure and monitor.* Step 5 is measuring and monitoring, which is how to track progress and improve over time. The key to success in this step lies in the ability to translate data into information, information into knowledge, and knowledge into action. Through sequential actions, Version 1.0 will transform itself into Version 1.1 and so on.

The Final One-Half Core Competency of the ACO

We listed five core competencies earlier in this chapter, though we promised five and one-half. The final half core competency is the most difficult to describe and arguably the most difficult to achieve. The current activities-based transactional delivery model with activities-based reimbursement is not going to be terminated one weekend and replaced with a new care delivery, organizational, and economic model by the next weekend. The transition will be gradual, and, for some period of time, organizations that pursue this strategy will be living a paradox in which they will be asked to simultaneously support two opposing and even contradictory realities. Short-term reality must acknowledge that success in today's competitive delivery and economic model requires behaviors that are antithetical to those required for success in the future model. Leaders and key participants in ACO experiments will have to live with one foot in each world.

Ignoring this paradox will only produce organizational anxiety, confusion, and cynicism, given that both truths simultaneously exist. Trying to *resolve* the paradox is an exercise in futility for the same reason. Instead, the paradox must be *acknowledged directly* and *managed sensitively in the context of your competitive market.* This is the most important role and the most difficult challenge for leaders who are pursuing this strategy. There is no proven recipe for managing the paradox, but the first step is clear: Acknowledge that it exists.

Organizational Questions

The organizational questions raised in this chapter include the following:

- What do we believe about the future of healthcare delivery in our community?
- What do we want our future to look like?
- How is our future likely to be most different from our present?
- How should we be engaging those within our organization about our future?
- What questions do we need to answer in order to select the best strategic course for us?

Category of Readers	Key Concepts	Actions to Consider
Category A (interested)	• What is an ACO?	• Educational forums on ACOs for board, managers, and physicians
	• Requirements for an ACO	• Executive, board, and physician leadership strategic retreat
	• Core ACO tenets: effectiveness and efficiency	• Attend national ACO meeting with other system leaders
Category B (engaged)	• 6 goals of an ACO	• Executive, board, and physician leadership strategic retreat
	• 5½ ACO core competencies	• Outreach to system physician leaders
	• Physician employment vs. alignment	• Initiate high-level ACO assessment
Category C (committed)	• 10 ACO elements and attributes	• Initiate a conversation with other external entities regarding interest in ACO
	• ACO payment and delivery strategies, mindful of market dynamics	• Initiate a detailed ACO status assessment
	• Steps for building an ACO (see Chapter 9)	• Begin to develop a physician organization or physician hospital organization

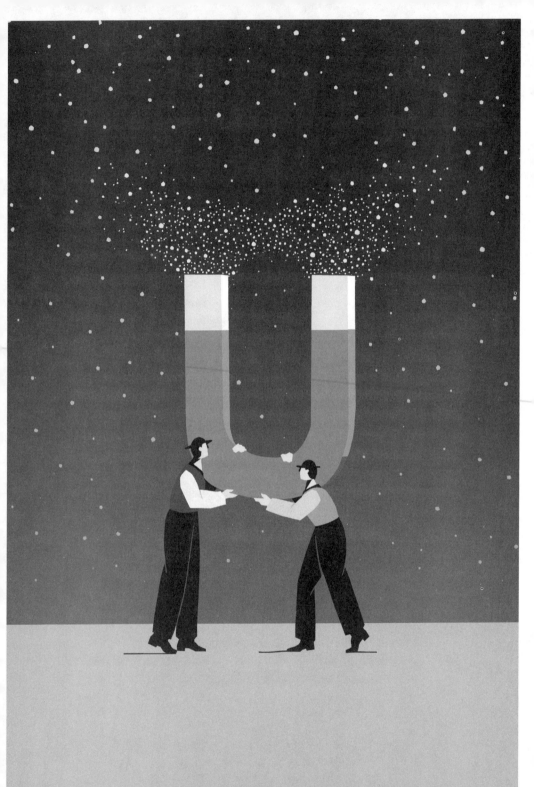

3

Accountable Care Organization Anatomy

with Charles Buck, Esq., Partner, McDermott Will & Emery LLP

We have employed physicians and independent physicians, and they are both important resources for our community. We are deeply committed to the operating intentions of accountable care with respect to clinical integration and operating efficiency. We simply have to find an effective way of organizing our physician relationships so that we can partner with all of them to achieve optimal outcomes for the patients we serve together.

—Grace Hines
Vice President, Corporate Strategy
Sentara Health

Accountable care organization (ACO) *anatomy* refers to the structure of the ACO. As noted in Chapter 2, the term *organization* in ACO is really a misnomer. The ACO is not itself an entity; rather it is a contractual relationship, dealing with delivery and financing strategies and tactics, between an organized healthcare delivery system and the Centers for Medicare & Medicaid Services (CMS) or other payers. Much like Medicare Advantage or Blue Cross Blue Shield of Massachusetts's Alternative Quality Contract, these contractual strategies and tactics need to be connected to some entity.

In this chapter and elsewhere in the book, "ACO structure" refers to the structure of the delivery system that participates in the ACO arrangement. This definition acknowledges that an ACO, *per se*, does not have a structure. It is our view that the organizational structure—the anatomy—of the delivery system is the foundation for an ACO. A well-designed and appropriately customized organizational structure sets the foundation for ACO leadership and management to make and execute decisions intended to integrate and coordinate care. The ultimate goal, of course, is to produce superior clinical outcomes in a cost-effective manner. While a solid, well-designed foundation cannot guarantee success, a weak foundation would almost certainly ensure failure.

Integrating Hospitals and Medical Groups

We assert that, at a minimum, an ACO must fully integrate one or more acute care hospitals and a set of physicians (i.e., a physician organization) who, as discussed more fully later, operate in the manner of a multispecialty group practice. In this context, operating as a multispecialty group practice means that the physicians recognize themselves as being members of an entity that has a shared destiny. Within that entity, they have accountability for their own actions, for the actions of their fellow specialists and employees, and for the collective clinical and business outcomes achieved by the group.

In an ACO, the hospital(s) and its physician organization are analogous to the anchor tenants in a shopping mall. Other "tenants" might include, for example, a skilled nursing facility, a long-term acute care hospital, a rehabilitation hospital, or even a health plan. While all occupants can benefit from participation in the ACO (the mall), we assert that the ACO cannot function without a hospital and a physician organization as its anchor tenants. The Patient Protection and Affordable Care Act of 2010 (PPACA) does not require the inclusion of an acute care hospital in a Medicare ACO. Yet, it is difficult to envision an ACO operating effectively without the hospital as a full partner. It is highly doubtful that the organization would be able to meaningfully integrate and coordinate medical care across the full care continuum, reduce avoidable costs, and manage the economic arrangements required to deliver that integrated care. Furthermore, without access to the capital and management expertise of the hospital—and the hospital itself having "skin in the game"—success would be doubtful.

Indeed, we suspect that medical groups that attempt to go it alone as ACOs would be naturally inclined to return to the destructive and unsuccessful practice of purchasing or leasing hospital beds on the margin from other organizations. This arrangement would not generate enough incentive for the hospitals to reduce their overall cost footprint and provide the level of innovation or collaboration required in an ACO strategy. It would likely result in great antagonism between the medical group and the hospital.

Another important point to keep in mind is that in a significant number of communities across America, the hospital is not only the anchor of the healthcare system but also, as the largest local employer, the keystone of the community's economic stability. "Squeezing the hospital" for savings will only destabilize the local economy and ultimately undermine the goal of improved community health. We hasten to add, however, that an ACO dominated, or controlled, by traditional hospital interests would also be unlikely to succeed. The requirements of the PPACA and common sense demand that the ACO organizational structure foster shared hospital–physician decision making.

Organizing the Components of the ACO

Broadly speaking, there are three options for organizing the various components of an ACO:

1. a particular component of the ACO could be owned or controlled by the ACO or the system that operates the ACO;
2. the various components in an ACO could be tied together through common ownership of the ACO itself (i.e., a joint venture); or
3. the various components of the ACO could be tied together through contractual arrangements (e.g., a comprehensive affiliation agreement or, at the other end of the spectrum, a simple contract to purchase or lease services from a vendor).

Whether long-term acute care hospitals, rehabilitation hospitals, dialysis centers, or infusion centers are "owned" by the ACO, are part owners of the ACO (along with the hospital and physician organization), or provide services on an as-needed basis for the ACO will depend on local market conditions, past and current relationships, and sound business modeling. We believe, however, that a well-functioning ACO will need the capability to provide the full continuum of integrated care to a defined population of patients — be they children, the elderly, or those with acute or chronic illnesses. Regardless of how the various components become integrated into the ACO, they must participate meaningfully in strategic, operational, and financial decision making on the design of care, the delivery of care, revenue and cost management, and the distribution of shared savings.

Resources

ACO resources can be categorized into three primary groups: (1) physicians; (2) inpatient facilities; and (3) entities that provide ambulatory care, services, and programs. A reasonably complete list of these components is shown in Exhibit 3.1.

This list brings to mind an important observation: Over the past 50 years, hospitals have matured, organized, and become managed organizations. The ambulatory environment, historically the domain of physicians, has remained largely unmanaged.

To appreciate the role that physicians must play in an ACO, it is useful to quickly review the evolution of physician–physician and physician–hospital relationships over the past 25 years.

The Evolution of Physician–Physician Relationships

Physician practice models remained remarkably stable for the first three-quarters of the last century. With the exception of the large multispecialty group "clinics," physicians generally practiced in solo or small group practices. These "independent" physicians related to one another primarily through their hospital affiliation and their local, regional, or state medical societies. Most physicians were generalists, either medical or surgical, and their subspecialty practice had relatively little distinction.

The last quarter of the twentieth century saw the explosion of specialization. Orthopedists became hand, upper extremity, trauma, spine, total joint, foot and ankle, or sports medicine specialists. Cardiologists became electrophysiologists, congestive heart failure specialists, or diagnostic or interventional catheterization physicians, to name a few.

Exhibit 3.1 List of ACO Resources

Physicians Organized as	Inpatient Facilities and Services	Outpatient Facilities, Programs, and Services
Independent primary care physicians (patient-centered medical home)	General hospital	Medical office
Independent specialist physicians	Psychiatric hospital	Urgent care clinic
Faculty group practice	Children's hospital	Minute clinic
Captive group practice	Specialty hospital	Ambulatory surgical center
Independent group practice	Inpatient rehabilitation facility	Ambulatory care center
Physician hospital organization	Skilled nursing facility	Durable medical equipment
Physician organization	Long-term acute care facility	Dialysis center
Independent physician association	Hospice facility	Infusion center
Employed physicians	Short-stay infirmary	Freestanding diagnostic center
Federal qualified health center	Information technology services	Employer-based clinic
Foundation model		Alternative care center
		Medical spa
		Home health service
		Alternative care program
		Federally qualified health center
		Elderly, adult, or child day care
		Pharmacy services
		Care coordination services
		Disease management services
		Patient registry services
		Information technology services

As advances in science and technology enabled physicians to provide increasingly complex care in lower-acuity settings, individual practices narrowed in scope and unit prices for procedures plummeted. As unit reimbursement increases slowed, practices re-expanded their scope to maintain volumes, and their practices began to encroach on other specialists' practices. Cardiologists, interventional radiologists, and vascular surgeons began competing for the same interventional procedures.

At the same time, nonprocedural primary care physicians began to use hospitalists for inpatient practice, becoming more and more estranged from the hospital and many hospital-based specialists and isolated from each other and from many of their clinical colleagues.

The net result of the subspecialization and isolation has been a precipitous decline in professional identity within the medical community. Collegiality has been replaced with competition and fragmentation. In addition, many of the newest generation of physicians are seeking predictability, work–life boundaries, and a more balanced lifestyle. All of these factors have contributed to the re-emergence of physician employment by either hospitals or physician organizations such as group practices, faculty practices, or independent physician organizations. We have made several observations regarding the management of physicians and the achievement of outcomes, whether they are employed by a physician organization, a hospital, or a healthcare system:

1. While greater clinical integration can be achieved without economic/financial integration, achieving a meaningful clinical integration is difficult without some economic incentives to support it.
2. Greater integration is a key driver of improved clinical outcomes, economic performance, and, perhaps most important, provider satisfaction.
3. Migrating from a loosely coupled to a tightly coupled management system is extremely difficult and takes significant investment of time, energy, and financial and social capital. (See sidebar.)
4. Transforming care enough to significantly improve outcomes and resource utilization is much more difficult than achieving "clinical integration," at least as defined by the Federal Trade Commission.

5. The emerging generation of physicians is more comfortable with standardization and more capable of practicing medicine as a true team endeavor.

Inside delivery systems a number of new models are emerging, the most significant of which is the redefinition of "employed physician." The past decade has seen a re-emergence of practice acquisition, albeit on different terms than were common at the end of the twentieth century. Payments for practice "goodwill" are now rare, and hospitals and systems are now much more conscious about protecting themselves from the business and the legal risks associated with guaranteed compensation arrangements. Productivity-based compensation and other performance-based strategies are now the norm. What has not changed, however, is that acquisitions are often pursued for defensive purposes, without a clearly defined clinical strategy: The acquisition is based solely on short-term economic gains rather than longer-term improvements in affordability, access, and quality of care.

As the economics of independent group practice make organic, internal growth of clinical practices less achievable, hospitals have been forced to either employ physicians or subsidize the recruitment of new physicians by independent groups or physician organizations to maintain their required or desired workforce. It makes little sense to a 64-year-old physician to recruit a young associate; ensure her base income for a period of time; invest millions in practice infrastructure support such as space, computers, and support staff; and, as a result, dilute practice volume (at least temporarily) and personal income if the established physician anticipates retiring in the relatively near future.

Whatever the impetus, the net effect in many systems has been an *ad hoc* and reactionary approach to employing physicians, with many of the employed physicians exhibiting few, if any, of the desired characteristics of those typically recruited into a group practice. Moreover, these employment arrangements lack the leadership, culture, ethos, or infrastructure commonly associated with mature group practices. They also fail to build any meaningful sense of belonging to a professional organization, lack internal brand identity, and engender little sense of loyalty to either the delivery system or to a set of professional colleagues and collective outcomes. Rather than operating as a multispecialty group practice, these physicians operate as a loose confederation of professionals under independent contractual agreements with their employer.

It should come as no surprise that physicians in these types of employment arrangements frequently underperform at many levels. They lack the drivers that are embedded within the group practice model and culture. In addition, many of these practices are managed by professional hospital administrators who are unfamiliar with operations in the ambulatory environment. The downward pressure on physician reimbursement rates and the increasing restrictions on generation of significant ancillary income have further accelerated the trend toward employment as the preferred option for many physicians.

As payers continue to ratchet down reimbursement, the disconnect grows between physician compensation and the market's willingness to pay. Until ACOs align compensation packages and external market rates, ACOs risk even larger levels of cross-subsidization.

Multispecialty Group Practice Models

Over the past five years, there has been a near-universal strategy to migrate these dysfunctional physician employment relationships into structures that operate as true multispecialty group practices. This has required health systems to build internal leadership capable of working effectively with professional managers to produce desired clinical outcomes. As we discuss more fully later, we believe that a multispecialty group practice model is the necessary core of the ACO physician organization. What is frequently underestimated, however, is the energy and effort required to create this level of functionality in a physician practice. The large, integrated multispecialty practices most commonly referenced as the "industry standard" took many decades to develop, and most grew organically rather than by acquisition or aggregation.

In addition, most were founded by a forceful leader or team of leaders who shared a singular and compelling vision, and most were unhampered by the economic conditions present today. Simply putting a disparate group of hospital-focused physicians together with a group of ambulatory-based physicians, calling it a group practice, and expecting the group to function as a seasoned multispecialty practice is like putting eggs, cheese, and mushrooms together in a bowl and expecting an omelet to spontaneously emerge. Within this setting is precisely where the greatest tensions between preservation of autonomy and the benefits of group practice play out. As will be discussed more fully later, building a strong physician organization will be one of the primary challenges for many institutions pursuing the ACO strategy.

The Evolution of Physician–Hospital Relationships

The fundamental difference between the management of hospitals and medical staffs can be understood by examining each one's traditional organizational model.

Traditional hospitals, apart from the independent members of the medical staff who provide professional services within them, are *tightly coupled systems* that operate under a *management model* in which there are clear lines of authority, unambiguous delineation of accountabilities, and recognizable consequences (both positive and negative) for individual and collective actions. What this means is that a declaration of intention on the part of the hospital's chief executive officer has a reasonable chance of producing some action within the organization, although it may not necessarily be the desired or intended action. The "carrot and stick" inherent in traditional management models create incentives, rewards, and sanctions that are strong drivers of behavior. Compared to nonmedical corporations of similar size and complexity, hospitals generally appear relatively loosely coupled. But compared to the internal structures of their medical staffs, hospitals are actually tightly coupled.

Traditional medical staffs, on the other hand, are *loosely coupled systems*, analogous to the graduating class of a university or the members of a professional association. A university's student body is relatively loosely bound to the institution, coalescing at key assemblies, sporting events, and graduation ceremonies. At the same time, each student enjoys his or her own major, curriculum, friends, extracurricular activities, membership in a fraternity or sorority, and so forth. In brief, the traditional medical staff is best described as a collection of more-or-less independent physicians who fundamentally *work alone together*. Any resemblance of a medical staff to a team would be a track team, in which each member is competing in his or her own event, can win without a team victory, and is even likely to find himself or herself competing against teammates. Contrast that to a soccer team, in which the only way for the goalie to win is for the entire team to collectively score more goals than its opponent.

For many institutions, the only formal construct that unites the medical staff is the medical executive committee (MEC), presided over by the president of the medical staff or the MEC chair. In contrast to orders issued by a hospital CEO, a declaration of intention by the MEC chair generally produces deafening silence followed by astonishing inactivity. The medical staff typically suffers from being able to influence physician behavior only through severe sanctions, such as limiting or suspending privileges to practice within the institution. Because of their severity, these sanctions can only be justified in the case of flagrant and repeated policy violations. To further complicate the picture, the sanctions must be levied by a group of peers who may have economic dependence on the errant colleague for their livelihoods, representing an even greater barrier to action.

While yesterday's environment permitted and even encouraged a supplier–customer relationship between the hospital and its medical staff, today's environment requires a partnership relationship. Unfortunately, advances in science and technology, perverse reimbursement strategies, and in some cases compliance requirements have inhibited partnership relationships, fostering barriers or competition between the parties. Increasingly, physicians today are either *hospital dependent* (e.g., hospitalists, intensivists, emergency physicians, anesthesiologists, certain surgical specialties), *hospital independent* (e.g., primary care physicians, dermatologists, medical and surgical specialties such as sports medicine and endocrinology), or *hybrid* (e.g., gastroenterologists, cardiologists, many surgical specialties, some orthopedists, obstetricians).

Mutual need has kept hospital-dependent physicians reasonably tightly aligned with hospitals or healthcare systems. Hospital-independent physicians have little or no need to maintain relationships with the hospitals in today's environment. But it is the hybrid physicians with whom the hospitals have had the most contentious relationship. Many find themselves in direct competition with one another for patients because of their investments in diagnostic and imaging ventures or ambulatory surgical centers. This has been a source of great conflict over the past 25 years. Now, with changes in reimbursement, many physicians are seeking to reduce their financial risk, recoup their capital, and relinquish their entrepreneurial ventures.

It gets even more complicated. It is now common to find that the doctors who most vocally defend the "independent private practice of medicine" receive sizable stipends for managing and covering the hospital's critical care unit, catheterization laboratory, or stroke program. These arrangements further obfuscate the boundaries between voluntary or independent practice and employed medical staff. A hospital's medical staff has so many different relationships—voluntary private, employed, contractor, joint-venture partner, co-management partner, gainsharing participant, faculty practice, independent practice association (IPA), physician hospital organization (PHO), to name just a few. This tempts one to ask, "Just *which* medical staff are we talking about?" And one is also prompted to ask, "Just what does membership on the medical staff even *mean* to a primary care physician who hasn't practiced within the hospital's walls for more than a decade, and what does this mean to how we structure our ACO?"

ACO Structural Models: The Spectrum of Potential Options

Analogous to hospital and physician organizational models, the full spectrum of potential ACO structures includes tightly coupled organizational models, loosely coupled organizational models, models that lie between the two extremes, and models that combine elements of all three. In this section, we describe four archetypal models. We also present an innovative model that is quickly catching on among ACO innovators. It will become clear that for those systems not already operating as integrated delivery systems, only the intermediate models are practical for an ACO.

Joint Venture or Contractual Affiliation Model

The most loosely coupled option would create the ACO as either:

1. a joint-venture partnership entity that comprises enterprises that have an ownership stake in the business and a contractual relationship with the joint-venture partnership to provide clinical services (see Exhibit 3.2a) or
2. a series of contractual arrangements among the independent components of the ACO under which they agree to operate an ACO (see Exhibit 3.2b).

This federated model offers the benefit of relative ease of initiation, because it operates more like an "association" or "affiliation" of relative equals integrated through a series of internal service, contractual, and business agreements. The board (a fiduciary board in the case of a true joint venture, or an advisory board in the case of a

Exhibit 3.2a ACO Joint-Venture Partnership

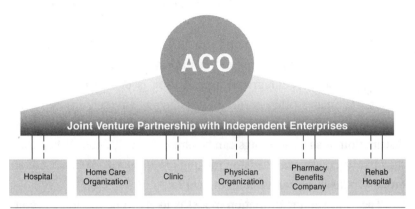

Note: Solid lines indicate ownership stake; dotted lines indicate contractual relationship

Exhibit 3.2b ACO Contractual Affiliation Model

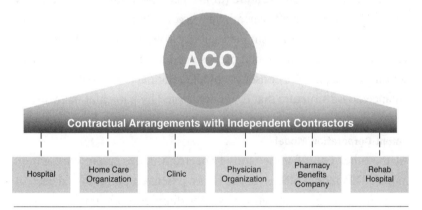

purely contractual arrangement) of such an entity would be populated by designees of its "affiliates."

The primary challenge in any affiliation model is balancing the need and desire of the individual parties to protect their parochial interests, on the one hand, and the need for the ACO to be a nimble, effective organization, on the other. In our experience, affiliation and joint venture models are frequently burdened by a governance structure that does not sufficiently limit the need for consensus-based decision making to major actions, therefore creating a high risk of deadlock and inaction. This is contrasted to the parent corporation model in which the component entities surrender ultimate control to the parent corporation, thereby reducing the risk of consensus paralysis.

This more loosely integrated structure often defaults to deal making between the participating entities in order to achieve consensus. But when a loosely integrated organization is unable to reach consensus, stalemates often ensue. Issues such as strategic investments, increase or reduction of the joint-venture partners, funds flow, and distribution of shared savings can be particularly difficult. When used selectively, consensual decision making has its merits. When used too broadly, consensus can gum up the works.

The joint venture/affiliation model is likely to be too loosely coupled for effective decision making in an ACO, unless the participants structure an affiliation/joint venture that delegates significant authority to the board of the joint venture (or the steering committee for a purely contractual arrangement) whereby the board is empowered to take most actions on the basis of a simple majority vote. For the affiliation/joint venture structure to work, the parties need to limit the scope of major actions that require the consensus of all participants and to create a governance/board structure that is not dominated by parochial interests.

Parent Corporation Model

At the other end of the coupling spectrum is the parent corporation model. This model places the ACO as a parent corporation and each of the participating organizations as subsidiary corporations to the parent. This model could be illustrated as shown in Exhibit 3.3, where each rectangle represents a participating subsidiary corporation, such as the hospital, physician organization, home care organization, pharmacy benefits company, and rehabilitation hospital.

The benefits of the parent corporation model lie in the clarity of decision making (the parent) and the capacity for enterprise integration. The challenges of the parent company model are that, depending on how authority and accountability are distributed, the participating organizations can be required to yield to the parent corporation an uncomfortable amount of authority.

Exhibit 3.3 ACO Parent Corporation Model

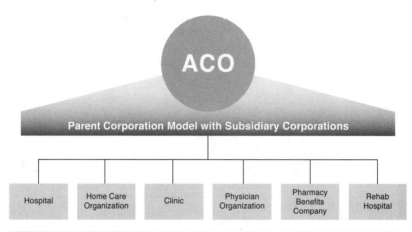

While in theory this model appears viable, in practice it would be analogous to a hotel partnering with a florist, a limousine service, and a music booking agency to form a new corporation whose sole business was wedding planning and production. None of the partners could survive with a business that functioned exclusively in that limited market. For the same reasons, a parent corporation whose sole business line is ACO contracting and delivery is impractical for the present or foreseeable future. Therefore, having a parent corporation that is an ACO (i.e., a corporation whose sole purposes are to contract for and deliver ACO-style care) is not really a viable option.

Subsidiary Corporation Model

Depending on the distribution of authority and accountability, the subsidiary corporation model offers some of the advantages of both the parent corporation and the joint-venture models. Much like the joint-venture model, management of the ACO can be controlled by its participating members, offering the ACO reasonable but limited authority over strategy, operations, and resources. Like the parent corporation model, however, certain powers over decisions (e.g., large capital investments, dissolution of the ACO, elements of business planning) are retained by the parent corporation. The parent also has the authority to step in if the subsidiary becomes paralyzed or ineffective. (See Exhibit 3.4.)

Exhibit 3.4 ACO Subsidiary Corporation Model

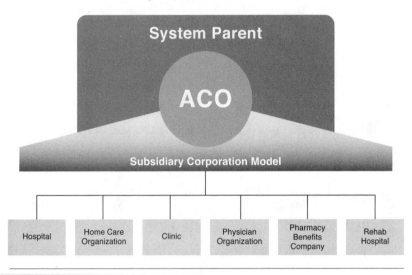

Organizing the ACO as a subsidiary corporation provides a reasonable structure for addressing a unique challenge faced by multi-modeled HMOs in the 1980s and 1990s—that is, it is difficult for an organization to function under two simultaneous and fundamentally different ideological and operational models. Bluntly speaking, from an economic perspective those components of the parent corporation that operate as the ACO will be faced with a near-term incentive to keep people out of the hospital and will naturally seek "parental" resources to support that goal. But the other components of the parent corporation have a near-term incentive to keep hospital beds filled and will be seeking resources to support *their* goal. The subsidiary corporation model enables the parent to invest in both models, just as some holding companies concurrently market competing products.

We expect that the ACOs organized under this model will likely be preexisting integrated delivery systems already subject to common control who see themselves as embracing a new strategic and clinical vision.

Operating Division Model

This model creates the ACO as an operating division of the system parent corporation. Here, the ACO operates as a division of the

Exhibit 3.5 ACO Operating Division Model

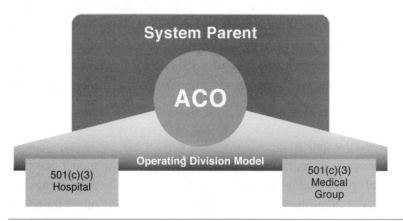

system, but it is not organized as a separate corporate entity (see Exhibit 3.5). The governing body of the ACO is the governing body of the system, although the system could establish an ACO steering committee. Moreover, the management team of the ACO is fully integrated into the management team of the system and will often overlap with the management team of the various other components of the system.

In this model, the ACO is one line of business inside the portfolio of business lines that operates within the parent corporation and, as such, will ultimately be affected by the overall system strategy. This is generally viewed favorably when an operating division is the recipient of strategic resource investments from the parent and less favorably when those resources are invested in sibling divisions.

In the operating division or subsidiary models, the level of parental control will naturally be determined by the needs of the organization, personalities of leaders, local conditions, and so forth, so that these models can operate anywhere along the continuum of loosely to tightly coupled systems. Regardless of the model chosen, oversight, control, authority, and accountability must be explicitly spelled out (in charter documents or other governance documents) to avoid conflict and resentment during the design and implementation phases of the ACO.

The first decision an organization that participates in an ACO will need to make is to define its corporate structure (this is discussed further in Chapter 9). Whichever model is chosen, the ACO must be structured to make the business cases and share accountability for managing care and allocating resources. These two principal functions will separate the winners in this strategy from the losers.

An Innovative Option

At this early stage, there is no "best" option, but one model deserves special consideration. It has been successfully deployed in a growing number of controlled physician practices and is well suited for adoption with respect to an entire ACO. This model combines some of the more desirable features of the subsidiary corporation and the operating division models.

The *legal* structure used in this model is an operating division model (i.e., there is no separate legal entity). The *functional operating* model, however, is that of a subsidiary corporation. That is, the ACO division operates with a governance structure that is designed to mimic that of an independent corporation. Instead of a fiduciary board, however, the ACO division is governed by two leadership committees in which leaders of key components of the ACO actively participate. One committee is the strategy and business development committee, which serves most of the functions of a traditional board. That committee establishes policy; selects the managers; sets strategy; and makes business decisions such as capital investments, revenue cycle vendors, internal funds flow, compensation strategy, and information technology investments (to the degree negotiated with the parent corporation.) The other committee is the clinical operations committee. It focuses on care integration, clinical operating efficiencies, clinical office management, population management, workflow, and the development of clinical protocols. It, too, has representation from system leadership. The two committees meet together at least quarterly and jointly develop strategy and budget, subject to approval by the parent company management. This model is shown in Exhibit 3.6.

Exhibit 3.6 ACO Functional Operating Model

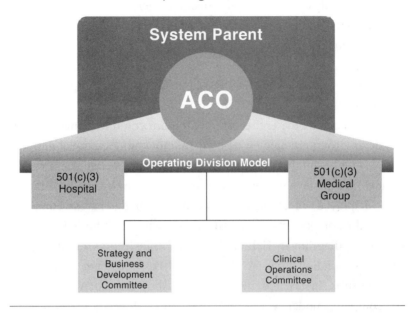

Department and division chiefs, facility leaders, medical directors, and professional and other clinical managers are distributed across the two committees according to interests and capabilities. To the degree possible (while still achieving appropriate standardization), day-to-day management is left up to the ACO component parts.

One key feature of the operating division model, however, must be clearly retained: At all times the system parent has the authority to step in and make decisions, especially if the two leadership committees demonstrate an inability to work together effectively.

ACO Building Blocks

Broadly speaking, the ACO has four major structural components, each of which can be integrated into the ACO through one of the models discussed earlier. The four broad categories are as follows:

- Physicians in a tightly organized physician organization
- Hospitals—in general, acute care, specialty, pediatric, psychiatric, rehabilitation, and chronic

- Other facility-based service entities, such as ambulatory surgery centers, dialysis centers, and infusion centers
- Other non-facility-based services, such as home care, pharmacy, and physical and occupational therapy

As noted earlier, while the PPACA provides that a physician group could serve as a Medicare ACO, it is inconceivable that a meaningful integration across the entire care continuum could be achieved by a physician group practice on its own. Without an operational partnership with a hospital or healthcare system the physician group would be unable to achieve meaningful performance improvements. Graphically displayed, in a manner consistent with the parent company model, the components of an ACO are shown in Exhibit 3.7.

In the diagram in Exhibit 3.7, solid lines represent subsidiary corporate relationships, while dotted lines represent contractual relationships. In essence, the solid lines show the extent of the parent company model, while the dotted lines show the extension of the parent company model through the affiliation model. We expect that most ACOs, as a reflection of local market conditions and historic circumstance, will operate as a combination of solid and dotted lines. As stated, in our view, the subsidiary corporation and operating division models present the best opportunity for success. This is especially true with respect to the tie between the physician organization and the hospital. Unless those two fundamental building blocks of the ACO have a "corporate" relationship to the ACO or its parent to ensure tight-enough alignment for meaningful clinical integration, joint decision making, and economic risk sharing, we think constructing an ACO that will meet the challenges of the evolving market will be an uphill battle.

System Physician Organization

We use the term "physician organization" to describe all the physicians who are connected, in at least some portion of their practice, to the ACO. As depicted in Exhibit 3.7, physicians could be brought in to the physician organization through a variety of models. A relatively

Exhibit 3.7 Components of an ACO

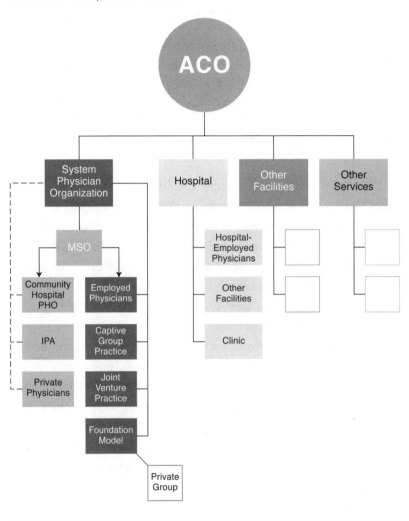

complete list of such models, from most integrated with the ACO to least, includes the following:

- direct employment by a hospital or other ACO component;
- employment by a wholly controlled, but with a separate legal entity, group practice;

- a joint-venture group practice owned in part by a component of the ACO (e.g., a controlled group practice) and in part by private practice physicians;
- a foundation model arrangement with a private group practice;
- a physician hospital organization or an independent practice association (IPA) in which the ACO participates;
- a management services organization model; and
- a contractual affiliation other than a PHO, an IPA, or a medical service organization (MSO).

As a physician organization moves toward the less-integrated end of this spectrum, the challenges of operating in a tightly coupled, effective fashion will increase, as will the legal barriers to such action. On the other hand, moving toward the less-integrated end of the spectrum opens the possibility of broader participation in the physician organization. A physician organization that restricts itself to the more highly integrated models may find it difficult to build a physician organization of sufficient size and breadth.

In most ACOs, the physician organization, as a function of history and necessity, will need to operate across several points on this spectrum. It will need to integrate employed physicians who are captive to the system with independent physicians who voluntarily elect to join the physician organization for at least part of their practice. As stated, the physician organization must, by definition, operate as a tightly coupled organization with respect to the *design and operations of the clinical practice* while at the same time potentially permit a more loosely coupled portfolio of *economic relationships* to enable the physician organization to attract a broader group of high-performing participants (e.g., high-performing specialists). The most important operating principle is that, in agreeing to participate as a member of the physician organization, each physician or physician practice explicitly agrees to adhere to a set of fundamental practice principles. These principles will include patient-centered and evidence-based care; efficient resource utilization; and adherence to identified care pathways, protocols, and operational systems designed and directed by the physician organization to which the individual or group voluntarily belongs. This operating principle can be seen in Exhibit 3.8.

Ideally, the physician enterprise is organized to encourage and enable all interested physicians to actively participate in the design and implementation of clinical delivery. It must also be structured in a way that actively monitors physician compliance with clinical practices and takes corrective action to effectively address those who fail to comply with such agreed-upon clinical standards. Failure to introduce and fully support (in word and deed) that important principle from the outset will only breed organizational cynicism, spur the development of unproductive habits, and produce suboptimal results. It is important to reiterate here that there can be no exceptions to rules until an organization creates those rules and sets the expectations for adhering to them.

There is no perfect recipe for leadership and management of the physician organization. But in our experience, the model that seems to achieve the best outcomes is based on a productive partnership between physician leadership and professional management. Physician leadership is most heavily represented in the organization's governance structure, setting strategy, direction, and policy and approving capital investments and operating budgets. Carrying out those tasks is then delegated to the professional management, who is explicitly accountable to the physician governance leadership. The professional managers must be able to analyze the organization's practices and make the rational and compelling case for action or change. We have found that this is most effectively carried out when the professional managers are selected by and accountable to the physician leadership. Physicians are much more accepting of direction provided by professional managers that they have had a hand in choosing, especially if the direction is one that is not preferred by some or all of the physicians.

Employed Physicians

Because the physician organization must operate as a tightly coupled organization with respect to the design and operations of the clinical practice, we believe that most successful physician organizations will have at their core a large group of employed physicians who operate in

Exhibit 3.8 ACO Physician Organization Principles

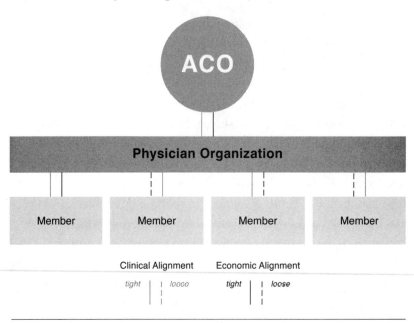

the manner of a high-functioning multispecialty group practice. Such a multispecialty group practice does not necessarily require a separate legal entity, but it must be grounded in a large group of employed physicians who practice in a collaborative manner. These physicians could be employed in a separate legal entity; indeed, we think that such a separate entity will often reinforce the culture and operational environment that needs to be established. However, the physicians could also be employed by a hospital or another ACO component.

Whichever model is chosen, the governance over the practice of the employed physicians must be vested, in the first instance, in a leadership committee (when the physicians are employed by the hospital) or a board (when the physicians are employed by a separate legal entity). In either case, the governing body is the heart of a high-functioning multispecialty group practice. (This is analogous to the earlier discussion regarding the leadership committees or board of the ACO itself.) While distinctions between governance and management are often ambiguous in small physician group practices, in a group practice large enough to serve as the core of an ACO's physician organization (e.g., more than

100 members) the governance and management functions need to be separated. Our emphasis here is on governance. Management should be delegated to experienced, professional lay managers.

In short, the physician organization must have, at its core, a group of employed physicians (not necessarily employed by a hospital or health system) who operate in the manner of a multispecialty group practice. This means that

- the physicians are members of a leadership committee, a governing board, or another body that plays a meaningful role (subject to ultimate oversight and authority at the ACO/parent level) in the direction of the clinical practice;
- the group practice can make decisions and hold individual physicians accountable for executing those decisions; and
- members of the group practice collaborate on providing clinical care.

With such a core, a physician organization can relatively easily extend its reach through one or more of the models described in the following section.

Medical Foundation Model A flexible new model that is emerging out of today's quest for greater integration is a "reinvention" of the medical foundation model. While traditional foundations emerged in California as a work-around for the legal corporate practice of medicine restrictions, a number of systems today are creating "new model" foundations that offer unique flexibility and opportunity. Under this model, the foundation, which is essentially a group practice controlled by the system, enters into a professional services agreement with private group practices under which the non-employed physicians provide medical services through the foundation.

In most cases, the group practice that is the foundation could, and should, be the group practice that forms the nucleus of the physician organization as described earlier. This model permits physicians to retain some degree of economic autonomy as employees of their private group practice, yet it allows the system to fully integrate them from a clinical perspective because the physicians provide medical services through the

Example of an Aligned Group Practice: Children's Hospital of Atlanta

An excellent example of an organization that has been effective in transforming its physicians under employment into an aligned group practice is Children's Hospital of Atlanta. While its issues are relatively typical of hospitals across America today, its solution was atypically effective in aligning its employed physicians.

Children's Scottish Rite campus is served by a large number of committed private physicians along with a growing number of employed physicians across a wide range of specialties. By late 2008, the number of employed physicians at the hospital had grown to nearly 200 and tensions between the physicians and hospital administration had also increased significantly. The employed physicians felt disenfranchised from the hospital and lacked sufficient unity to resolve the situation. Four issues dominated the employed physicians' concerns:

1. The absence of a forum for physician input into system strategic planning, clinical resource planning, and management decisions that affected patient care
2. The feeling of isolation from each other and significant missed opportunities to collaborate on patient care
3. The feeling of a significant number of employed physicians that they were professionally "lost" in the hospital organizational structure
4. The experience by most employed physicians of not having sufficient influence on the providers of hospital administrative services that support their clinical practices

At the same time, hospital administrators were experiencing the following:

1. The absence of a platform for the development of a unified physician strategy
2. The inability to manage an overly complex web of disparate "one-off" physician relationships
3. The lack of a vehicle for effective mutual business planning and execution
4. The sense that their physician counterparts lacked a holistic perspective on programmatic demands on the capital "envelope" across the system

Finally, the independent community physicians expressed their own set of issues:

1. The sense that the system was unwilling (at least historically) to partner with community physicians to achieve mutually held goals
2. The (incorrect) assumption by many that the system intended to eventually employ as many physicians as possible
3. The insufficient collaboration among various private medical groups and with the hospital

With this background, Children's leadership invited a group of physicians to join it in a "Continental Congress" (described further in Chapter 9) to design and implement a different organizational model for integrating its employed physicians. The process produced an innovative structure in which pods of similar practices were created, each supported by its own local clinical operations council. Each pod is led by a physician–professional manager dyad. The physician leader of each pod serves on a practice-wide strategic leadership council to set strategy, policy, and standards and to manage business operations of the entire practice (much like a traditional physician practice board does). That council is chaired by the president of the practice, who is appointed by the hospital in conjunction with physician leaders in the practice and who works in partnership with the executive director of the practice. (See Exhibit 3.9.)

When asked about the model, Carolyn Kenny, Children's executive vice president for clinical care, pointed out that the real value was achieved in the process of designing the model: It was during the six-month design process that attitudes shifted, relationships were built, trust was established, and optimism developed. "Everything shifted when the physicians joined us at the design table," says Kenny. "While the end product is an institutional structure that enables the hospital and its employed physicians to optimize clinical integration and operational efficiency, the real value lies in the new relationship more than the structure."

Children's took a unique approach to the assessment and design process. Not only did the hospital involve its governing board as active participants, it also invited the president of the medical staff, a private

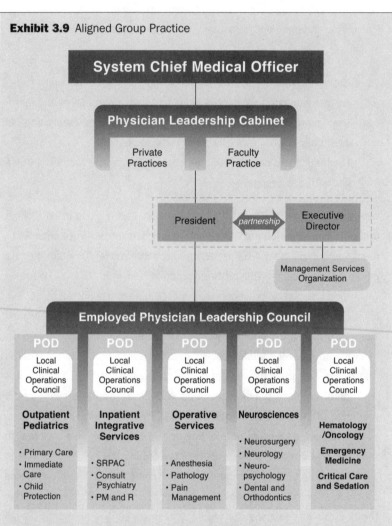

Exhibit 3.9 Aligned Group Practice

System Chief Medical Officer

Physician Leadership Cabinet

Private Practices

Faculty Practice

President ←*partnership*→ Executive Director

Management Services Organization

Employed Physician Leadership Council

POD	POD	POD	POD	POD
Local Clinical Operations Council	Local Clinical Operations Council	Local Clinical Operations Council	Local Clinical Operations Council	Local Clinical Operations Council
Outpatient Pediatrics	**Inpatient Integrative Services**	**Operative Services**	**Neurosciences**	**Hematology /Oncology**
• Primary Care			• Neurosurgery	**Emergency Medicine**
• Immediate Care	• SRPAC	• Anesthesia	• Neurology	
• Child Protection	• Consult Psychiatry	• Pathology	• Neuro-psychology	**Critical Care and Sedation**
	• PM and R	• Pain Management	• Dental and Orthodontics	

Note: PM and R: Physical Medicine and Rehabilitation; SRPAC: Scottish Rite Pediatric and Adolescent Consultants

physician, and other private physicians to actively participate in the process. This demonstration of full transparency had two unexpected effects on the outcome. First, there was absolutely no resistance from the private staff. Second, a number of private physicians are now considering joining the employed practice because they can see that the new model increases the sense of partnership between the hospital and the physicians.

Additional insights are offered by Daniel Salinas, MD, the hospital's chief medical officer: "Children's Healthcare of Atlanta, with multiple practice models among our medical staff, long understood the need for greater clinical integration and alignment of physicians across our system in order to improve quality and the delivery of care for our patients. We focused first on aligning the physician practices we employ. Through that process we invited the participation and input of those not directly employed by us, and we were able to crystallize our overarching understanding of physician alignment at Children's, regardless of practice model. 'Physician-led, professionally managed' has become the apt description of how Children's is bringing together physician leadership and administration to drive systemic improvements and innovations to help us achieve clinical and operational excellence. Our shared passion and commitment to improving the lives of children became a strengthened guiding principle that united us in a way that we never fully understood before. From that common understanding emerged what we now call the Physician Promise, which is our joint commitment to each other of what we need and what we promise in return in order to deliver on our vision for pediatric care in Georgia."

foundation. Support staff and MSO functions are generally managed by the foundation, though they can be managed by each participating group or can even be subcontracted back to the system, if preferred. In this model the foundation sets clinical standards and monitors and manages clinical performance. As employees of their individual practices, the physicians retain control over individual compensation arrangements. Incentives, rewards, and penalties attributable to the ACO arrangement are created by the governance and management of the foundation. This model looks like Exhibit 3.10.

Joint-Venture Group Practice Model The joint-venture model contemplates a group practice owned, in part, by an employed physician organization (or another entity within the system) and, in part, by independent

Exhibit 3.10 ACO Medical Foundation Model

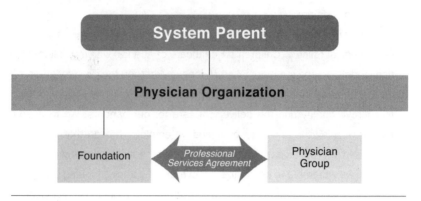

physicians who choose to joint venture with the employed physician organization. How such an arrangement works in practice will depend to a large degree on the relative ownership/control of the joint venture between the physician organization and the private physicians. Majority control by the physician organization/ACO may result in a more tightly aligned relationship. Less than majority control will probably result in the joint venture being more of a contractual "affiliate" to the physician organization. This model is graphically represented in Exhibit 3.11.

Contractual Arrangements Model The most common contractual methods for expanding the reach of the physician organization are the PHO/IPA and the MSO models. These are traditional and well-understood models that we will not focus on here, except to point out the significant challenges of incorporating these models into a true physician organization. There are significant legal and operational barriers to integrating physicians, through a PHO/IPA, an MSO, or another contractual relationship, into the physician organization. These models are best thought of as vehicles to give physicians an opportunity to test-drive participation in a physician organization before they enter into one of the other models.

Conceived in the late 1980s, PHOs were initially used as single-signature contracting vehicles to enable hospitals and their affiliated physicians to accept capitated contracts. As capitation failed to gain

Exhibit 3.11 Joint-Venture Group Practice Model

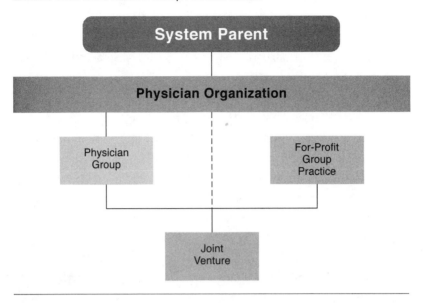

momentum in the early 1990s and all but disappeared from many markets in the late 1990s, the role of the PHO came into question. Some evolved into MSOs, and others simply became dormant vestiges of managed care. But with the emergence of the ACO, many organizations are reconsidering the clinically integrated PHO as their preferred physician–hospital management structure. One such contemporary PHO is being developed within Detroit Medical Center, an organization in the throes of accelerating organizational change. (See sidebar.)

Governance of the Physician Organization
Regardless of the model selected, the governing body of the physician organization must be able to establish, adjudicate, and enforce policies and standards that apply to all participating physicians. If the physician organization is an entirely independent economic business enterprise (as might be the case under the affiliation model, for example), these policies will necessarily include strategic business-related issues such as overall direction, strategy, capital investments, and operating budgets. If the physician organization is not an independent

Example of a Contemporary PHO: Detroit Medical Center

The philosophy of the PHO at Detroit Medical Center (DMC) (2010) is "each doctor's decision regarding his or her practice structure is fully respected and supported. Private physicians, faculty doctors, and employed staff are all considered equal, and no participant is being asked to change his or her practice structure."

In the DMC model, the PHO board will be composed of 24 physicians, 12 members representing private physicians, 6 members representing University Physician Group (faculty practice), and 6 members representing DMC executive and medical leadership. The PHO start-up is partially funded by a $1,000 initial membership fee. The goal of DMC's PHO is to integrate private physicians, faculty physicians, the medical school, and the Medical Center. Its challenge will be to effectively integrate a broad set of diverse interests (i.e., teaching, research, clinical care, hospital management, medical school management, and practice management) within a large governing body of which half will effectively represent even more widely divergent interests of private physicians.

The art of this PHO anatomy will be in constructing the reserve powers of the anchor organizations—the Medical Center, the Medical School, and the faculty practice. If the faculty practice is reasonably tightly coupled, its six representatives will be able to effectively represent a unified set of interests. The 12 private physicians on the board will almost certainly represent widely divergent interests of a large number of private physicians. Without the unifying construct and shared destiny of the ACO to serve as a fiduciary integrator, decision making within this relatively large board will be difficult.

economic enterprise (as would be the case under the divisional model and, to a lesser extent, the parent company model), the operating budget will be developed in partnership with the parent organization's management team. In either model, the strategic direction and allocation of resources must ultimately support the business and strategic goals of the ACO.

With respect to the clinical enterprise, the focus of the governing body will be on the establishment of clinical, quality, and service standards, such as access, productivity, efficiency, patient satisfaction, compliance, and quality outcomes. This type of practice culture will predictably be challenged by independent physicians who, virtually by definition, place high value on independence and autonomy; this runs counter to the ultimate goal of the ACO physician organization, which is to reduce non-value-added practice variation to optimize clinical and business outcomes.

"Autonomy" is preserved in the individual physician–patient relationship and the sanctity of what transpires between patient and caregiver in the examination room, but not in those approaches to care in which there is demonstrable evidence that certain policies or protocols lead to superior clinical and business outcomes and improvement in the health status of a population. When it comes to the design and delivery of care management, there must be strict adherence to practices, guidelines, and protocols that have demonstrated value— whether in producing quality outcomes, reducing resource utilization, or (ideally) both.

Roles of Governance A fundamental role of governance is to establish the policies and mechanisms that will enable physician and professional managers to hold practitioners accountable for adhering to practices developed by their physician organization.

Another role of governance, which is a parallel role to that of ACO governance, is to develop the operational model for internal funds flow within the physician organization. Principles and strategies must be developed and deployed for distributing clinical, administrative, research, teaching, and strategic funds and the potential shared savings among the participating practitioners/resources—that is, physicians, nurses, psychologists, optometrists, podiatrists, and the like. While this is often a formidable task, models developed by integrated delivery systems and multispecialty group practices that do not operate on a strictly production model have worked. Many examples can be used to help physician governing bodies develop reasonable internal funds flow and income-distribution models. Their utility and applicability depend highly on the flexibility and generosity of spirit of the participating physicians.

Clearly, the most contentious issues in ACOs are likely to be those surrounding the distribution of revenue and shared savings bonuses to the clinicians. No single best formula exists that accurately identifies the contribution of individual physicians or even groups of physicians to either group practice clinical outcomes or operating efficiencies. However, many methods can be used to help physician governing bodies develop reasonable internal funds flow and income-distribution models. Most attempt to put a value on the clinical, administrative, research, teaching, and strategic contributions that various resources make to improve end goals, such as quality and efficiency. See Chapter 7 for more details on recommended funds flow design and mechanics.

At the end of the day, the physicians must accept either the perspective that efficiency and quality outcomes are team endeavors or continually battle over who contributed what to performance. Suffice it to say that myriad models can be introduced that are innovative, responsible, rational, and fair. None is perfect. The funds flow and allocation of shared savings or other performance incentives and rewards will, of course, vary depending on the ACO reimbursement model. Keep in mind that the Medicare pilots intend to operate initially within a fee-for-service reimbursement model. Regardless of whether the ACO is operating in a traditional fee-for-service or a partially or fully capitated environment, the focus must be on ensuring that appropriate care is always provided to each patient whenever needed. At the same time, non-value-added interventions must be eliminated, and the organization must never fall prey to the temptation of preventing sick, needy, costly, and vulnerable patients from participating. Depending on whether or how CMS risk-stratifies patients, these needier members may paradoxically offer the greatest opportunity for improving the cost trends, potentially contributing disproportionately to operating savings. This is covered in greater detail in Chapter 7.

The final role of governance is its fiduciary responsibility to the practice. While each member of the governing body brings the perspectives and insights of a particular discipline, specialty, or work group, the foundational purpose of the governing body requires that members remain focused on the overall interests of the physician organization rather than on individual departments or specialties. At the risk of sounding overly altruistic, the fact is that the shared destiny of the clinicians requires short-term trade-offs and compromises in order to optimize long-term performance and success of the ACO. Unintended and undesired inequities that emerge in the course of events will need to be adjudicated by the governing body.

Roles of Management As noted, the primary role of governance is to establish overall direction for the practice and establish operating policies that enable members of the physician organization to hold one another accountable for performance. Management's first role is to translate that strategy into action through coordinated, integrated operating and care delivery models that optimize clinical and business performance.

A second role of management is to ensure that the clinical practices are adequately supported by technology and service practice supports, such as revenue cycle management, supplies, malpractice insurance, and other essentials. Management's responsibility is to set clear expectations and provide performance feedback to ensure that the *preferred* way of getting the work done is always the *easiest* way of getting the work done. (This is discussed further in Chapter 5.) Simply providing data is not enough. Unless data are processed and analyzed, they do not become information that can be used to take action. Finally, analysis of the information in conjunction with tight feedback loops yield knowledge that can then be used to further refine the organizational design. This underscores the axiom introduced in Chapter 2: All systems are perfectly designed to produce the outcomes they produce. Transforming raw data into information and finally knowledge enables organizations to continuously refine their design in the service of performance optimization.

The overarching management strategy is to continually transform a loosely coupled system into a more tightly coupled system. Some physicians are well suited for this; others are not. It is best to be up front about expectations for physicians who are considering this type of practice model: Generally, those ill suited to a more tightly coupled system will opt out before they find themselves practicing in an environment that makes them feel uncomfortable. It is wise to take an important lesson from the flight attendant who performs a destination check just before closing the aircraft door: "This is a reminder that you are on Flight 314 headed for Chicago; if Chicago is not in your travel plans, this would be an excellent time to depart this aircraft." Those who elect to participate in this type of practice must recognize that individual and collective performance is more closely managed within a more tightly coupled structure.

Autonomy, however attractive, will not be a highly supported individual value in this type of practice environment. It will be replaced by a willingness to be a full and active participant in designing and supporting the practice model. Finally and most important, the practice must be managed in such a way that supports and advances the goals of the ACO, of which it is an essential component. Those who find such a proposition undesirable would be well advised to "depart the aircraft" before the door is closed.

Hospitals Within the ACO

Governance and Management

Volumes have been written about the governance and management of hospitals. This section focuses on one important aspect of contemporary physician–hospital relationships, which, unfortunately, have eroded badly during the past quarter century. Primary care physicians have increasingly withdrawn from active participation in the hospital setting, while specialists have competed with the hospital for what feels to them like a zero-sum game for reimbursement dollars (especially those related to lucrative ancillary services). The net effect has been the progressive disengagement of primary care providers and the growing tension among overlapping specialists and between specialists and hospitals.

To further heighten the tension, advances in science and technology have enabled increasingly more complex care to be provided in less resource-intense environments outside the hospital. As a general observation, as care migrates to less resource-intense settings, patient satisfaction improves. Perhaps the most discouraging consequence of all this has been a profound breakdown of collegiality and professionalism among physicians. This lack of collegiality is one of the major contributors to the escalation of the ubiquitous deal making that has taken place between hospitals and physicians over the past 25 years. Many hospitals, while preferring to work collaboratively with most or all of their specialists in a given field, have had to choose among them because of the lack of collegiality and civility among competing individuals and groups. The net effect is that physicians have been significantly underrepresented in hospital strategic planning and operations management. This is a deficit that must be overcome if an ACO is to succeed.

The Transition from Hospital to Healthcare System

With continued industry consolidation, shrinking volume, eroding margins, and the loss of once-reliable investment income in the past few years, hospitals have had to protect their already thin margins to support the renovation of aging facilities and investments in new technology. This focused need, along with the tension between the hospital and its medical staff described earlier, has kept many hospitals and hospital systems from making the transition from hospital systems to healthcare delivery systems. When they do make this transition, hospitals find themselves as the logical conveners of new, integrated models in which they may no longer be the central player. Given the competitive healthcare environment between hospitals and physicians that has evolved over the past 25 years, learning to share accountability and authority with physicians is not something that comes naturally or easily to many hospital leaders. Shared accountability and authority goes well beyond appointing five physicians to the hospital's board or hiring a chief medical officer or vice president of medical affairs. It means actively inviting the physicians to the strategy table as full contributors, despite their lack of formal management training or ownership of institutional assets.

As a result of this, many hospitals are reorganizing their leadership models around physician partnership. While the role of the medical executive committee (MEC) remains, its functions are more clearly defined around credentialing, establishing medical staff policy, and performing peer review. For hospitals that adopt this shared-leadership model, the MEC is no longer the sole imprimatur of the physicians. As hospitals redefine their boundaries outside of their traditional walls, many are beginning to design and implement management models that fully engage formal physician managers—not as observers or advisors, but as full partners in decision making. There is mounting evidence that when hospitals reorganize their leadership and management functions in this way, physician leaders step to the plate and actively participate in the difficult decisions that healthcare delivery systems need to make.

A good example is Saint Agnes Medical Center in Fresno, California. By late 2008, tensions between the hospital and its medical staff had reached a feverish pitch. Trust had eroded, hospital leadership had undergone significant turnover, and local competition among physicians and between physicians and the hospitals had reached a breaking point. Under the joint direction of Thomas Anderson, an innovative and bold interim CEO, and Dr. Charles Farr, the well-respected and thoughtful president of the medical staff, Saint Agnes asked nine physicians to join the hospital's senior managers in what they called their "integrated leadership team" (ILT). This group expanded the previous senior management team; it did not replace the existing medical executive committee function. Instead, it was chartered as the new senior management team of the hospital. From its inception, the ILT became the strategic and operational decision-making body for the hospital.

Within a year, the ILT had significant impact on the hospital. Decisions about key clinical services that had been politically deadlocked for months were resolved, along with decisions about coverage and capital investments. Physician integration, as measured by The Bard Index®, had improved remarkably. As one member of the ILT noted, the greatest tribute to the ILT was that over the course of the year no "stupid decisions" had been made. "The ILT has fundamentally transformed the culture and the performance of Saint Agnes Hospital," says Stacy Vaillancourt, Saint Agnes's vice president for strategy. "The physicians are now engaged as partners in the strategy, operations, and destiny of our medical center."

Another strategy that has worked particularly well has been to replace the rotating elected physician departmental leadership structure with appointed physician leaders. These leaders are paid a fair-market-value stipend for their time and effort and operate with clear performance expectations in their management roles. The appointed chiefs, in turn, join the senior management team of the hospital and play an active role in the design and implementation of hospital strategy and operations. This model is, of course, a logical precursor to the joint management model required within an ACO. While the focus today is primarily on the inpatient environment, over time this will include partnership in the management of the ambulatory environment as well.

As physicians migrate to a more tightly coupled management structure that is physician led and professionally managed, the hospitals are also migrating to a more shared-management structure. They are beginning to redefine themselves as healthcare delivery systems and are actively inviting physicians to the leadership and management table.

Other Facilities in the ACO "Mall"

Many other services will be required by the ACO, including pharmacy, dialysis, home care, and urgent care. Because of the relatively bounded span of each service, sound business modeling can determine how each component should be integrated into the ACO (i.e., subject to common control, as a joint-venture partner, or through contractual arrangement). The two exceptions are care coordination and information technology. Of all the services required for operating within the ACO, these two services are absolutely critical to success, and both should be fully embedded within the core management and operational structure of the ACO *at every level*. These functions are addressed in more detail in chapters 4 and 6.

In general, there is no best management practice, and any model developed by an ACO will evolve over time beyond its initial design. Experience continually teaches us that the initial design should focus on the development of core values and principles rather than on envisioning each and every situation that might develop. With strong guiding principles, the managers will be able to craft solutions to unanticipated situations and use them to develop case-law guidelines. The needs of the specific patient population being served will play a big role in determining the appropriate model. Ultimately, the decision about how to design the ACO may depend on a set of leadership intangibles, including the skills and interests of leaders in the local medical community and their capacity for effective partnership. Management books strongly advise leaders to design their management models around functions rather than around people. Experience teaches us that the answer is always some blend between the two.

Clearly, facilities that participate as partners will need to have leadership representation on the governing body of the ACO. Those who participate in a meaningful way within the operations of the ACO should be included in the management structure as well, particularly those facilities and resources that need to get involved in innovation and integration of their historic operating structures and systems. These other participating facilities would certainly play a role in the operating councils, and this topic is covered in great detail in Chapter 4.

Governance Principles for the ACO: Transitioning to Physiology

The core functions of any governing body are to establish policies; select and evaluate the performance of executive management; ensure legal compliance; and provide input, oversight, and approval of performance standards, capital investments, and operating budgets. The ACO model also requires that the governing body establish the principles of funds flow among the entities within the organization and the principles that govern the distribution of potential shared savings among the participating entities. (Under capitation, these could become shared losses.) The PPACA requires the governing body to handle this role. So does common sense. Funds flow within any practicing organization is best left to the governance or leadership of that organization (see the discussion later regarding the physician organization).

If the subsidiary corporation model is selected, the following principles might help guide the formation and initial structure of the board. If one of the suggested hybrid models is used, the following principles would apply to the operating committees. These principles are stated as reserve powers of the parent board, and great care should be taken to limit these powers to a minimum so as to not impair the flexibility and innovative potential in the ACO:

- The parent company board should retain a "must agree" relationship with the ACO board's selection of its executive director and its medical director.
- The parent company must approve the removal of either ACO executive.
- The parent company board should retain the power to approve the addition of any new partners in the ACO and must agree on their participation in the governance of the ACO.
- Capital investments over a certain threshold should require approval by the parent board.
- The parent company board should approve the ACO's strategic plan and budget.
- The parent company's board should be informed of any unresolved tension between the parties that make up the ACO.
- The ACO board chair should sit on the parent company board.

If selecting the divisional model, the following principles might help guide the formation and initial structure of the leadership bodies:

- The parent company board selects, provides oversight for, and fires the ACO executive director and medical director.
- The parent company board approves all additions of partner organizations within the ACO.

- The parent company board approves the strategy, budget, and capital budget for the ACO.
- The parent company's executive leadership team (e.g., chief executive officer, chief financial officer, chief operating officer, chief medical officer) sits on the ACO leadership committee.

Management of the ACO

Executive management of the ACO requires a balance between physician leadership and professional management. If both are present in a single individual, the ACO can and should be under the direction of a sophisticated physician leader. If not, it is strongly recommended that the executive leadership function be shared by an experienced and committed physician leader and a seasoned professional manager, each of whom has demonstrated the capacity to operate effectively within a shared leadership structure and together seem compatible enough to operate as a team. More details about management activities are addressed in Chapter 4.

Moving into Physiology: Organization of ACO Operations

There are a reasonable number of alternative functional and management models that can be considered for ACO operations. Each model will support ACO development, and each could be a logical structure for a given set of circumstances. All evidence suggests that CMS is seeking to promote alternative models to learn the benefits and challenges of each through a series of measured ACO experiments; these are explored in Chapter 4.

The clinical operating structure of the ACO could be a series of integrated councils that report to the chair of the clinical operations committee. The composition and focus of the councils could be constructed using many different organizing principles. We present two examples within the hybrid organization model presented earlier in this chapter. The ideal model for a given ACO will probably be determined by the leadership strengths already present in the system and the medical group because the capacity to integrate is so critical to success.

The first example of potential clinical integration councils is organized around the principle of core clinical and support functions (see

Exhibit 3.12 Clinical Integration Council Organized by Core Functions

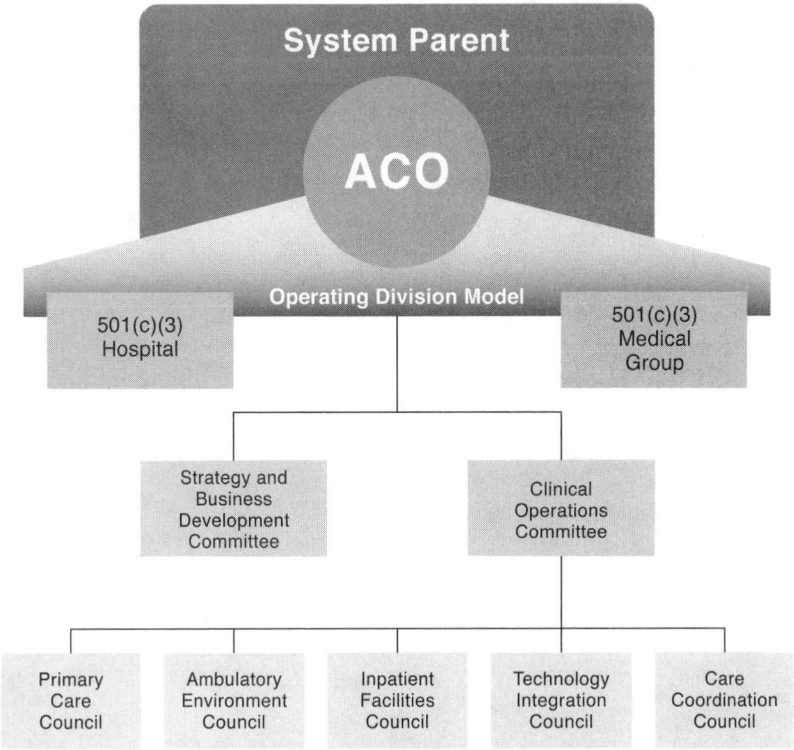

Exhibit 3.12). The second example is organized around care coordination needs for particular cohorts of patients (see Exhibit 3.13).

In both examples (exhibits 3.12 and 3.13), each council comprises representatives of all programs, functions, facilities, or resources appropriate to the focus of the council. Many functions will be represented on multiple councils, and the leaders of each integrated council will probably serve collectively as the clinical operations committee. Note that all councils are, by design, integrated bodies: We advise caution lest an ACO unwittingly re-create the types of dysfunctional and disintegrated silos that are disabling healthcare systems across America today. For example, it would be a poor choice to be designed around a "physician council" or "nursing council" or "emergency care council."

Exhibit 3.13 Clinical Integration Council Organized by Patient Cohort

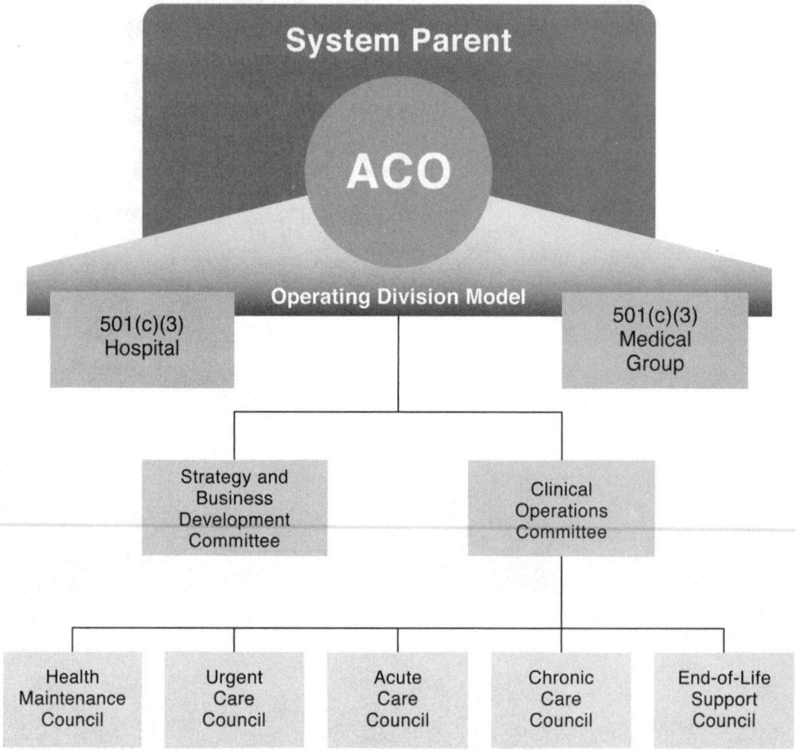

Each of these models has benefits and challenges, and none is perfect. While also imperfect, an innovative model is offered for your consideration as we advance our discussion to ACO physiology in Chapter 4.

Organizational Questions

The organizational questions raised in this chapter include the following:

- What external resources should we consider as potential "tenants" in our ACO mall?
- What do we see as attractive or unattractive about the alternative ACO structural models?

- What body should our ACO use as its physician organization, and how should it be organized?
- What governance principles should we consider to guide the leadership of our ACO?
- What management principles would serve our ACO well?

Category of Readers	Key Concepts	Actions to Consider
Category A (interested)	• Traditional and contemporary medical staff organization	• Reevaluate physician roles in hospital leadership and consider alternatives
	• Components of an ACO	• Redesign employed-physician practice model
	• Contemporary hospital organizational models	• Assess compensation model for employed physicians
Category B (engaged)	• Innovative contemporary physician organization models	• Begin building or refining your system's physician organization
	• Governance and management of the physician organization	• Consider physician governance, requirements, and eligibility
	• ACO corporate models	• Review potential corporate models with board
Category C (committed)	• ACO legal structure models	• Create legal ACO corporate structure
	• An innovative contemporary management model	• Develop a road map for building ACO functionality (see Chapter 8)
	• Governance principles for the ACO	• Charter a "Continental Congress" (see Chapter 9)

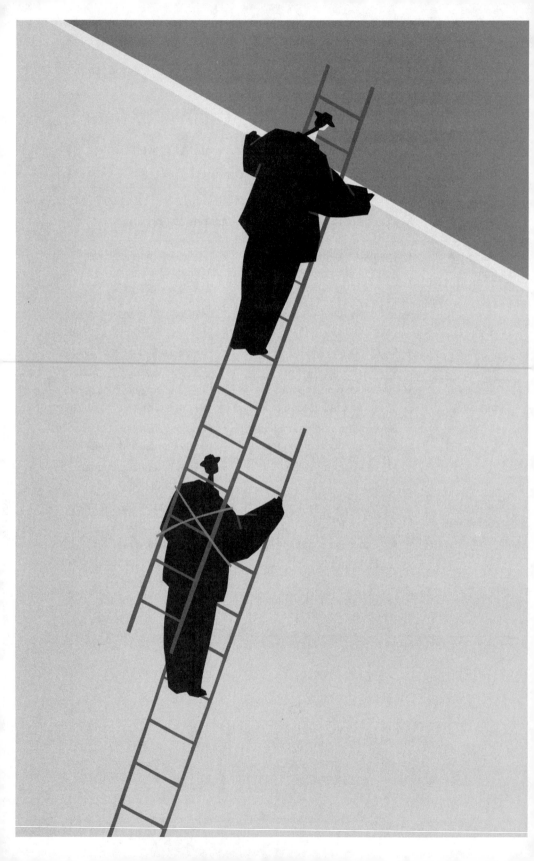

4

Accountable Care Organization Physiology

> We have all the right components for an ACO but as a system we need to sharpen our discipline around clinical effectiveness. We must engage everyone in the system to build the skills, systems, and commitment to delivering the right amount of care and the right care in the right place at the right time in the most efficient manner possible. That's our next opportunity.
>
> —Daniel Silverman, MD, MPA
> Chief Medical Officer
> Sinai Hospital of Baltimore

Accountable care organization (ACO) *physiology* refers to the systems, processes, and operations of the ACO. In brief, physiology describes the ACO functions—the who, what, when, where, and how of decision making, organizing, tasking, delegating, creating accountabilities, and so forth. It provides for measuring, managing, giving guidance and feedback, developing and implementing incentives and rewards, and choosing staff for promotions. Physiology enables a disparate collection of components to function effectively as a care delivery system. While there is some overlap with both anatomy (structural relationships) and sociology (culture), physiology focuses more on tasks and activities than on legal and operating structures or human behavior.

The Three-Legged Stool of Physiology

Success in the ACO model requires the seamless integration of three perspectives during decision making at all functional levels, from vision and strategy to day-to-day operations. Those three perspectives are the optimization of care delivery, or clinical effectiveness; the efficiency of resource utilization; and the management of risk. The significance of risk management (actuarial, financial, and clinical) varies depending on the reimbursement mechanism in a particular ACO. If using a predominantly fee-for-service model, the risk management will focus primarily on clinical risk management and performance optimization. If using a global payment or capitation model, risk management will focus on clinical, financial, and actuarial factors. Risk management will be addressed more fully in Chapter 7.

ACO physiology operates in two separate but integrated domains.

The first domain is enterprise operations, which serve as the infrastructure of the ACO and design, build, and maintain the platform for care delivery. Examples of enterprise operations include personnel recruitment and retention, revenue cycle management, supply chain optimization, and information technology (IT) platform selection and deployment. It also includes cyclical processes such as capital allocation and budgeting, which occur every year or quarter. Enterprise functions are critical to the overall performance of the ACO.

The second domain is delivery of care to the patient. This is the domain of the doctors, nurses, and other caregivers. This also seeks to optimize clinical effectiveness and efficiency but requires medical expertise that most professional managers do not have. The converse, of course, is also true: Most physicians are not fully competent in systems operations management. Even those physicians who have moved into management are unlikely to have operated at a scale or complexity necessary for optimal integration within an ACO. As we described in Chapter 3, the operating dictum must be "physician led, professionally managed."

Using this model, the hierarchy of management within the ACO looks like this:

- Governance sets broad parameters for the organization.
- Management designs the delivery of care.
- Doctors, nurses, and others on the front line deliver care within those parameters.

See Exhibit 4.1 for a graphical representation.

The Key to ACO Physiology

In Exhibit 4.1, the rectangles at the bottom represent care areas, the most crucial parts of the ACO structure. In most hospitals today, those areas of care might be clinical areas such as cardiology, obstetrics/gynecology, and oncology. This "silo" model represents the old way of organizing care.

For the ACO, managers and caregivers need to think about the needs of patients, and *how* they will be treated, rather than about their specific clinical conditions. Looking at *care requirements* rather than *clinical diagnosis* is the start of a well-functioning ACO. It moves care out of today's transactional, fee-for-service model. That could very well be the most important decision leaders make as they craft their ACO strategy. To get there, leaders will need to completely abandon traditional ways of organizing care.

The Physiology of Care Delivery

Again, the mission of the ACO is to create an innovative system of care and payment that results in measurably improved clinical outcomes and resource efficiencies. The strategy involves both care delivery and payment reform. The primary responsibility of senior management is to design an organization that systemizes and supports care delivery so that *the most efficient and effective way to deliver care is also the easiest way for those who give and receive the care.* As discussed later in this chapter, architect Louis Sullivan's famous dictum "Form ever follows function" is an excellent guide.

Exhibit 4.1 Hierarchy of ACO Management

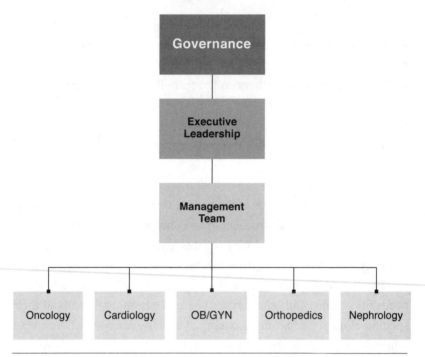

In its most effective form, ACO care delivery must be envisioned as population-based concierge medicine. Most healthcare in America is fragmented into units defined by physician, practice, specialty, department, floor, unit, clinical discipline, or institution. The reimbursement system has further driven the fragmentation to molecular and even atomic levels through coding, modifiers, documentation, and billing compliance and practices.

Senior managers in the ACO need to fight fragmentation and consolidate care into a seamless, integrated service for physicians and patients. This will result in a radically different type of clinical organization. The past decade has spawned integrated clinical service lines in areas such as cardiology, neurosciences, and orthopedic care. In many hospitals these are deemed, in occasionally self-congratulatory fashion, "centers of excellence."

These service lines are often developed in response to market opportunities rather than the unmet clinical needs of the institution's patient population. There are valuable lessons to be learned from the integration that these centers of excellence have provided. They are the true "focused factories" of care envisioned over a decade ago by Regina Herzlinger, a Harvard Business School healthcare economist. While they are still initiated in response to patient demand, none fully integrate the holistic needs of the patient. And they are certainly not care delivery systems or ACOs.

That being said, it is possible to use a center of excellence within an ACO as long as all parties are willing and able to create effective points of integration between the ACO and the focused clinical service line. The center of excellence cannot stand on its own; it must be a totally integrated part of the ACO, much as traveling on an interstate toll road can be part of a larger trip that includes city and county roads.

Looking at Patient Cohorts, Not Conditions

Any cross-section of the patient population can be envisioned as creating a set of customer needs. Taking a strictly patient-centered focus, interactions with the healthcare system are triggered by a predictable and limited number of needs:

1. *Maintaining good health.* This activity includes routine vaccination, medical screening, annual health review, and education.
2. *Diagnosis and treatment of a self-limited minor illness.* These illnesses include earache, sprained ankle, laceration, urinary tract infection, and bronchitis. These are illnesses that, for the most part, can be diagnosed and treated on an ambulatory basis and, when resolved, have few if any sequelae. Self-limited minor illnesses represent the vast majority of patient-initiated interfaces with physician offices, urgent care centers, emergency rooms, and retail clinics every day.

3. *Diagnosis and treatment of an acute, major, non-self-limited illness that requires some level of coordinated care, typically in a hospital or related facility.* These illnesses include appendicitis, cholecystitis requiring cholecystectomy, major fracture requiring surgical stabilization or repair, endovascular procedure, and total joint replacement. For the most part, once the acute illness has been resolved, there are few, if any, chronic sequelae, though the initial care requires coordinated scientific and technological resources generally available in a hospital.

4. *Ongoing maintenance, periodic surveillance, and intermittent inpatient or ambulatory treatment for a chronic illness with episodic and unpredictable exacerbations.* These illnesses include asthma, diabetes, congestive heart failure, and multiple sclerosis. For these patients, close monitoring and tight control have demonstrated the greatest clinical and economic benefit. The fragmentation of today's healthcare system hits these patients the hardest.

5. *Chronic care for those unable to care for themselves, either in a confined or ambulatory setting.* These patients require ongoing nursing and social support, which either are provided by committed family members or require external resources. This cohort includes end-of-life and hospice care, dementia, end-stage renal failure, advanced Parkinson's disease, and many congenital diseases.

Each of these needs defines a set of patients who can be aggregated more by care requirements and system interfaces than by clinical diagnosis. In brief, the choreography of these patients' clinical courses resembles one another reasonably closely. In this method of organization, then, a patient with diabetes and a patient with congestive heart failure may have more in common with one another than patients with dyspepsia and ulcerative colitis—two diseases that would have been categorized together under traditional discipline distinctions. The two latter conditions are both gastroenterologic ailments, but they typically have vastly different clinical courses.

Exhibit 4.2 shows how, in this new way of thinking, patients might be categorized into cohorts on the basis of the intensity of care they need.

Exhibit 4.2 Placing Patients into Cohorts

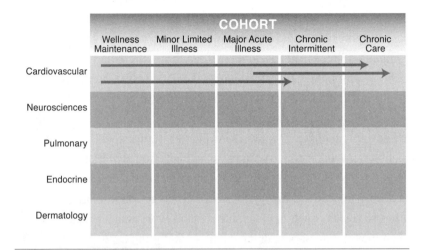

In the ACO model, care for each of these five cohorts must be thoughtfully designed and carefully executed. The care can then be applied across many different clinical diagnoses. Each arrow in Exhibit 4.2 represents the course of a single clinical diagnosis. For instance, a successful system of care designed for an asthmatic population could be adapted to provide ongoing care for patients with multiple sclerosis, because these cohorts of patients have similar system interface needs and navigate the care system in similar ways. The system must be designed to provide for care at all stages for the patient, including assessment and diagnosis; ongoing proactive surveillance between primary and specialty care; and the provision of advice, guidance, reassurance, or clinical intervention.

Designing Effective Care for the Patient Cohort

As stated several times in previous chapters, all systems are perfectly designed to produce the outcomes they produce. If we accept that the ACO is committed to optimization of clinical outcomes and efficient resource utilization, then it follows that the critical ACO competence is *care design* followed closely by consistency of execution. Hard work, commitment, team spirit, and strong credentials are all useful in delivering excellent clinical care. But the crucial element—the one that will separate the long-term winners from losers—is effective care design. Moreover, putting together a group of highly committed people in a poorly designed system will only generate angry, frustrated, cynical, and resentful caregivers. If anything, the better the team, the more essential the need for thoughtful and effective care design.

In our model, the management team that organizes care for each cohort will be headed by a council made up of up to eight to ten people. These individuals can come from diverse professional backgrounds, such as nurse educators, specialist physicians, social workers, and nurse practitioners. But once again, the team must have a crucial skill: It has to deeply understand the needs of its particular cohort of patients. The leadership team must demonstrate the ability to transfer its knowledge to all the other members in the cohort care group.

System designers will need to be competent in and committed to defining the resources that contribute to health, assessing resource waste, standardizing resources, and configuring resources as first-order design principles to improve quality and efficiency. For that reason, we recommend that the members of the integrated leadership councils be individuals who demonstrate competence in clinical integration design and delivery. Then, going back to the structural models introduced at the end of Chapter 3, a thoughtful delivery system organizational structure might look like the illustration in Exhibit 4.3.

In the Exhibit 4.3 model, the people represented by the gray rectangle above integrated clinical councils (the smaller rectangles) are senior ACO delivery system managers responsible for coordinating and integrating resources within that defined cohort/aggregation of patients. By using the leaders of the integrated councils as the senior management team of the ACO delivery system (along with nonclinical senior managers who support care delivery, such as human resources, finance, and legal), care can be integrated across the identified cohorts of patients. Over time, patients will naturally migrate from one cohort to another as their conditions improve or worsen. The senior management team must design smooth transitions between cohorts for patients as their overall health changes.

Exhibit 4.3 Delivery System Organizational Structure

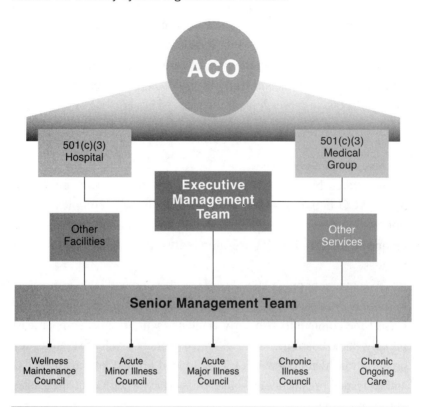

Membership in each of the councils would be determined by the needs of the patients in the cohort and the resources within the ACO. By making care integration the core design principle and major focus of ACO senior management, leadership sends a powerful signal to everyone in the system about what is important to the organization and the community of patients it serves.

This model is intended to be more illustrative than prescriptive. You do not need to follow it exactly. Where it has been implemented, it has been effective, but no design or system of care is universal. You must look at the specific needs, intended outcomes, and core capabilities within your own delivery system. This represents a starting point for organizational planning in your institution. Moreover, as we have noted several times already, whatever initial design you implement, it is only Version 1.0. It should be expected to evolve over time as experience increases your understanding of care design.

The most important element in this potential design is grouping patients together based on the type of care they need, rather than the specific nature of their ailments. With this care delivery structure in mind, let's take a closer look at the roles of governance and management in the ACO hierarchy (see Exhibit 4.1).

The Role of ACO Governance

As illustrated by the potential structural models shown in Chapter 3, the ACO delivery system will necessarily be a complex operation made up of many sub-enterprises. Its composite origins create unique challenges for its governing body—the board of directors or trustees.

As a matter of pragmatics, board membership will include directors or trustees from each of the participating organizations as well as members of the community. An early challenge will arise because, at least initially, some board members will have stronger loyalty to their legacy organizations than to the ACO. This divided loyalty between the ACO and its legacy organizations is likely to surface when the board creates initial governing policies. There will be a natural bias toward preserving as much decision-making authority at the component organizations as possible. The evolving ACO model, however, requires a great deal of flexibility from all participants during its formative period: Board members will have to tolerate higher levels of ambiguity than might be expected in an independent start-up organization.

Board members must be guided by three duties:

- *The duty of obedience*. This ensures that the organization, under its charter and applicable laws, does not attempt to perform acts that it is neither allowed to perform nor is capable of performing.
- *The duty of care*. This is the level of attention required of a trustee, which is commonly considered "the duty to be informed" about the activities and performance outcomes of the ACO.

- *The duty of loyalty.* This requires that all directors act solely in the best interests of the ACO members and the patients served by the ACO.

The need for the board to support executive leadership in designing and implementing integrative models and systems requires that the board take the time and effort to fully understand the ACO's mission and vision. The board must itself become integrated enough to provide the level of support needed by its executives. This will go well beyond approving reports, budgets, and plans; it will require active support. The board is likely to be called upon to do the hard work necessary to bring the participating organizations together. This will require board members to work closely with their legacy boards during the initial phases of development and to help those boards understand the unique needs for integration within the ACO. In short, this will be a working board, and members will be expected to put in significant time and commitment.

Another challenge is that unlike most healthcare boards, the ACO board will probably *not* choose the leaders of the ACO. Initial leadership of the ACO may be the CEO of the hospital or his/her designee and the leader of the physician organization or his/her designee. This will require the board to develop unique mechanisms for managing the performance of the ACO's executive team, because each executive is likely to report to two divergent governing bodies (shown in Exhibit 4.4). The hospital CEO will report to the ACO board and to an external community hospital or parent board. Similarly, the physician leader will also report to the ACO board and to an internal board composed of physicians elected by the membership of the physician organization. If the physician organization is structured as a 501(c)(3) charitable organization, that board will also include community members. This creates a dynamic tension that the ACO board will need to manage actively.

Therefore, it is incumbent upon the ACO's board to keep its focus on the goal of the ACO: to create an innovative system of care and payment that results in measurably improved clinical outcomes, high degrees of patient satisfaction, and resource efficiencies. The ACO

Exhibit 4.4 ACO Executives Reporting to Two Boards

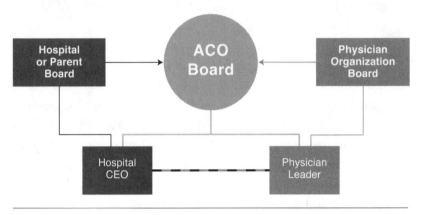

board will also need to pay close attention to the partnership relationships among the leaders of the ACO and intervene if there is any evidence of emerging tension.

Executive Management: Adding Up to a Perfect 10

Dyad or paired management teams are not uncommon in healthcare delivery systems. Paired management teams that function well together are much rarer. In the ACO, it is absolutely imperative that the appointed pair function at a consistently high level. The two prerequisites for effective functioning are as follows:

1. The two leaders must be complementary in such a way that together they create a "perfect 10." Ten can be reached by 5 and 5 or any combination that adds up to 10, including 9 and 1, as long as all facets of leadership (see Exhibit 4.5) are covered and both parties are comfortable with the distribution of responsibilities and activities within the relationship.
   Any tension that develops at the executive level will create potentially destructive friction throughout the organization. It is highly unusual to find an organization capable of performing significantly better over the long term than the condition of the relationship between its executive leaders.

Exhibit 4.5 ACO with Three Leaders and Two Boards

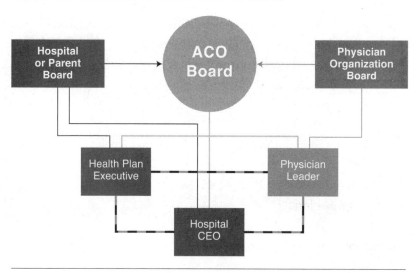

2. The members of the pair must respect each other's contribution to the leadership function such that, at a minimum, 7 plus 3 equal 10 rather than 8 or even 6. In the best case, the relationship will exhibit synergy, and 7 plus 3 might add up to 11. However, anything less than a full 10 means the relationship itself will consume time and energy that is better used in guiding the organization.

To achieve a collective 10, the complementary leadership team (not necessarily each individual) must be competent in visioning, strategic and financial planning, analytic assessment, and business planning. They must also engage others; make the compelling case for action; communicate through active listening, processing, and storytelling; organize and coordinate action; identify and solve problems; measure and evaluate performance; and give and receive feedback. Independently, each must demonstrate the most important competence—partnership with the other.

Given that it is unlikely that an ACO will be developed *de novo*, there is a high probability that the ACO's leaders will already be members of the delivery system. Mitigate the risks of management conflict by selecting two individuals who have already demonstrated a propensity for working together. The midst of making a crucial decision is a bad time to discover incompatibilities within the leadership team.

For some systems, three people will form the leadership team: the hospital CEO or his/her designee, the physician organization medical director or his/her designee, and the leader of a provider-owned or captive health plan (see Exhibit 4.5). The health plan executive could bring, at a minimum, competency in risk management, care and disease management, claims processing, and claims-based data analysis to the executive leadership team. This could be a real strategic asset for the organization.

The Paradox of Physician Management

Singling out physician management in a treatise whose singular message is "integration" seems, at first glance, inconsistent. Instead, it should be thought of as paradoxical. The paradox refers to the discussion in Chapter 3 about loosely and tightly coupled systems.

Physicians naturally favor autonomy and self-determination. This is surely an echo of something they learned throughout clinical training. Physicians in training received a powerful message when their senior resident scolded them for relying on the x-ray analysis of the board-certified faculty radiologist rather than reviewing the film themselves. As scientists, physicians are taught to trust no one else because the clinical buck always stops with them.

When physicians become leaders in their healthcare organizations, this cultural bias often dominates their management philosophy and style. For this reason, as well as the competitive distrust rampant in today's environment, many physicians are uncomfortable letting others make management decisions that affect their practice. Unfortunately, this attitude is an important contributor to the fragmentation of care in today's healthcare ecosystem.

Here's one way to deal with this natural mistrust.

Over the past 30 years of consulting experience, we have made one observation often and consistently enough to treat it as a "truth":

Physicians are most comfortable ceding control to a peer when they experience a true personal relationship with that individual. We call these relationships "line-of-sight" relationships, because both parties are peers and know each other well; they usually develop as a result of adjoining practice relationships where each party can literally observe the other's practice. The emphasis here is on *relationship*. The strength of the relationship is comforting to the physician being managed. Physicians need to be assured that if things get too onerous as a result of a particular decision, they can go to their supervisor (a peer) with whom they have a line-of-sight relationship and use their personal relationship to resolve the concerns. More often than not, they'll be able to persuade their colleague to reverse or modify the decision without personal embarrassment or loss of face.

This creates two diametrically opposed truths that can be difficult to integrate. A core tenet of ACO organizational design is to give managers a broad span of control to promote standardization. This offers the greatest opportunity for cross-functional integration across disciplines, sites, and professions. Yet it flies in the face of the physicians' need for line-of-sight management relationships, and their unwillingness to cede control to non-peers. By giving a manager broader control, the people he/she manages no longer have a line-of-sight relationship.

Solving this problem requires a simultaneous loose–tight management design in which clinical delivery teams maintain elements of local responsibility for day-to-day operations, while larger strategic decisions are ceded to the integrated leadership councils. Higher-level strategic decisions tend to focus on care delivery models, clinical pathways, protocols, standardizations, IT support solutions, delegated partnership and team roles, solutions, and so forth. Local operational decisions, on the other hand, tend to focus on coverage and details such as hours of operation, urgent care coverage, office-based patient flow, internal communication, and selection of support staff. There is no single recipe for success, but high-functioning organizations have found effective ways to honor both loose and tight design elements within their organizations.

More than 200 years ago, Benjamin Franklin observed that it takes a strong partner to be a good partner. This caveat is still true today. With few exceptions, physician leaders and professional managers must both be strong partners for their partnership to succeed.

Physicians in an effective delivery system have to be organized so that a small number of committed and competent physicians are entrusted by their peers to make, implement, and enforce decisions on behalf of the group. The consensual culture of too many physician practices results in a vote of 99 to 1 being considered a "tie," thereby requiring an alternative decision that can work for everyone. Those consensus decisions are often suboptimized to gain broad acceptance. This will not work in an ACO. Entrusted physician leaders must be *formally authorized* by the physician organization to act on behalf of the organization. These physician leaders must develop relationships with those they manage such that their subordinates ("peers") feel that their voices are at least being represented during decision making.

That last point is crucial. At a meeting at Kaiser Permanente, the integrated healthcare organization in California, a group of surgeons sought to redesign the surgical booking process to improve its efficiency. The most vociferous opponent was a urologist who advocated strongly for an alternative model from the one being favored by the rest of the group. Ultimately, a vote was taken and his option was not selected. But after the vote, the urologist was an enthusiastic supporter of the new system. "This was great," he told his colleagues. "You gave me every chance to raise my issues, defend my option, and attempt to sway all of you. I wasn't able to, so I accept your decision" (Bard 1990). This is how it has to work.

All too often, healthcare leaders ask for input from physicians or other groups, but when the ultimate decision fails to reflect the input given by each member, the result is a sense of almost personal betrayal. Over and over again, we hear, "Why did she ask for my opinion if she wasn't going to listen to it?" The fatal mistake here is the failure to communicate the decision-making process. Leaders must reinforce the simple fact that being *solicited* for an opinion doesn't mean the opinion will be *adopted*. It only means it will be considered.

Effective leaders always circle back to participants and acknowledge their personal contributions and reiterate their peer's point of view, even (or especially) if that perspective isn't reflected in the final decision. When both steps are followed, physicians feel they have been heard and are much more likely to comply with decisions, even those with which they don't agree.

Contrary to common belief, physicians do not always have a need to operate in their own way. What they do need is an opportunity to participate in clear and transparent processes that guarantee that their insights, knowledge, and perspectives are considered during appropriate decision-making processes. Then, they demand a sound rationale for the final decision—the "case" for why that particular option or solution was selected. It is good discipline for healthcare organizations to set a reasonable standard around decision making: Invite perspectives and points of view, and always share the rationale for the final decision. By setting the rules of the road in advance, organizations can avoid getting trapped in unnecessary and unpleasant conflict resolution.

Another problem frequently seen in physician decision making is the self-defeating battle for consensus. In an ill-fated quest for collegiality, often the only decisions considered are those to which every member can subscribe. The result, usually, is a suboptimal decision. Building consensus often means regressing to a mean and arriving at a least-common-denominator solution. By pleasing everyone, the outcome is optimal to no one.

The solution to this problem lies in the increasing reliance on evidence-based decisions. In the ACO model, an evidence-based solution (clinical or otherwise) trumps every other. Proven best practices must be adopted without debate. Evidence-based clinical, business, and management decision making is the antidote to the tyranny of consensus.

Once a reasonable physician management structure is designed, it is important to construct and share the decision matrix so that everyone in the enterprise clearly understands the limits and boundaries of the decision-making authority. Without up-front clarity, decision making will be marred by friction that will ultimately test the integrity of the system.

Finally, while there is no "right" decision-making process, it is safe to conclude that the traditional organization of physicians by specialty or geography will simply perpetuate the current level of fragmentation—one that is inconsistent with the goals and values of the ACO. Whenever possible, the system should be designed around *fiduciary,* rather than *representative,* decision-making bodies. Each participant should always be representing the interests of the whole enterprise rather than the interests of his or her work unit, practice, discipline, specialty, and so forth.

Getting the Design Right

Remembering our bias in favor of form following function and our belief that organizations are perfectly designed to produce the outcomes they produce, we argue that to achieve a higher level of integrative function, organizations will need to be designed differently than they are currently. Chapter 3 focused on the structural components of the design; this chapter focuses on the operational features required for success.

A few principles derived from the discussion earlier should be considered drivers of organizational design in the ACO:

1. Aim for the broadest span of accountability and authority at each operating level.
2. Organize around function or outcome rather than discipline or profession.
3. Play it simultaneously loose and tight. Include broad expertise and perspective for analysis and input into decisions while using tight management-team decision making.
4. Require that all decisions be accompanied by a rational case for the outcome along with a summary of alternative options considered.
5. Share the decision-making case with all stakeholders.
6. Select leaders on the basis of expertise and merit rather than discipline, profession, longevity, or political acceptability.

7. Ensure that workgroups that make decisions always include members who can implement those decisions.
8. Introduce all major changes as trials rather than long-term solutions; doing so will decrease resistance immeasurably.
9. Explain that input into decisions is *avidly requested*, while compliance with decisions is *actively required*.
10. Whenever possible, create systems and process that are self-initiating (hard wired) rather than rely on individuals (be they patients or providers) to initiate them.

Making Work Groups Work

Whether an *ad hoc* committee or a senior leadership team, the sole purpose of work groups in an action-oriented organization is to inform and make decisions. This includes identifying issues, problems, opportunities, and challenges; analyzing them; and providing perspectives to assist those with decision-making authority. Whenever a work group devolves into a book club, action is impeded.

Decision making in a complex, adaptive organization is also complex. It entails the integration of multiple data points, perspectives, points of view, and insights. As a result, most significant decisions require acceptance of reasonable trade-offs between options. The "best" solutions represent the "best overall package," broadly balancing benefits and burdens to achieve desired outcomes. Perfect solutions are rare. It's most prudent to abandon the search for a perfect solution: Attempts to thread the eye of the needle generally require too much time, energy, social capital, and resources for the outcomes they generate. It is fascinating that people who comfortably accept trade-offs for major personal life decisions (who, after all, works in the *perfect* organization, lives in the *perfect* house, or married the *perfect* mate?) push to find the "perfect" solution in an organizational setting, casting aside the flexibility they demonstrate in every other aspect of their lives.

The sole function of a work group, then, is to inform and, where appropriate, to make decisions. Once work groups lose their focus on decision making, they devolve into debate societies, town meetings, book clubs, and gripe sessions, favoring endless debate over action. Work groups that follow a simple format seem to achieve better results than those that are less disciplined. Here are the five easy steps:

1. Start by describing the problem or opportunity being addressed. Identify it in terms of what isn't happening that should be or what is happening that shouldn't be.
2. Envision how things should work when the problem is solved. Create a shared vision of the resolution.
3. Identify what information will enable the group to identify a solution and what standards will be used to evaluate that information.
4. Generate and evaluate options and apply the criteria.
5. Choose the option that meets the greatest number of criteria or has the fewest flaws.

Use the full decision process as the content for communication back to the organization. Communicate frequently, clearly, and proactively throughout the organization, with particular emphasis on those parts of the organization most affected by the decision and those individuals who have contributed the most input into the decision-making process. When communicating, remember that the organization is composed of visual, auditory, and somatic learners; use all three modalities to touch everyone.

The Physiology of Primary Care

Primary care is the centerpiece of the ACO. Primary care practices are currently envisioned as demonstrating the attributes and capabilities of the patient-centered medical home (PCMH); this concept is in sharp contrast to the gatekeeper models of the 1980s and 1990s and the tri-age models of the past decade. While the earlier models were designed to limit the care provided by the system, the current PCMH model is designed to expand the services provided within primary care.

The goal of the ACO is to create a system of care to optimize clinical outcomes and patient satisfaction across the continuum of care while generating the efficiency of resource utilization to achieve those outcomes and generate cost savings. From this perspective, several core principles should guide care design at both the global or population level and the episodic or individual level.

The Patient-Centered Medical Home

The first principle is that every patient cared for by the ACO should have a contact who serves as the patient's portal to the entire healthcare system. Traditionally, this role fell to the primary care physician (PCP). But the PCP is in a bind today. Clinical demands have mushroomed. Reimbursement has been stagnant or declining. Costs, especially related to revenue cycle and compliance management, have steadily risen. And demands for outcomes and reporting have escalated. Is it any wonder that fewer medical school graduates choose primary care as their specialty? Some reports indicate that only 2 percent of today's medical school graduates are identifying primary care as their professional goal (Newton and Grayson 2003). It is clear to everyone who provides or receives care in the current ecosystem that the role of the PCP must significantly change. The PCMH is one response to the current crisis in primary care.

It is difficult to envision an ACO in which the principle point of access is not primary care—particularly, primary care that embraces the medical home model as the assessor, organizer, provider, and manager of care. The locus of care coordination can be at the ACO enterprise level, or it can be embedded within primary care in the medical home model, though the latter will likely be more efficient and more effective. Either way, care coordination must be integrated, robust, and part of the core DNA of the ACO.

Much has been written about the PCMH, so we address it only briefly. In essence, this model transforms the PCP's role from *provider* of all care to *designer and manager* of a team of care providers, including physicians, physician extenders, nurses, social workers, navigators, care coordinators, nutritionists, clinical educators, public health population analysts, home care providers, psychologists, clinical pharmacists, volunteers, and support staff, to name but a sampling of the participants in medical homes. Collectively, this group takes responsibility for providing care to an identified group of patients. When the model is working effectively, participants identify their job as a "care provider," regardless of their specific role. The physician's role, therefore, expands from care provider to care designer and team manager.

The PCMH model, of course, can only function when the payer community, operating out of enlightened self-interest, sees the long-term value in this type of care. The primary care provider must clearly get reimbursed for coordination activities that are part of care management and for value-added encounters that are not face-to-face and therefore not traditionally reimbursed. In this model, care provision transforms from a reactive and responsive operation, triggered when a patient calls or comes in the door, to a proactive and managed one. In brief, each patient must be evaluated to assess short-term needs and assigned a customized "program" or *care plan* that is consistent with the five needs of the patient-cohort model described earlier.

Each patient should have an identified access point into the system, and the system should have an identified relationship manager for the patient. The importance of this role underscores our bias toward patient enrollment in the ACO rather than the retroactive-attribution technique that is currently being considered by the Centers for Medicare & Medicaid Services (CMS). Clearly, each patient should have a unique and integrated electronic health record that is accessible and used throughout the system and by any partner or vendor who provides care within the ACO. As each patient completes a periodic health needs assessment, a care plan is created, much like a student's course curriculum: The patient's "major" is identified as maintaining beneficial wellness, managing a chronic illness, or returning to health. Short-term "subjects" are also identified to contribute to the overall care plan.

Each patient is assigned a health delivery team, usually in primary care, and one member of the team is assigned as the patient's navigator and point of contact. Every patient is entered into appropriate registries so that his/her care can be tracked on an individual and a population basis. The navigator's job is to manage the care itinerary proactively, providing periodic surveillance, initiating the team's response when a need is identified, initiating interventions when medical advances indicate a new or improved approach, and serving as the point of contact if a question or need arises. Speedy patient access to the team, making certain that today's concerns are dealt with today, is critical to the success of the PCMH. Whenever possible and appropriate, the navigator and all care providers are guided by common care pathways and protocols. Navigators can access anyone on the team for judgment and support as needed.

Whenever care is needed beyond the scope or capability of the medical home team, outside care providers must be guided by the common pathways and protocols. They must have access to the same electronic health record and must provide care that is consistent with the objectives created by the patient in conjunction with the medical home team. When using a center of excellence or service line model for focused care (e.g., a heart failure program, a musculoskeletal institute), initial patient enrollment and initiation of care should take place within the medical home. That way, the patient is well along the structured care pathway before interfacing with the specialists in the service line. All care within the system or with a partner/vendor of the system must be coordinated through the patient coordinator, and centers of excellence should remain *focused factories* that interface seamlessly and comprehensively with the patient's medical home.

Care Coordination as a New Specialty

It seems inevitable that a new clinical specialty will emerge; this is the second principle that will guide care design. Similar to nurse educators, maternal–fetal medicine subspecialists, geriatric nurse practitioners, or orthopedic physician assistants, a group of clinicians will become experts at navigating and coordinating resources to improve care. But to see this role as strictly administrative undervalues it. For example, these new specialists will need to be able to accomplish the following tasks:

- Design clinical itineraries
- Partner in the development of care pathways and clinical protocols
- Establish clinical priorities
- Participate in systems design for managing care, including IT supports
- Manage transitions from ambulatory to inpatient settings and back again
- Interface with other care providers, including home care
- Interface with school-based programs and other community-based resources
- Interface with employer-based programs
- Work with pharmacists and pharmacologists
- Work with payers to design payment methods that reward quality, productivity, and efficiency improvements
- Design products, services, and bundles of resources that patients, purchasers, and payers want to buy
- Possibly provide clinical care when appropriate and needed

Clearly, a clinical background will be of great value in the role. It would not be surprising to see the care coordinators further sub-specialize according to the five care pathways identified earlier in this chapter. There will be clinical coordinators for wellness care, acute minor-illness care, chronic maintenance, and so forth. Coordinators in the lower acuity end will operate at the population level, and those at the higher acuity level will operate at both the population and the individual levels. Clinicians who develop these areas of expertise will be highly sought after as critical members of clinical teams because they operate at the intersection of care delivery and resource utilization. They should be the first to recognize a problem or an opportunity to better integrate care, improve outcomes, or reduce waste. Because the role combines some elements of hands-on care with systems design and organizational management, the new specialty is likely to be an attractive career for motivated and competent healthcare workers; these individuals are likely to begin their careers as physician extenders. Over time, the new field will likely develop its own training programs. This will be yet another valuable consequence of healthcare reform and another step in the direction of developing a healthcare *system* in America rather than merely an *ecosystem*.

The Physiology of Specialty Care

Much has been written about the role of primary care in the ACO; little has been written about the role of the specialists. Some medical specialty societies have expressed great interest in the model; others have been dismissive; and still others have expressed anxiety and concern. Extending the strategy of the patient-centered medical home, some have suggested that within the ACO a clinical specialty area such as a center of excellence or clinical service line could even serve as the patient's medical home.

While it is true that a small number of patients—generally, children and young adults—have single chronic conditions, such as significant developmental disorders, multiple sclerosis, inflammatory bowel disease, certain cancers, or hemophilia, few older patients have such focused, single-dimensional needs. It seems unlikely that a single specialty could meet the breadth of needs of a patient longitudinally. Therefore, it seems reasonable to assign each ACO member a primary care–based medical home. Patients will get referrals as required to medical specialists in clinical service lines, clinical institutes, or centers of excellence. For some specialists, this harkens back to the gatekeeper model. Given the platform of quality and efficiency, the model will only work if the specialists fully participate in those goals and therefore organize themselves around those two objectives. Rather than worrying about primary care medical homes withholding referrals, specialists should be focusing on how they can offer value in the new model.

The obvious exception to this model is the care of children. It's possible that, over time, pediatrics will be carved out of the CMS general program and will contract independently as a pediatric ACO. Given their reliance on Medicaid reimbursement for survival, pediatric centers across America are considering options for how best to provide care to children inside of healthcare reform. Another exception could be women during pregnancy, who might benefit from a specialty medical home. Centers of excellence that partner with the ACO must mirror the attributes of the ACO itself with respect to care coordination, disease registries, and other factors.

One model being considered by some advanced tertiary and quaternary care centers is an "Intel Inside" branding model. Much in the manner that Cleveland Clinic has actively marketed its intellectual property and technology through Cleveland Clinic Heart Centers, some advanced medical centers are considering developing transparent portals through which they can effectively attach to ACOs as the advanced care provider for the ACO. This will require the deployment of IT that, effectively, enables the advanced care center's IT platform to operate seamlessly with a wide variety of other platforms and will require such tertiary care centers to fundamentally redesign many of their delivery functions. In this regard, the balkanized nature of many academic medical centers could be advantageous to ACOs, because the ACOs may be able to contract with specific departments within academic medical centers—say, the nephrology department for kidney transplants or the orthopedic department for joint replacements—without necessarily being required to contract with the entire academic medical center.

For the majority of specialists who operate at the secondary care level, a small number of organizational models could be used to serve the needs of patients within the ACO. The physicians who practice within the specialty will require some form of membership in or relationship with the participating physician organization, as described in Chapter 3. Compensation, funds flow, and distribution of potential shared savings will be the responsibility of the governance of the physician organization. Therefore, our examination of the role of specialists in the ACO focuses more on physiology and culture than on anatomy.

The most frequently asked question among specialists over the past year, clearly echoing back to the health maintenance organization (HMO) era, is whether specialists can belong to more than one ACO. The Patient Protection and Affordable Care Act does not address this issue, so the answer must be guided by pragmatism, common sense, and a little foresight. Certain specialty practices couldn't possibly stay solvent if they were forced into a yes-or-no decision about joining a single ACO. It is unlikely that a group of nephrologists, head and neck surgeons, urologists, or oncologists could limit their practice solely to an ACO unless the ACO had many more covered lives than required. On the other hand, a cardiology or gastroenterology practice could probably practice solely within the ACO because of the nature of their practices. These specialists care for patients with long-term needs and others for whom they provide routine diagnostic tests.

At the outset, it is far more likely that specialists will practice within *and* outside the ACO. Pragmatics may make it difficult to practice in more than one ACO because that would require investment and active participation in multiple IT platforms, care pathways, centers of excellence, physician organizations, and so forth. With the judicious use of information exchanges, however, this obstacle could be mitigated. Most specialist physicians will more likely devote some of their practice effort to an ACO and the rest to traditional managed care or fee-for-service environments.

Five options for integrating specialty care in an ACO seem viable at this time. We explore each one in this section.

Model 1: Equal Opportunity Players

In this model, specialties aggregate into large regional consortiums of single-specialty providers and contract as a single entity with all regional ACOs. At the same time, they also contract with other non-ACO provider organizations and provide independent community and hospital-based referral care as independent practitioners. In this model, Specialty Consortium A might be gastroenterology, Specialty Consortium B might be endocrinology and diabetes, and Specialty Consortium C might be orthopedics. More likely in this model certain specialists would focus their attention within one ACO so that they could develop peer relationships and optimize integration within the organization.

This model, of course, assumes that there is more than one ACO within a geographic area. This is only likely to be true in mid-to-large urban and suburban markets. One of the challenges of this model is integrating and maintaining the infrastructure of a large specialty practice. Over the past few years, many "supergroups" have broken up because of their inability to develop and support the ethos of a true group practice. These groups aggregated for contracting purposes and never developed common approaches, practices, and values required for long-term success. Also, this model, which focused on contracting clout, often failed to achieve the benefits of operational efficiencies and economies of scale. (See Exhibit 4.6.)

Model 2: All for One, One for All

In this model, regional specialties aggregate into a single, large, non–primary care multispecialty group practice independent physician organization that contracts as a single entity with all regional ACOs. It also contracts with other non-ACO provider organizations to provide independent community and hospital-based referral care as an independent multispecialty group practice. Once again, we would expect that a designated cadre of specialists would primarily serve one ACO in order to develop primary relationships with its clinicians, care coordinators, care protocols, and so forth. The challenge of this model is in building the integrity and infrastructure to support a large multispecialty group practice from scratch. While some regional specialists are considering this model, it seems impractical from an operational point of view in many markets. (See Exhibit 4.7.)

Model 3: Choosing Sides

In this model, small, independent single-specialty group practices would contract individually with local ACOs through the ACO's physician organization. The arrangement could range from employment by the physician organization to subcontracting with the ACO's physician organization, possibly through a professional services agreement or memorandum of understanding. In this model, the specialists would serve as exclusive

Exhibit 4.6 Model 1: Equal Opportunity Players

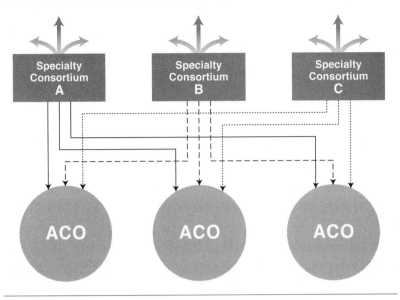

Exhibit 4.7 Model 2: All for One, One for All

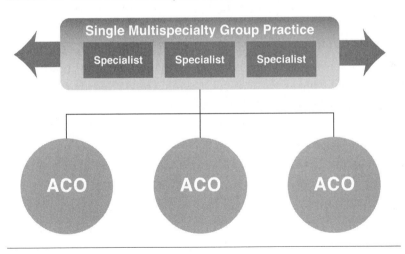

providers for their specialty within the ACO. The specialists' practices would be confined solely to the ACO. This may not be practical in the near term. (See Exhibit 4.8.)

Exhibit 4.8 Model 3: Choosing Sides

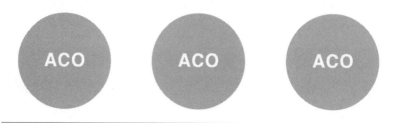

Model 4: Playing the Field

In this model, small, independent single-specialty group practices contract individually with one local ACO to serve as the exclusive provider for the ACO's specialty services. But these groups also maintain independent external practices outside of their ACO relationship. Of all the models, this seems to be the likeliest model to meet the needs of the ACO while also meeting the economic realities of a specialty practice. The challenge in this model is that the specialists could easily find themselves participating in two different approaches to care: a tightly managed and highly integrated approach within the ACO and a more traditional approach outside the ACO. While this may appear schizophrenic to the outsider, many excellent specialists found little difficulty in practicing in different environments during the HMO era, so this model has demonstrated historic success. (See Exhibit 4.9.)

Model 5: Family Ties

In this model, certain specialty groups join the ACO in partnership with PCPs to together create a mutually exclusive multispecialty group practice physician organization. The physician organization then contracts with non-ACO clinicians for those specialties (such as cardiac surgery, neurosurgery, and radiation oncology) that are unlikely to be included in the group practice. The challenge of this model is that creating a well-integrated multispecialty group practice through aggregation rather than organic growth has proven difficult for many physicians, as noted earlier in this chapter. (See Exhibit 4.10.)

Exhibit 4.9 Model 4: Playing the Field

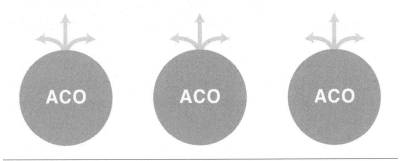

Exhibit 4.10 Model 5: Family Ties

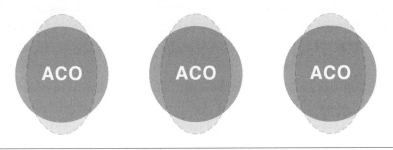

Questions have been raised about compensation for specialists. Compensation will be determined by the organization model of the larger delivery system, not by the ACO. Ultimately, if specialists are members of an integrated group practice, compensation will likely include base pay, some sort of an incentive, and some sort of a performance-based reward. However, it seems unlikely that the volume-based compensation models that have emerged over the past decade will be useful in an ACO delivery model. Each practice will dictate a different compensation model.

The Role of Hospitalists

Hospitalists and related hospital-based physicians, such as laborists, intensivists, nocturnalists, and surgical hospitalists, are the newest and the fastest-growing class of physicians in the United States. These physicians are hybrids between PCPs (focusing on care for the patient in the inpatient setting) and specialists for hospital care management. They are employed through many economic structures—from direct employment to contracts with local hospitalist, primary care, or multispecialty groups to contracts with regional and national hospitalist firms through medical services agreements. Numerous studies have demonstrated the benefits of hospitalists on clinical performance improvement, including hospital mortality, and on resource management, including length of stay and cost per discharge.

Hospitalists are especially useful in perioperative care of relatively routine surgical procedures. In that role, they are frequently praised by specialists, such as orthopedists, for their postoperative management of routine procedures. At the same time, hospitalists are commonly criticized by PCPs for failures of communication and ineffective handoffs between the inpatient and the outpatient setting. This area of hospitalist work will require the greatest redesign. This area also will provide the greatest benefit. There is, for example, growing evidence that hospitalists who introduce themselves to patients (and then behave) as their doctor's "associate for hospital care" produce high patient satisfaction. In brief, those who present themselves as a component of an integrated system of care often generate high satisfaction among patients.

The need for seamless handoffs between settings and care providers within the ACO is critical for optimization of integration, clinical quality, and resource management. Great care must be taken in the design and implementation of hospitalist programs to ensure that the benefits are achieved and the common pitfalls are avoided. This begins with the hospitalist working closely with the care coordinator and primary care medical home to develop a true system of care.

Designing Care Pathways

There is clearly no best practice for care design. The only commonality among care design models is that they all begin with the premise that care will be designed and, wherever possible, will be standardized within a care system.

Task Force

The process generally begins with the appointment of a multispecialty and multidisciplinary task force led by an experienced care designer. This can be an important role for the care coordinator, as discussed earlier. This task force undertakes a thorough review of publicly available, evidence-based best practices. It polls caregivers to evaluate which of the best practices are largely agreed upon by the providers. Some members of frontline operations management must be included on the task force to evaluate which best practices could reasonably be implemented, supported, and standardized in the ACO. That initiates the design process.

"Design by committee" is generally best avoided in organizational settings. But comprehensive, integrated care design must be developed by all of those who will be delivering the care. That makes design by committee an imperative. There are three benefits of design by committee:

1. Through the process of design, those within the system will learn and better appreciate how the care must be integrated. In brief, the design process *is* the integrating process. (See the parable of "The Tower" in Chapter 5. This parable can be useful in initiating the design process.)
2. It is an opportunity to build relationships that are critical for successful integration.
3. Given that there is no single best practice design, trade-offs will need to be made. Ultimately, the best model will be the one that (a) can produce the outcomes needed and (b) has the commitment of those who must make it work. These two conditions can only be met if those responsible for the success of the system are those who helped design it and accepted the inherent trade-offs associated with each design element.

The final point that needs to be made here is that the complexity of integrating care requires an ongoing approach. As with the ACO itself, the initial design will be Version 1.0, and it must evolve over time. The initial design team should reevaluate the process quarterly for the first year and make modifications on the basis of their view of internal processes and clinical outcomes. Then, as advances in science and technology develop, the design committee should reconvene to evaluate whether the care pathway should be modified to include any of the advances.

Longer term, as the organization becomes more comfortable with a standardized approach and staff becomes convinced that standardization produces better clinical and business outcomes, the "clinical flywheel" will spin more quickly. Care delivery will continue to evolve and improve. When the improvement curve levels out and further change produces only marginal improvements, the approach is considered finalized. Until, of course, advances in medicine and technology warrant a return to the design table.

Exceptions to the Rule

Those who design care processes will want to be reassured that provisions are made for those patients or circumstances requiring exceptions to the rule. It is wise to be reminded, yet again, that there can only be *exceptions* to rules when there are *rules* to begin with. While not scientific, our observation confirms that standardizing some aspects of care processes improves outcomes significantly: All aspects of the care process need not be improved to reap significant benefit. The "rule of 80/20" applies here: Standardizing 20 percent of the care processes generates 80 percent of the potential benefit. That seems a reasonable goal for standardization.

When Gordon Bethune assumed leadership of Continental Airlines, he focused on baggage handling and on-time arrivals, generating a great deal of resistance from Continental's ground crews around the world. Those in the field were quick to remind him of the tornadoes, floods, snowstorms, hurricanes, fog, or rush-hour traffic that could unpredictably delay planes. He cleverly devised the perfect antidote to the excuses. He demanded a standardized process only for airplanes taking off and landing between 10:00 a.m. and 2:00 p.m. on clear days without weather delays. Adoption of that limited standardization transformed Continental Airlines from worst to best in the industry in baggage handling and on-time arrivals. It was proof that standardizing a small percentage of operations generated the bulk of the benefits. Healthcare can learn from this experience.

For these reasons, care delivery can only be designed by those who deliver the care and are ultimately accountable for it.

Specifications for Design Standardization

While actual delivery design is beyond the scope of this book, several design specifications for standardization of care design deserve emphasis:

1. The ACO must have a detailed and regularly updated registry of all of its members.
2. The system must have a way of contacting each member.
3. Every member (from vigorous 20-year-olds to ailing 90-year-olds) must have

   a. a clear, understood, and implementable care itinerary, map, or plan (both short-term and long-term);
   b. an identified care navigator who is familiar with the member and operates proactively to keep the member integrated in the system;
   c. an accurate, up-to-date electronic health record that is available to every individual who provides care to the member;
   d. a clear understanding of the goals and purpose of the ACO and some level of personal commitment to that mission;
   e. regular touch points with the system, by design; and
   f. periodic reevaluation so that the member's care plan can be updated.

4. The ACO must integrate business operations with clinical care design and patient-centeredness at every level of care and delivery to simultaneously optimize all three goals.
5. Clinical risk management must be integrated into the design and delivery of care.

6. Electronic decision support integrated into the health record must be available to all caregivers.
7. Leadership must believe that well-designed standardized approaches to care delivery can produce superior outcomes, and delivery systems must avidly recruit those who share that point of view.
8. Those who practice within the ACO must be willing to practice healthcare as a "team sport."
9. Wherever the system is not designed to transfer important information or insights from one care provider to another, it must be shared manually until the discontinuity is fixed.
10. Everyone in the delivery system is a care provider, so everyone is responsible for improving care and resource utilization.

Organizational Questions

The organizational questions raised in this chapter include the following:

- What care delivery model do we want to use to design our system of care?
- What governance principles will serve us well?
- What management principles will serve us well?
- How do we want to design and implement our primary care medical home model?
- How do we want to integrate specialty care into our delivery model?

Category of Readers	Key Concepts	Actions to Consider
Category A (interested)	• Tripartite requirements of clinical effectiveness, efficiency, and risk management	• Initiate infrastructure supports for clinical effectiveness
	• Roles of governance in an ACO	• Engage physicians in designing and managing core integrated clinical functions
	• Executive management in an ACO	• Engage physicians in designing and co-managing operational efficiency initiatives for reducing length of stay, resource utilization, etc.
Category B (engaged)	• Cohort model of patient needs	• Focus on building and integrating physician and professional management in the ambulatory environment
	• Physician leadership capabilities in an ACO	• Initiate IT supports in physician offices across the system
	• Specialty care models	• Introduce, manage, and reward the introduction of care pathways in common clinical areas
Category C (committed)	• Drivers and enablers of organizational performance	• Focus on strengthening inpatient and ambulatory care coordination across the system of care
	• Designing a patient-centered medical home	• Design, build, and implement medical home pilots in partnership with payers
	• Redesigning and coordinating care	• Designate a leadership team to coordinate and manage ACO activities

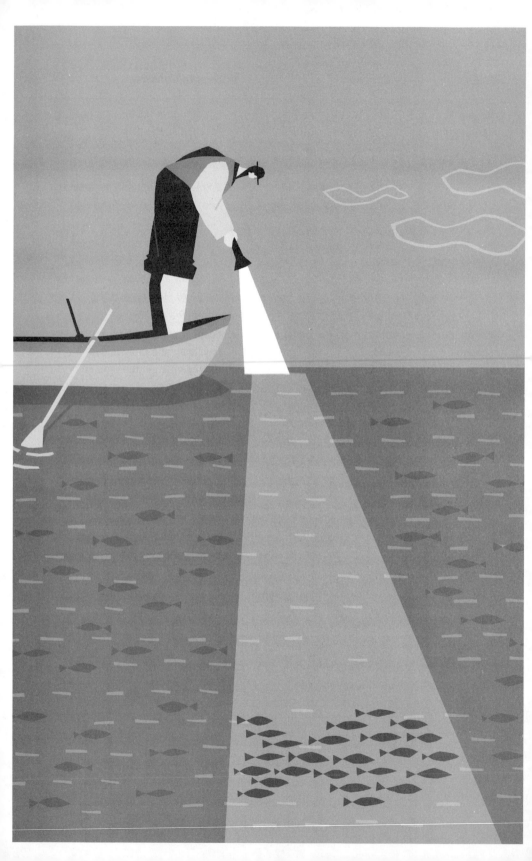

5

Accountable Care Organization Sociology

When it comes to performance, strategy is significant but culture is critical. Sometimes, to get results, you just have to change the rules.

—Lynda D. Curtis
Senior Vice President and Executive Director
South Manhattan Health Care Network
Bellevue Medical Center

The *sociology* of the accountable care organization (ACO) is its culture. Because it is well accepted that culture inevitably trumps strategy, the ACO, as a strategy for linking reimbursement to clinical outcomes, patient satisfaction, and operating efficiency, will fail if it does not have a supportive culture. More specifically, ACO leaders must be sensitive to the culture during two separate and distinct phases of ACO development and deployment: one when building the ACO, and another when operating as an ACO. Each phase has a distinct set of leadership requirements and a unique set of necessary cultural supports.

This chapter explores the influence of culture on ACO strategy and operations and, more specifically, suggests some cultural attributes that are likely to be beneficial in the development and operational phases of a successful ACO.

Defining Culture

"Culture" is most often defined as the set of observed behaviors within a defined society. *Organizational* culture is the collection of assumptions, values, and beliefs, and their derivative adaptive individual and collective behaviors displayed within an organization. Collectively, these behaviors create a set of habits that enable complex adaptive organizations to carry out their missions. One way to think of culture is as the way people in the organization behave when no one is watching.

These assumptions, beliefs, and values are deeply held—sometimes within the deep subconscious—by formal and informal organizational leaders. Every organization has formal leaders, those whose names fill the little boxes within the organizational chart. Every healthcare organization also has a set of informal leaders who are *de facto* leaders by virtue of having followers. These unofficial leaders are able to influence others. In healthcare organizations, these people typically fall into the following categories:

- Former official leaders who have what is commonly referred to as *legitimate power* through their emeritus status
- Distinctively competent individuals whose power base is referred to as *expert power*
- People who are in a position to either withhold or provide something of value to others, which is referred to as *coercive* or *reward power*
- People who have a close personal or professional relationship with the formal leaders, which is referred to as *associative power*
- People who influence others because others, for whatever reasons, genuinely want to please them, which is referred to as *referent power*

The formal and informal leaders' deeply held assumptions, beliefs, and values are most commonly projected as "informed truths" rather than personal beliefs. These informed truths are rarely identified, infrequently questioned, and almost never challenged, despite the fact that they play such an important role in producing outcomes. Their connection to outcomes is clear: These truths form the bedrock of organizational direction and design. The direction and design, in turn, preprogram outcomes. The fact that many healthcare leaders refer to culture as "soft and fluffy" belies the culture's influence on performance outcomes. More often, the culture is a reflection of leaders' perceived inability to influence the organization, which is a powerful misperception. Many of us tend to be dismissive of that which we do not understand.

Cultures evolve and adapt over time, and most demonstrate historical relevance and value at some time in the organization's life cycle. When evolutionary cultural attributes work at cross-purposes to the organization's goals, and leadership is strong enough to recognize the dysfunction and open enough to identify and challenge the underlying beliefs and assumptions, the maladaptive attributes of the culture get extinguished. This is most often observed when new leadership is introduced, because new leaders are able to see what others who are more deeply immersed in the culture cannot. The familiar metaphor of the "frog in boiling water" supports this observation. A frog immersed in tepid water and heated to boiling will be unable to recognize incremental changes in water temperature and will allow itself to literally boil to its death. A frog placed in boiling water will immediately feel the heat and jump out. When leadership is unable to reshape the culture to be adaptive to current needs, either the organization falters or fails or new leadership is brought in.

Culture does not produce results; rather, culture *supports* or *impedes* performance. Cultures have valences or scale: Some cultures are relatively weak, while others are strong. But cultures do not have vectors or specific directions; they are neither good nor bad. Instead, they are either *supportive of* the outcomes that an organization is seeking to achieve, *unhelpful* (neither supportive nor disruptive), or *impediments to* the outcomes being sought.

Often, the reason organizational behavior is difficult to change is partially a result of the collective organizational habits that have developed as responses to unrevealed and unchallenged assumptions, beliefs, and values. Everyone knows that habits are difficult to break. Motivation for changing habits can often be tied to one of two forces: a *burning platform* or a compelling vision. Experience in healthcare organizations suggests that the ideal time to introduce change is when there is recognition that the platform is heating up and will eventually combust, and a rational vision is developing to respond to the rising heat. The vision need not be compelling; it simply needs to be attractive enough to represent a reasonable alternative to the anticipated future state. Organizations that wait until the flames erupt often experience non-goal-directed and reactive "jumping off the platform" rather than purposeful and organized action.

When changes in science and technology; economic conditions; and patient, purchaser, payer, and provider desires and demands create enough of a discontinuity that the evolved habits are no longer adaptive, organizational habits are forced to change. But when individual and collective behavior needs to change significantly, it is difficult to initiate and sustain the changes without exposing the assumptions, beliefs, and values that support the current undesired behavior and impede adaptive behavior. Authoritative imposition is the alternative, and that usually does not come with insight and engagement.

The Simple Rules of Complexity Science and Organizational Culture

Complexity science teaches us that complex adaptive organizations, such as hospitals, airports, city governments, and universities, maintain their internal integrity by adopting core "simple rules" that specify three organizational conditions:

1. What is required
2. What is prohibited
3. What is allowed

The power of simple rules can be appreciated by recognizing that scientists have been able to reproduce the complex flocking

Exhibit 5.1 Computer-Simulated Simple Rules of Bird Flocking Behavior

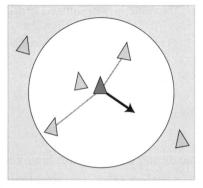

Separation:
Steer to avoid crowding local flockmates

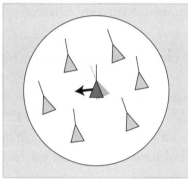

Alignment:
Steer toward the average heading of local flockmates

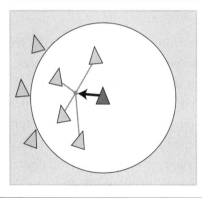

Cohesion:
Steer to move toward the average position of local flockmates

behavior of birds in flight by programming only three simple rules into a computer simulation (see Exhibit 5.1). (The name of this computer simulation is a New York–inflected "Boids.")

The power of simple rules can also be illustrated by an example most of us face every day—driving home during rush hour. To ensure each driver's timely arrival, traffic movement is optimized if drivers follow three simple rules:

1. Drive the same speed as the car in front of you.
2. Maintain a constant distance from the car in front of you.
3. Drive the same direction as the car next to you.

Anyone who has ever driven home during Boston's rush hour knows that while these simple rules make perfect sense, the actual simple rules followed by Boston rush hour drivers are quite different:

1. Switch to what appears at any particular moment to be the fastest moving lane of traffic.
2. Continually minimize the distance between you and the car in front of you to prevent other drivers from observing Rule 1.
3. Never signal your intentions with your blinkers as that will only goad advancing drivers to follow Rule 2 and prevent you from accomplishing Rule 1.

What appears reasonably orderly from an airplane at 1,000 feet is utter chaos on the ground. Traffic gets snarled, the pace slows, and fender-benders proliferate. Such is the power of simple rules.

As a final example, the simple rules that define airport behavior changed dramatically after the terrorist attacks on September 11, 2001. Watch at any airline terminal and you will observe that, when compared with traveler behavior before the terrorist attacks, travelers today are much less likely to draw attention to themselves, become aggressive or argumentative with airline personnel, act playful with airport staff, or initiate conversation with fellow travelers.

Simple rules are implicit, not explicit. Unlike contracts, memoranda of understanding, service agreements, written policies, or organizational bylaws, simple rules are unstated. However, they are deeply embedded within organizational design and direction, having been derived over time from the assumptions, beliefs, and values of current and previous leaders. Once they are exposed, the impact of these simple rules can be found in foundational elements of organizational *direction*, such as its vision, strategy, and employee performance expectations. These simple rules can also be discerned in foundational elements of enterprise *design*, such as organizational structure, compensation, incentives and rewards, and resource allocation. Quite simply, the simple rules infiltrate the entire organization at all levels and become part of its DNA.

Now, if we accept the premise stated in Chapter 2 that all organizations are perfectly designed to produce precisely the outcomes they produce (Hanna 1988), then it follows that these powerful yet invisible rules predetermine organizational performance. We have seen this in many organizations that have hired our firm to run a unique program called Changing the Rules®. These organizations are often able to expose their deeply embedded simple rules and reevaluate them in light of current needs, aspirations, and goals. Many organizations describe the outcome of the endeavor much like clearing the fender-bender off the side of the road: Suddenly traffic begins to flow again. A few examples will prove useful. *Explicit rules* found in a healthcare organization define where smoking is and is not permitted, where mobile phones may or may not be used, and where public parking is and is not allowed. *Simple rules* are deeper and usually invisible to those within the system.

Healthcare Examples of Simple Rules

One simple rule identified by a well-known and well-regarded Midwestern healthcare system was "Compliance requires consensus." To those within the system, this meant that an individual could not be held accountable for adhering to any expectation or action if she was not explicitly included in the process that led to approval of that behavior or action. While at the surface this meant that many decisions were, in effect, optional for those who did not participate, the impact was far greater. The organization was forced to develop complex and highly inclusive processes in which all those expected to comply were included. The system soon found that it was almost impossible to make even simple decisions because of the time and effort required to include everyone in approving, recommending, and informing decisions. It found itself deeply mired in non-value-added processes. Its conference rooms even evolved, getting large enough so that hundreds could "participate."

Despite all the time and effort, the process didn't work. While consensus was usually reached, in reality it was often "faux consensus" because everyone felt pressured to "get on with" decisions that were being promoted strongly by leaders. No one wanted to be the one individual among hundreds who broke consensus. Leaders within the organization were fully aware of the problem. They observed that after difficult decisions, the parking lots were full of disgruntled participants who disagreed with the decision they had just "supported." When the organization decided to pursue an aggressive quality agenda, leaders recognized that this type of faux consensus would not suffice.

Another healthcare system revealed a simple rule of "Differences of opinion are best resolved through compromise." At first glance, this seems reasonable. But the organization recognized that resolving differences through compromise rather than through data analysis and business modeling undermined its strategic planning efforts. When it comes to strategy, compromise is often the least effective decision-making option. The organization's "compromise" strategy was just that.

Finally, a large hospital system in the South revealed this simple rule: "Revenue drives margin." All organizational attention, energy, and resources were invested in securing high-revenue inpatient volume with little attention paid to efficiency of resource management. But as the competitive environment changed and reimbursement started to fall, system leaders began to realize that resource management was the best strategy for generating margin.

Efforts at managing efficiency were resisted at every level because of the concern or excuse that the efficiencies would be viewed unfavorably by the high-revenue-generating physicians.

Challenging the Current Simple Rules to Enable the Evolution to the ACO

Organizational transformation from traditional fee-for-service delivery systems to accountable care organizations will require significant reprogramming of structures, systems, processes, programs, and, most important, people's attitudes and behaviors. This reprogramming will inevitably challenge subconscious as well as conscious assumptions, beliefs, and values. More important, however, is that at the organizational level, it will challenge existing simple rules. As it does, passive and active resistance will escalate. Each organization will need to explore and potentially challenge its own simple rules to enable it to evolve into an ACO.

In a later section of this chapter, we suggest some new rules that might supplant commonly existing rules. But we strongly advise each organization to engage in a process of exposing its own simple rules and evaluating which support, which are benign, and which impede the ACO delivery model. Questioning the *validity* of a simple rule is akin to revising history. Questioning the *utility* of the rule in light of the organization's current strategy is helpful. Every rule had value when it was adopted.

In addition to the simple rules that operate at the organizational level, there are simple rules that operate at subgroup levels. These subculture simple rules are generally compatible with organizational simple rules. When they are not, the incompatible rules usually get extinguished, often when departmental or divisional leadership is replaced. The important observation about subcultures in healthcare organizations is that they are often incompatible enough with one another to inhibit the level of collaboration and integration necessary for producing required ACO-related outcomes.

Because many healthcare organizations face common challenges and much cross-fertilization of leadership occurs across the American healthcare landscape, it is not surprising that many provider organizations' simple rules are similar. We list some of these relatively ubiquitous simple rules below. While many seem obsolete and naïve in the current healthcare environment, all had validity at the time they were adopted:

- Hospitals have unlimited resources.
- Volume drives performance.
- Physicians are hospitals' customers.
- High admitters set the rules.
- Technological capabilities are more valued than cognitive abilities.
- Financial success in healthcare is achieved at the negotiating table.
- Healthcare is transactional at every level.
- Economies of scale are achieved through size.
- Healthcare providers operate in a zero-sum game.
- Standardization is good for healthcare systems.
- Standardization is bad for physicians.
- All healthcare is local.
- Hospital managers understand ambulatory care management.
- Physicians understand hospital management.
- Physicians must preserve autonomy.

Just as there are neither good nor bad cultures, there are neither good nor bad simple rules. Like culture, simple rules can either support or impede the intended goals and outcomes of the organization. But because results in healthcare are produced by people and because simple rules are the silent drivers of behavior, it stands to reason that the unstated rules preprogram organizational performance. They either drive behavior that advances an organization toward its goals, generate behavior that is neither helpful nor harmful, or support behavior that is contrary to the organization's quest to achieve goals.

Changing the Prime Directive in Healthcare

Each organization has its own unique constellation of simple rules. Experience teaches us that only a few of them (generally five to ten) will have the greatest impact on the ability of the organization to change successfully when change is required. Because of the noted cross-fertilization within the healthcare industry and the relatively common mission across institutions, a number of these key simple rules are shared by many organizations.

We believe that one overriding, powerful, and ubiquitous simple rule that permeates healthcare in America should be singled out for a provocative challenge as organizations envision becoming an ACO. Its origins date back to Hippocrates, the father of Western medicine, and its impact has been deeply embedded in virtually every facet of healthcare design and delivery for the ensuing 2,500 years. While eminently supportable at so many levels, it is this simple rule that is likely to be the most significant impediment to the design and execution of ACOs.

That simple rule is "I am accountable."

This has been introduced and reinforced to every physician from the first day of medical school, and physicians continue to live by it until their last day of practice. But in the American healthcare ecosystem, individual accountability is at the heart of fragmentation, discontinuities, and failures of integration. Because no individual can possibly be accountable for the overall health of a patient in today's complex healthcare environment, each contributor to the patient's health must necessarily define logical and reasonable boundaries of accountability. This enables each caregiver to accept accountability for some (necessarily bounded) aspect of the patient's healthcare needs. The PCP is accountable until the patient is referred to a specialist or the hospital; the anesthesiologist is accountable until the patient reaches the post-anesthesia care unit; the surgeon is accountable during the operative and perioperative period; and so forth.

It is ironic that the most integrated healthcare program or system in many communities is hospice care, which is focused on the dying process. The point is that each provider, each setting, each department, each location, and each time horizon represents its own autonomous and individually accountable universe of care; there is no overarching system to provide integration at the transitions. Moreover, the culture of individual accountability goes beyond clinical care to affect the legal system, the reimbursement system, technology support, and most other aspects of care delivery and reimbursement. In summary, this core cultural attribute of personal accountability profoundly shapes today's healthcare ecosystem and creates resistance to the development of system accountability for care—the ultimate goal of the ACO.

So while the rule "I am accountable" appears entirely admirable at many levels, it has had a profoundly deleterious effect on the integration of healthcare in America. This is in contrast to organized national systems of care. As a high-level administrator from Great Britain's National Health Service (NHS) once observed, "From the time the [pregnancy] test tape turns blue until the end of life, we are responsible for every patient" (Reid 2009). While few would argue that the NHS is the perfect system, at least it is a system of care that is authentically concerned about childhood and adult immunizations, sanitation, malnutrition, obesity, and the like. To put it crassly, the system, collectively, either pays now or pays later for an individual's care, and later is always more resource intense. In brief, there is an integrated system of care that recognizes that a pound spent now on childhood immunization may save two pounds later in life.

Many simple rules within hospitals, medical practices, and healthcare systems will need to be reevaluated to support the design and implementation of ACOs. But the core rule that will be called into question is "I am accountable." It must be replaced with "*We* are accountable." Once this single rule is in place, it will promote a profound cultural shift within organizations and between those who provide and receive care. It will overcome one of the most profound challenges to systems thinking and design. This simple rule—when it is fully operational as opposed to merely a public-relations label, as "patient centered" is often used—preprograms an organization's capacity for systems thinking.

An appreciation of systems thinking can be obtained by studying the computer game "SimCity," which was introduced by Will Wright in 1989. It is a computer simulation of a complex, adaptive organization (a city) and illustrates the impact of non–systems thinking and design. Basically, the players work together to build the infrastructure of a city and learn in the process how schools, public works, fire and police, sanitation, parks and recreation, economic development, housing prices, interest rates, and yes, healthcare influence one another as a city grows and develops. While it is a gross oversimplification to say that a mayor's job is to integrate all these functions, it is fair to note that cities, at least, have mayors who can attempt to integrate and influence these functions. Healthcare systems, except those that are truly integrated, don't have mayors. As a result, for example, there is often little understanding within healthcare systems today about how a shortage of primary care access affects the overall cost of healthcare or how the absence of a diabetic management program affects productivity and competitiveness in the community.

The Impact of Changing the Prime Directive

Quite obviously, "We are accountable" is the antidote to "I am accountable." "We are accountable" sets a new framework for accountability from the individual to the system. It also redefines the boundaries for opportunities and problem solving. Because of the ubiquitous nature of the "I am accountable" rule, most problems are identified as either "inside or outside of my sphere of influence and/or control." This either/or perspective limits problem definitions and solutions to those controlled by an individual or a group.

While many operational problems can be solved within a reasonably bounded arena, most strategic opportunities and problems span traditional organizational boundaries of autonomy and control. The most fertile domains of innovation in many organizations are the "white spaces" on the organizational chart. Organizational cultural barriers often make it difficult or impossible to broaden the definition and analysis of a problem and consequently narrow the range of potential options. "We are accountable" is designed to break down internal silos and barriers and thereby encourage innovative solutions, improved outcomes, and optimized resource use. When a provider adopts the ACO strategy and creates the potential for shared savings across the organization, other people's problems suddenly become everyone's problems. The question shifts from "Is this *my* problem?" to "How can I help solve any organizational problem to maximize impact on clinical quality, patient satisfaction, and resource utilization so that *everyone* benefits from the solution?

Once "We are accountable" is a core driver of organizational design and delivery, the following attributes will begin to emerge in the healthcare delivery system:

- Everyone who participates in the system will see himself as a "healthcare provider."
- Traditional healthcare hierarchy will be replaced by problem solving across all levels.
- Healthcare executives and physicians will have the novel experience of being on the same side of the table.
- Healthcare providers will hold one another accountable for performance outcomes.
- Patients may begin to comply more readily with their treatment regimens.
- Opinion will be trumped by a quest for data, information, knowledge, and evidence.
- Data and evidence will enable leaders to make the compelling case for change.
- Generosity of spirit will replace traditional turf battles in organizational problem solving.
- Those who participate in the delivery of care will have real input into the design of care and thus will feel more empowered and experience greater ownership of the results.
- Responsible experimentation will be the norm rather than the exception.
- Leadership paralysis will be replaced by decision making.

- Teamwork among members will begin to resemble a soccer team more than a track team.
- Feedback loops between decisions and results will be tightened, promoting quicker change.
- Growing "systemness" will create new options for problem solving.
- Rather than feel like helpless cogs in an unfeeling system, patients will be able to have useful input into the design of their own care.
- Proactive care and wellness treatment will replace patient-initiated care.
- Rather than feel shunted from one care provider to another in an unfeeling system, patients will feel they are in a seamless system of care with smooth handoffs.
- Patients will choose to remain within the system rather than feel forced to do so.

Clearly, simple rules are invisible and powerful drivers of organizational behavior. And in healthcare, changing one simple rule can have an enormous impact.

Changing Simple Rules Is Not So Simple

No leader who declares, "Effective Tuesday the rules are changing" should expect to see any meaningful or positive change by Wednesday. That approach has about the same effect as when the prison warden proclaims, "The beatings will continue until morale improves." Really changing the rules that underlie an organization is a more complex process than that.

The first step in the process of cultural change is the development of a clear and shared picture of the organization's desired future. It must be clear enough that everyone in the organization is capable of envisioning the same future.

The second step in the process requires organizations to make their set of invisible simple rules explicit and open for discussion. Simply naming them is a start. Members will be able to see them in a different way. And once they can talk about them, they can evaluate and possibly change them.

The third step in the process is to evaluate the current rules in light of the desired picture of the future. This requires the organization to ask itself whether it is likely to achieve its desired picture operating with its current rules or whether some of the rules need to change. Once identified, the rules can, over time, be extinguished in favor of new, more effective contemporary rules. Over time, these new rules get reinforced through myriad systems such as performance management, performance review, rewards and incentives, annual awards, and so forth. Only then does an organization really have a new set of simple rules.

The fourth and final step in the process, then, is the reinforcement of these new rules.

Exhibit 5.2 is one way to represent the cultural change process visually.

There is no "right" time to impose change. Often, however, the "best" time to introduce change is when there's enough evidence that undesired and untoward outcomes are looming and likely to happen and that a reasonable picture of an alternative future is emerging. The perfect example of both conditions is healthcare reform in the United States.

In the following section, we offer 24 additional simple rules (including changing the "I am accountable" rule) that healthcare organizations might want to consider as they transform into ACOs. They are presented here in order to frame important organizational conversations about cultural support for new models of care. In addition, six parables are offered that have proven extremely useful over the past 15 years to organizations that are undergoing significant or transformational change. Their application is described as well.

24 New Simple Rules and 6 Parables for the ACO

In this section, we suggest 24 simple rules that can have profound effects on healthcare organizations along with 6 parables that are intended to spark organizational conversations that could lead to change.

Purists may note that rules refer to requirements, prohibitions, and allowances, and as such, they should begin with "You must always"

Exhibit 5.2 Cultural Change Process

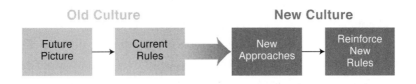

(a requirement), "You must never" (a prohibition), or "You may" (an allowance). Liberties have been taken here so that the rules are not all worded as strictly as these standards. In reality, most of these rules are recommendations (rather than requirements, prohibitions, or allowances) that organizations might want to consider in their quest for accountable care.

Simple Rule 1: We Are Accountable

As discussed, changing one ubiquitous simple rule—from "I am accountable" to "We are accountable"—can have wide-ranging effects on a healthcare organization. To underscore the power of this rule, we present the well-known parable of the stonecutters.

Parable 1: The Three Stonecutters

A traveler came upon three men working with stone. Curious as to what these workers were doing, the traveler approached the first worker and asked, "What are you doing?" Without hesitation, the worker replied, "I am a stonecutter and I am cutting stones." Still unclear as to the nature of the workers' task, the traveler approached the second worker and asked the same question. The second worker thought for a moment, gazed briefly at the traveler, and explained, "I am a stonecutter and I am cutting stones to earn money to support my family." Perplexed by the two different responses, the traveler approached the third worker and asked, "What are you doing?" Stopping for a moment, the worker stared at the stone in his hand, slowly turned to the traveler, and said, "I am a stonecutter and I am building a cathedral."

This parable shows that three men—all working at the same site and performing the same task—had three different perspectives of what they were working toward. One of the most profound impacts of changing to "We are accountable" is that everyone involved in the organization begins to feel that her job is providing healthcare. This is crucial to adopting the ACO strategy. Until everyone in the healthcare system sees himself or herself as "taking care of patients," it is impossible to appreciate the nobility of countless mundane, job-related activities.

Under the transactional, revenue-driven fee-for-service model, dollars became the most important yardstick in providing healthcare. In the ACO, when "We are accountable" becomes one of the unspoken simple rules, a new spirit begins to prevail in the workplace. Instead of looking at spreadsheets and reimbursement, employees start to look at more meaningful measures of accomplishment. Instead of the old-fashioned sign in the factory "We have worked 37 days without time lost to an accident," employees will begin to see a virtual sign that shows their collective progress: "So far this year, we have helped eliminate 20 preventable infections, 10 deaths, and 15 lost limbs in the population we take care of."

Another parable helps underscore this change within the healthcare organization.

Parable 2: The Gift of the Washerwoman

King T'sao's rapidly failing health was a cause of increasing concern to his countrymen. The king's despair over the growing dissension among his six sons only heightened the citizens' concern over the future of their beloved nation. To escape the palace tension, Prince Li, the king's eldest son, journeyed far and wide throughout the countryside in search of wisdom and enlightenment, spending his last weeks in isolation at a mountainside hut. He returned to the city looking more like a peasant than a prince. As he entered the walls of the city, he paused by the river to reflect on the lessons from his journey. There, he was greeted by an old woman carrying a large basket of clothes to be washed by the river's edge.

Recognizing his anguish, she placed her basket by her side and took a seat next to the prince. The old woman inquired about the cause of his apparent despair. Without revealing his true identity he told her of his concern about the failing state of their nation and his yearning for better times. Prince Li finished telling his woes and fell into prolonged silence. After some time, the old washerwoman placed a deeply furrowed hand over his and begged him not to worry. "King T'sao has six sons, our Princes," she said. "They will rise above their differences to save our nation. Of that you can be certain."

Prince Li inquired as to the source of her deep conviction about the princes and the certainty that the sons would return the nation to prosperity. The washerwoman replied that despite her appearance, she possessed (from birth) great powers to predict future occurrences and her predictions had not been wrong in her 80 years of life. "Do not worry," she repeated, "our king's sons will save our nation."

Prince Li bid the old woman farewell and returned swiftly to the palace where he told his brothers of the strange encounter with the old washerwoman. The brothers were as struck by her apparent powers as Prince Li was. Prince Li was the eldest and therefore destined to be king. Yet Prince Su was the wisest and best educated. Prince Mueng was the strongest and most fit. Prince Cheng was the kindest and gentlest of the brothers. Prince T'ai was the most insightful and decisive and nearly always correct in decisions of great importance. And Prince Yu was the most generous and most beloved by the citizens.

Over the ensuing days, each brother reflected on the prediction of the washerwoman. On the grounds that each might be the leader who would reverse the fortunes of their nation after their father's death, each began to conduct himself with unusual dignity. And each, contemplating his brothers' potential role in saving the country, began to treat his siblings with unprecedented respect.

This new spirit of leadership among the princes was immediately apparent to the citizens, producing great optimism and hope. An air of excited anticipation settled over the land. A sense of calm could be felt among all of its people. New levels of productivity and innovation could be seen in every corner of the land, and the nation once again flourished.

Simple Rule 2: Broaden Input, and Narrow Decision Making

For many physicians, decision making is synonymous with consensus. Consensus certainly has utility, though, as noted in Chapter 3; it is often used in healthcare when alternative decision-making processes would be far more effective. The standard in consensus building is to have "general agreement" around a decision *and* to have no one involved in the process who cannot live with the decision. This process prevents anyone who feels strongly enough about an issue, for whatever reason, from keeping a group from finalizing a decision. Give and take, compromise, and horse trading are often required to achieve consensus. The process frequently results in a least-common-denominator result.

Consensus can be effective in making operational decisions that have no evidence-based or analytically derived "best" or "right" option and in a system that can tolerate a range of responsible options. But when the evidence or analysis favors one option over the others, consensus is either unnecessary (the best option is the best option regardless of how everyone feels about it) or is ill advised because anyone in the process can overrule the objective "best option." Hence, we recommend a simple rule: Those within the system who touch the issue or are affected by the decision should participate actively in the analysis and in the initiation of solution options. Then, it is up to managers to weigh the evidence, evaluate those options that can produce the desired outcomes, consider potential unintended and undesired consequences, and make a decision. Afterward, the managers need to explain how they arrived at the decision for all those who participated in the process.

Several approaches and tools can be useful here, including the following parable, which emphasizes the value of inviting broad input into important decisions.

Parable 3: The Tower

Long ago in ancient China, there lived a great and powerful ruler, King T'sao. King T'sao's people had enjoyed many years of peace and prosperity, which were attributed to his wisdom and to the wisdom of his counsel—a wise man known as Mu-Sun. As a tribute to the king, the people built a great temple, and at its center was a tower that was the highest point in all the kingdom. In this tower, Mu-Sun resided along with his disciples—the six sons of King T'sao who would one day carry on his rule.

The eldest son, Prince Li, had studied and meditated under the great master for many years, but he had not reached enlightenment. Sensing the boy's growing resignation, Mu-Sun called him to his chamber in the top of the tower: "Today," said the great master, "you will begin your journey to enlightenment." Mu-Sun then took the boy to a window in the chambers and asked, "Tell me, Prince Li, what do you see?"

The prince looked out the window; it was a view he had seen many times before. "Master, I see the clouds rising from the river in the valley floor. I see the ocean to the east and the mountains to the north, and the outlines of the villages and the roads between them." The master listened to the boy's response, then took his hand and began to lead him slowly down the steps of the great tower.

After they had descended halfway down the tower steps, Mu-Sun paused by another window and again instructed the boy to tell him what he saw. "Great wise one, I see the palace wall, and beyond it, the cows grazing in the fields. I see the roofs of the village houses and smoke curling from the chimneys there," said Prince Li. The great master only nodded and smiled, and they continued the descent.

When at last they reached the bottom of the tower, Mu-Sun took the boy into the courtyard and instructed him to look beyond the palace gate. "Enlightened one, I see three peasant children chasing after a rooster. An old woman is carrying her goods to market. A man is leading his mule down the road to the city. I see the dust rising in the air from the movement of their feet, and the river throwing spray over the rocks along the bank," said the prince.

The master walked with Prince Li through the temple gate and then sat with him under an old tree. "What did you learn today,

Prince Li?" The boy thought hard but could not answer, for he had seen the same views many times before. After a long silence, Mu-Sun continued: "The path to enlightenment is like the journey down the tower. What one sees at the top is not what one sees at the bottom. And what is seen through one's own eyes is only a small part of what can be seen through the eyes of many. Without this wisdom, we close our minds to all that we cannot view from our position, and so we limit our capacity to grow and improve. Never forget this lesson, Prince Li: What you cannot see can be seen from another vantage point."

We often present this parable inside client organizations when an issue requires multiple perspectives to reach the best resolution. The "best" alternative is usually one that can meet four criteria:

1. The solution *could* work.
2. The solution enjoys relatively broad commitment from those who need to make it work.
3. There is either data to support the solution or no "disconfirming" evidence to refute it.
4. Those in the organization have reasonable confidence in the organization's ability to effectively manage potential unintended and undesired consequences associated with that solution.

We remind leaders that every option has imperfections. Those who aren't committed to the option will only see the imperfections. Those who are committed will see what works. Finally, we instruct organizations to go beyond traditional cost–benefit or reward–risk analysis. We ask, if there are potential positive outcomes from the decision, what is the likelihood that those outcomes can actually be realized? If there are potential undesired consequences, what is the likelihood that those outcomes can be averted? And, lastly, if they do occur, what is our confidence that we will be able to effectively manage them?

Only by looking at the situation through these multiple perspectives can an organization choose a valid response to a problem.

Simple Rule 3: Use the Wide-Angle Lens

Simple rule 3 is a variant of simple rule 2. Virtually any organization can look at a recent problem definition and solution and ask whether that problem could have been identified closer to its source and, if so, whether the resulting solution might have been more comprehensive or more effective. The late Anthony Athos, esteemed professor of management at Harvard Business School, used to remind his protégés that the initial answer to "What is the problem?" is more likely to be a symptom of the problem than the identification of the problem itself. As in the parable of the tower, the use of a wide-angle lens invites more and offers the opportunity for creative and comprehensive solutions. The corollary to simple rule 3 is simple rule 4:

Simple Rule 4: Some Problems Just Need to Be Made Bigger

There is a strong tendency in healthcare organizations to use Newtonian problem solving, in which large complex problems are broken down into their component parts and each subsequent manageable component is solved separately. The total solution is the aggregation of each independent solution. This process is often useful for solving complex problems. But when there is a primary need for organizational integration, such as in the ACO, Newtonian problem solving may not offer the best solution. Some problems need to be made bigger, not smaller, in order to be solved effectively.

A simple example is a common problem faced by hospitals: throughput in the emergency department (ED). The ED relies on interfaces with the laboratory, x-ray, the operating room, critical care units, medical-surgical floors, and hospital bed management. It even relies on factors outside its institutional control, such as bed availability in rehabilitation hospitals and nursing homes. Throughput in the ED simply cannot be adequately improved without the problem being enlarged to include all those systems and factors that contribute to the problem.

Exhibit 5.3 The Funnel of Options

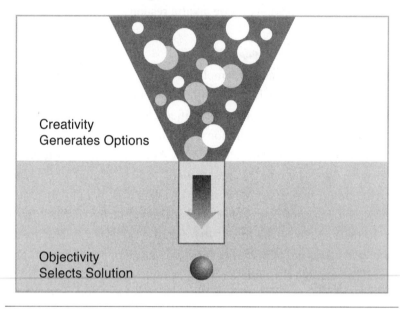

Creativity
Generates Options

Objectivity
Selects Solution

In short, this problem requires expansion of the *context*. The problem might be solved by improving ED registration or door-to-clinician time. But by using systems approaches, the problem of throughput in the ED might be best solved by recruiting more PCPs in the community, relocating their practices, or expanding their hours of practice—a completely different solution than would have been identified if the problem was being solved solely within the traditional boundaries of the ED.

Senior management's role in this kind of organization is to frame issues within as broad a context as possible and then facilitate a process that convenes those with potential insight and interest in the outcome (see the "The Tower" parable) to participate in evaluating the cause and generating options. From that point on, senior management must narrow the choices and select the best solution.

This process can be thought of as a funnel, illustrated in Exhibit 5.3. Creativity is used to generate options; objectivity is used to select solutions.

Simple Rule 5: Emulate Water, Not Fire

All that is needed to understand this simple rule is the following parable. It emphasizes creating thoughtful long-term solutions over expedient short-term fixes. It reminds everyone in the system that total accountability for care of a population is a long-term goal, not a quick fix.

Parable 4: The Wisdom of the River

Prince Li had spent many years traveling throughout his kingdom in search of wisdom that might aid him in leading his people. As successor to the throne, he had received word that his aged father was ailing, so he swiftly returned home to carry on in his father's place.

While on his journey, the prince had discovered a great many things. He now felt certain of his strength as ruler and fearlessly approached the palace, prepared to take the affairs of the kingdom into his own capable hands. As he approached the palace gate, he saw a stooped figure standing some ways off by the river. It was his old friend and master, Mu-Sun. He ran excitedly to greet him.

"Mu-Sun!" the prince exclaimed. "I have returned from my journey as a wiser man and am now prepared to lead as my father has done. There is much to do and little time to do it in. I shall wake like a rooster with the sun and will not rest until all is well in order!" The great master smiled warmly at the prince, then bade the young man to sit for awhile with him by the river.

Prince Li followed his master. He saw how feeble the master's body had become, and he knew that soon he would be leaving this world. Though he would miss him greatly, the young man felt that this was not a time for endings, but for new beginnings. And so he watched the palace gate with wild anticipation as the old man slowly piled wood and lit a fire. He held his tongue for all he wanted to say in his excitement, as the old master sat silently staring into the flames. They passed the night in this way, and it was not until the fire smoldered, cold in the morning light, that the master turned and spoke to the young prince who was soon to be king.

"The fire is gone and the sun is rising, Prince Li. Tell me, now do you understand what it takes to be a great leader?" The prince rubbed his eyes, tired from his long journey and a sleepless night, and looked out over the land. He thought back on all that he had learned on his journey but felt he could not give the answer his old master was look-ing for.

Mu-Sun continued, "Last night you returned home, strong, eager, and passionate like fire. The fire's flames can consume anything. Noth-ing can match its force. But observe now what has become of the fire, Prince Li." The prince saw the gray ashes shivering slightly in the morning wind. The fire had died. "Now observe the river," invited the old master. "It too is strong, but has a different strength. See how it slowly carves the stone of its bed. See how it runs ceaselessly and tire-lessly round the palace wall, growing deeper, broader, and ever more powerful. The fire is so fierce it consumes even itself. The river is for-ever flowing, providing life and sustenance to all. As it is with nature, so it is with rulers. Reflect on what kind of ruler you will be."

Simple Rule 6: Build Version 1.0 First

While all systems are perfectly designed to produce the outcomes they produce, all system design is inherently imperfect, representing the best package or best set of options, trade-offs, and alternatives at a given moment in a resource-competitive and complex universe. The rule of 80/20 offers excellent guidance—that is, 80 percent of the benefit is generally achieved in the first 20 percent of the time and effort invested. Striving for the perfect solution can exceed the group's attention span and require fussy, overly complicated design. When the goal is to build momentum for continuous improvement, it is better to build a prototype. As it is implemented, one can observe and measure the effects, and then use the lessons from the imple-mentation to drive additional improvement in both process and out-comes. This process resembles the river more than the fire in the last parable.

Version 1.0 of any process, program, protocol, or system should be the alpha test, searching for proof of concept rather than optimization of results. Too many organizations try to build Version 4.0 first. And that often produces paradoxically disappointing results because expectations are high that "the (ideal) solution" is on the way. But because all unintended consequences could not be anticipated, Version 4.0 falls short of expectations. It is far more effective to implement and refer to the initial solution as Version 1.0. That way everyone in the system understands that subsequent improvements or versions are fully planned.

This rule is often violated as healthcare delivery systems adopt electronic health records. Systems are often overdesigned, are too complicated for initial use, and too frequently require significant redesign as problems get revealed. In brief, focus on process optimization only after there is proof that the concept of Version 1.0 yields favorable results. Leaders will find that they have a great deal of internal support in their improvement efforts if they follow this simple rule.

Simple Rule 7: All Change Is a Pilot

There is much more resistance to a *change* than to a *pilot*. It stands to reason, then, that all changes are better introduced as the experiments that they are, with an ongoing intention to engage those within the system to assess and refine the pilot. Energy is far better spent on supporting subsequent improvement than on managing initial resistance.

Simple Rule 8: Make Compliance the Easiest Option

When the preferred action is also the easiest action, compliance is likely. Therefore, in system design, whenever compliance is necessary for those who provide *or* receive care, system design should focus attention on how to make compliance easy. This can be best achieved by helping people understand why compliance is important and then asking those who must comply to assist with the design. The more difficult it is to receive a flu vaccination, the greater the likelihood that many will go without it. Pharmacies across America have benefitted from that observation. Moreover, if you design a change so that it is easier to use than what came before, people will automatically gravitate toward the change.

Simple Rule 9: Good Design Trumps Great Attitude and Effort

A small group within an organization can often produce heroic results if they are committed to one another and to a common purpose. On the other hand, processes that cross work groups, sites, specialties, departments, and divisions (that is, the complex processes that ACOs are intended to improve) must rely on thoughtful design rather than on the attitude and commitment of a small group. Pretty good design will often generate better results than relying on Herculean efforts from a cadre within the organization. This concept is illustrated in the following parable.

Parable 5: The Fisherman's Tale

With renewed hope, Prince Li continued his journey to enlightenment; though his father was ailing, he felt certain that he and his five brothers would find the wisdom to lead their people. Thus, filled with excitement, he came upon a prosperous fishing village. The sun was just rising, and the fishing fleet was heading to sea. It was a glorious sight, the boats gliding on the wind. Full of pride for his family, Prince Li remarked to a fisherman who sat nearby, "My brothers and I shall be as those six great ships, and the prosperity of our kingdom will be as vast as all the riches of the sea!"

The fisherman looked out into the harbor and observed, "It is a large fleet indeed, with six of the finest boats on this coast. And each has the best nets and the strongest men. Yet each day my son with my leaky boat and his two slight cousins bring in twice the catch of all six of them combined."

The prince could not believe the fisherman's claim. "Look more closely and you will see the truth of my words," sighed the old fisherman. "See how poorly the big boats sail, how slowly they tack, and how unwieldy their nets are. They sail aimlessly, fishing the same banks day after day."

"Now see my small boat coming out of the harbor. It easily overtakes the larger boats and outmaneuvers them to the best fishing banks. Yet its nets are old and worn, and my son and his cousins must use every ounce of muscle, every bit of knowledge of the sea. They cannot become lazy with the size and power of their craft and must rely on one

another to bring in their catch. They know they cannot return with a poor catch, for they must first feed their families and have enough left to provide for the poor children of the village who rely on them for their sustenance. That was a commitment they made many years ago. They are driven by that motivation. Whatever is left thereafter can be sold for their own meager needs."

The prince sat with the fisherman in silence as the sun crossed the sky. As the sun sank slowly into the sea he watched the fisherman's boat sail swiftly in toward shore, followed by the fleet. The small boat's catch was magnificent, easily twice what the fleet of six brought in.

Simple Rule 10: Margin Triumphs over Revenue

As noted elsewhere, increasing competition, falling reimbursement, and technological advances have created a reactive focus on revenue as the key driver of financial performance and, therefore, success. No one would dispute the importance of revenue in healthcare. In an ACO environment, however, revenue becomes a supporter rather than a driver of success. Whether operating in a shared-savings model or a capitation model, the principal driver of success is margin, and margin production requires attention to unit reimbursement, mix, volume, and expenses. When unit reimbursement is fixed, the ability to influence margin falls on the other variables—mix, volume, and expenses. This trickles down to resource utilization (e.g., available bed days, clinic slots) and quality management, with an emphasis on clinical effectiveness (getting it right the first time, every time) and productivity. As a result, new metrics that emphasize margin per unit of available capacity and quality of care (e.g., revenue per available bed day, cost per available bed day) will emerge in time.

Simple Rule 11: The Most Important Partnership Is with the Patient

Ideological arguments about whether the patient is always right are of little value. The patient is certainly not always in a position to determine which treatment or prescription is best. But the patient is certainly capable of helping design care in such a way that he is best able to carry out the parts of the plan that he is responsible for. The system will simply work best when those who deliver and receive care are both intimately involved in the design of care. This should not be construed as promoting "one size fits all." Rather, simple rule 11 must be considered with its corollary—simple rule 12.

Simple Rule 12: Exceptions Require Rules

This rule has been stressed throughout this book. Rules always need exceptions. There will always be circumstances where a predesigned or standardized plan will fail. The reverse is also true, however: Exceptions require rules. The starting point for any care or support process must be "the rule"—the designed plan or pathway. In similar fashion, improvisation and innovation require standardization. Any exception to a formal or informal rule must be defensible in light of *both* the ACO's objectives and the patient's needs. Whether an organization implements a formal process for sanctioning exceptions is left up to the discretion of its leadership. But all exceptions must be defensible. And there can be no exceptions unless there are rules first.

Everyone in today's complex healthcare arena will face situations with conflicting expectations. The simple guiding rule is to do what's right and be able to defend the reasoning behind the decision. Those who follow the rule will always be able to either defend their actions or learn from them, even when the outcomes are undesirable. If there is no clear "right thing" to do, either course of action is probably defensible.

Simple Rule 13: It Actually *Is* Your Problem

Everyone in the healthcare delivery system is capable of recognizing a problem or an opportunity. Recognizing a problem means that an individual is responsible for it until it is *explicitly* handed off to those authorized to design and implement a response. The more explicit the process, the clearer the accountability. Put in simple terms, "You see it; you own it" until, like in a relay race, you have handed the baton off to the next person who is accountable for handling the situation. The words "it's not my problem" are never uttered in the ACO. This protocol applies equally to problems and opportunities.

Referring back to the parable of the tower, it should be clear that wisdom knows no hierarchy.

Simple Rule 14: Teamwork Is Not Optional

Teamwork in an ACO is critical to success. Those who cannot follow reasonable rules of teamwork have no place in an ACO. Historically, many hospitals and healthcare systems have endured or even encouraged a sense of "royalty" among physicians who admit heavily to the hospital. More recently, they have wittingly or unwittingly endorsed a caste system among physicians in which surgeons who perform high-revenue procedures enjoy the privileges at the top of the system. In this new model, royalty, privilege, and individualism can be toxins or viruses that ultimately threaten the integrity of the system.

Definitions of and expectations for teamwork should be explicitly shared throughout the ACO, feedback should be prompt and clear, and those unable to adopt the core principles of teamwork must be eliminated. Allowing some to operate using a different set of rules sends a clear and problematic message to everyone in the system and builds resentment and cynicism. Too many healthcare systems today make exceptions to the rule of teamwork, and that undermines leadership effectiveness at every level. Those in the ACO must be ready to participate in a true team-based approach to care.

Simple Rule 15: Mind the Gap

Anyone who travels on London's Tube has heard the familiar warning "mind the gap," which refers to the gap between the train door and the platform. Gaps in systems design represent discontinuities that undermine integrity, threaten integration, and create problematic breaks in continuity of care. All too often, gaps are used to attribute blame to individuals or work groups. Instead, they should be treated as what they are—design failures. Treating them as design failures produces two desired outcomes: it (1) closes the gap and (2) avoids the buildup of unnecessary tension or vibration within the system. While many gaps are closed by adding or redeploying personnel, some can be closed by adding programs and technology or simply by changing operating systems. If there is no obvious forum for addressing the gap, that is yet another design failure that must be addressed.

Simple Rule 16: Participation Is Both Voluntary and Mandatory

This paradoxical rule governs the expectations of those working within the ACO. The organization must be clear about what it expects of care-givers: Follow processes, care plans, pathways, and protocols. Everyone who participates in an ACO should be able to make a personal choice about participation—that is the voluntary part. After deciding to participate in the ACO, adherence to the processes, programs, care plans, pathways, and protocols is not voluntary—that is the mandatory part (see simple rule 14). Anyone who chooses to participate in the ACO chooses to participate in the activities and goals of the ACO. No exceptions.

Simple Rule 17: Enhance Personal Power by Giving It Away

Every leader has learned the paradox of power: If it is given away (used to empower others), then it is enhanced. Empowering others requires three critical steps:

1. A clear description of what "product" or "outcome" is being requested of the person being empowered, including a timeline, a format, and other attributes or parameters
2. Clear boundaries of what is allowed and prohibited
3. A clear offer of support or assistance if requested

Without following these steps, there is a greater risk that those you seek to empower will fail. Being vague and unclear about expectations only sets up others for failure. And failure is disempowering to *all* parties. This, then, introduces simple rule 18.

Simple Rule 18: Begin Design Efforts with Outcome Specifications

The first step in any design process is to clarify the goal: What are we trying to produce, and what must our work product be able to achieve? When a group of designers set out to create a vehicle that could carry seven passengers and their luggage and still fit in traditional parking spots and garages, they wound up with the minivan. For designers, clarity of outcomes specifications enhances rather than diminishes creativity. Less time and effort should be spent at the beginning envisioning a specific solution and more time and effort should be directed toward developing specific outcome specifications. Ironically, the more stringent the outcome specifications, the more creative the solutions can be; see Exhibit 5.4.

Simple Rule 19: Make the Case

Good managers don't just make the right decisions. They also communicate how they arrived at the decision. In the purest sense, this is what is meant by organizational transparency. Share the data, expose the reasoning, and reveal the options considered. In brief, as has already been stated in this book, leaders must make a rational case for the decisions. A good rule of thumb is that if the decision makers don't feel they can present a bullet-proof case for their decision, they ought to question their decision. When making the case, it can be helpful to acknowledge those within the organization who contributed input to the decision-making process, regardless of whether that input had an impact on the final outcome. Sharing credit for the decision-making process lends credibility and builds trust and confidence within the organization.

Simple Rule 20: This Sandbox Isn't Just Yours

The sandbox is shared by the group. And there are behaviors and norms expected of those who share the sandbox that are inculcated during childhood. If you have agreed to work in a team environment like an ACO, you have agreed that you can't always get what you want. Still, as Mick Jagger put it, you should be able to *get what you need*. If you are *never* getting what you need, you're probably playing in the wrong sandbox. If you are getting what you need *some* of the time, it's probably the right one.

Simple Rule 21: Treat Care as Science and Caring as Art

Everyone who participates in healthcare design and delivery has heard the adage that healthcare is more art than science. Anyone who has had the privilege of delivering care understands that both science and art are required for doing it well. As science and evidence-based

Exhibit 5.4 Outcomes Specifications for a Shared-Risk Arrangement

When designing a shared-risk arrangement, consider the following outcomes specifications.

Patient Population, Conditions to Cover
- What populations to cover (e.g., Medicare, Medicaid, large administrative services–only populations, individuals, or employees)
- What conditions to cover (e.g., chronic, acute, inpatient, outpatient)
- What benefit design, severity adjustment, patient incentives, and contract duration to implement

Physicians, Hospitals, and Other Caregivers to Include
- What provider panel and incentives to implement
- What services to carve out or treat out of network
- What contract duration to establish

Other Outcomes/Goals
- What utilization reduction targets to set, by year (e.g., reduce avoidable readmissions by 10%)
- What unit reimbursement and cost reduction targets to set, by year (e.g., reduce costs per ED visit by 15%)
- Where to steer/protect margins over time (e.g., steer margins to specialized, proprietary services)
- What capital investments to plan for, by year (e.g., new reports, new staff, construction of new tower)

best practices grow, we suggest ACOs begin with the premise that the design and delivery of clinical care be scientifically rooted wherever possible. In the words of Donald Berwick, CMS director, "Young doctors and nurses should emerge from training understanding the values of standardization and the risks of too great an emphasis on individual autonomy" (Berwick 2010). Where autonomy fits is in the caring component. Physicians must rely on their instincts and personal human traits to provide the artful caring component of healthcare. Learn from other systems that deliver care well.

Simple Rule 22: Accountability Must Match Authority

There is a delicate balance between authority and accountability in all organizations. They must match each other. When a nurse responsible for eliminating postoperative wound infections asks a physician to wash his hands and is rebuffed, accountability on the part of the nurse exceeds authority and authority on the part of the physician exceeds personal and collective accountability. This is never a good situation.

Conversely, when an executive is authorized to accept a risk-bearing contract that will affect the income of people other than herself, her authority exceeds her accountability and could lead to that executive taking on unreasonable risks. In these cases, the repercussions can be felt throughout the organization. Accountability and authority must remain balanced for an organization to maintain its integrity. Situations where they are out of balance tend to generate conflict.

Simple Rule 23: Always Play at the Highest Level Possible

This simple rule reminds system designers to make certain that all contributors within the system are able to contribute to the fullest extent of their capabilities and licensure. The resource efficiency achieved through such a strategy is useful, but it pales compared to the motivation and job satisfaction achieved by entrusting each player to give everything he can. Challenged employees are usually satisfied employees. Organizational psychologist Frederick Herzberg's motivation–hygiene theory from the late 1950s provided enlightenment about the factors in the work environment that promoted motivation. Contrary to popular assumptions, compensation and work conditions are strictly hygiene factors; professionals are motivated by challenges and personal and collective accomplishments.

Simple Rule 24: Keep Your Ears (and Eyes) Wide Open

Everyone who contributes to the success of an ACO ("I preserve the eyesight of diabetic patients," for example) is both a participant and a potentially critical observer. This rule invites and implores all those within the system to be observers of the system and its outcomes. When a critical observation is made, thoughtful inquiry will help ascertain the significance of the observation. Simple measurement will quantify the value of the observation, and analysis will begin to reveal the contributing factors and potential solutions. Observation, however, is not limited to that which is seen, as the following parable helps us understand.

Parable 6: The Voice of the City

Prince Li was to succeed his father as king, and the great master Mu-Sun had endeavored to help the boy discover the wisdom he would need to be a great ruler. Mu-Sun decided it was time to send Prince Li, having been confined to study and meditate within the temple tower, on a journey that might lead to new discoveries. Taking Prince Li as far as the palace gate, Mu-Sun instructed the prince to disguise himself as a peasant and then venture into the city and live there for one year. After the year, Prince Li was to describe the "voice of the city."

At the end of the year, Mu-Sun found the boy, sat with him on a rock at the edge of the river, and asked him to describe the voice of the city. "Master," replied the prince, "I heard the creak of oxcarts, and the rumble of voices, the roosters' crow, the dogs' bark, and the cows' low. I heard the rustle of wind over sheets drying and the constant roar of the river. All of these sounds and more make the voice of this city." The prince continued his report. When he had finished, the master left him, telling him to go back and listen to what more he could hear, as the prince had missed the most important voices in the city.

Confused, the boy returned to his dwelling in the city. He listened there for many days and many nights. He roamed the streets, wondering what sounds he could hear that he had not already heard before. Then, early one morning, he began to hear new sounds: the eager breath of children waking slowly in their beds; the worried hush of women bent low over coal fires; the steady, tired step of the old shopkeeper; and the angry snap of the washerwoman's brittle line. The closer he listened, the clearer new sounds became. "This must be the voice of the city," the young prince reflected.

The next day, Prince Li returned to the temple to tell his master what more he had heard. Mu-Sun commended the boy, saying, "To be a great ruler, you must hear not only that which is said but also that which is unspoken. Rulers cannot be effective when they listen but do not hear what is in the hearts and minds of the people. You must hear the unheard, for only then can you understand their true needs."

Using the 24 Simple Rules

As we have noted in this chapter, simple rules are extremely powerful influencers of organizational performance. Much of their power lies in their presence in the collective unconscious of the organization. The 24 simple rules presented here are neither prescriptive nor comprehensive. Feel free to pick and choose among them to find those that can help your organization. Even better, use them to start conversations among your leadership and membership to discover the hidden simple rules in your organization. Discuss the new ones you want to help define your emerging ACO.

Organizational Questions

The organizational questions raised in this chapter include the following:

- What are our organization's simple rules?
- What are our core underlying values, beliefs, and assumptions?
- How are our simple rules manifested in our organizational design and delivery?
- Where are they compatible or incompatible with an ACO strategy?
- Who should we bring together to explore old and new rules?

Category of Readers	Key Concepts	Actions to Consider
Category A (interested)	• Sources of power in organizations • Foundations of organizational culture: simple rules • Current common simple healthcare rules	• Perform an internal simple rules audit • Executive leadership team assessment of where your organization is culturally aligned with the discipline necessary for ACO performance • Design a strategy to introduce or advance a culture of performance
Category B (engaged)	• Foundations of organizational culture: simple rules • Leadership parables • How to change the rules	• Declare a leadership intention to pursue an ACO strategy • Perform an internal simple rules audit • Use the parables to engage those within the organization in a set of coordinated conversations about performance
Category C (committed)	• Foundations of organizational culture: simple rules • 24 simple rules • How to change the rules	• Perform an internal simple rules audit • Assess current rules against ACO attributes • Use the 24 simple rules to frame and facilitate a set of organizational conversations about the ACO

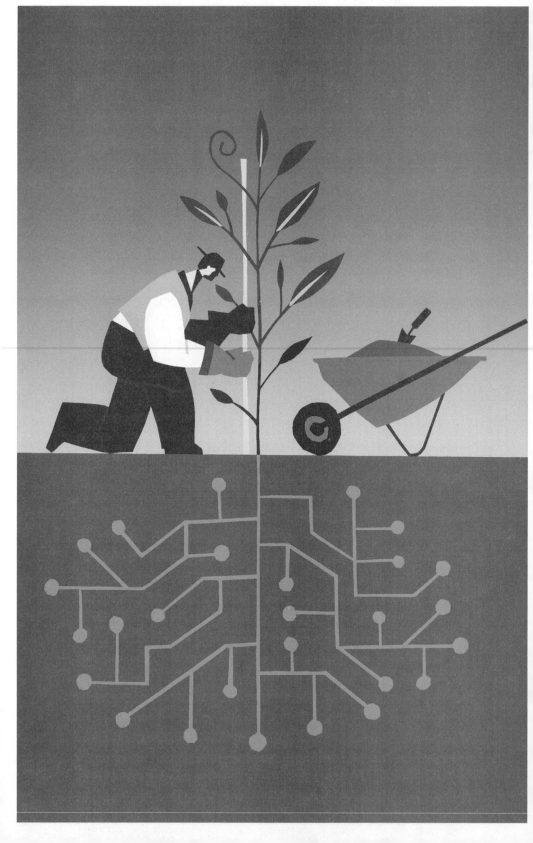

6

Technology for the Emerging ACO

Health information technology is absolutely critical to the accountable care organization. There's no way to track the health of a population without using technology. You need to measure performance across sites and across physicians. You just can't do that with paper charts.

—Micky Tripathi
President and CEO
Massachusetts eHealth Collaborative

Accountable care organization (ACO) skeptics have taken to calling the entire ACO movement "Capitation 2.0" or worse. They look at the elements of the ACO strategy—physicians taking on risk, efforts to control medical spending, and tighter networks—and see a repetition of the managed care era of the 1980s and early 1990s. They ask, "What's gonna be different this time?"

There are many differences between managed care as it was practiced 25 years ago and how ACOs intend to manage care going forward. One of the key changes is the vast improvement in health information technology (HIT). The state of the art 25 years ago was electronic reports of utilization of various services. But even that was limited. Labs could tell management how many LDL cholesterol tests were being done, but they couldn't say what the results were, how they varied across patient demographics, or which direction the entire population was trending.

Physicians who took on risk really didn't have enough information to make decisions about assuming that risk. For example, physicians often did not know the cost and quality impacts of referral decisions. They didn't have the tools to actively manage the health of the populations for which they were responsible. Almost inevitably, managed care focused on controlling costs by restricting access rather than on improving outcomes. So what will be different this time?

In this chapter, we assert that HIT will be a game changer for those physicians who fully commit to the core ACO goals of higher quality, lower cost, and greater service to the patient. HIT can help make a good system great by enabling providers to proactively reach out to patients with reminders, follow-ups, and health information appropriate to their particular health cohort. HIT will reduce the burden on the physician and her administrative staff. Gaps will shrink, particularly in the crucial areas of work flow and care handoffs between affiliated providers.

But building a great HIT system to support ACOs (and beyond) isn't easy or inexpensive. There are dozens of vendors competing for your IT dollars, most of whom make superlative claims for their products. More important, health information tools are merely that—tools to support the ACO strategy. They cannot substitute for a health system that has no mission, no immediate or long-term goals, and no strategy for reaching those goals. If these are missing in your organization, you must step back and work on those issues before doing HIT planning in a vacuum.

So where should ACOs start their HIT journey? We suggest five key steps:

1. Start with the electronic medical record
2. Understand meaningful-use standards
3. Plot the HIT plan
4. Avoid pitfalls
5. Move from analysis to work flow

A note about vendors: We don't recommend any particular vendor or consultant in the HIT space. However, in this chapter we quote several prominent vendors and consultants who have valuable experience to share regarding HIT implementation.

Start with the Electronic Medical Record

The basic HIT tool for the ACO, or any other healthcare provider, is the electronic medical record (EMR), also called the electronic health record (EHR). Simply stated, the EMR is a record of all health services received by the patient. Ideally, it can be accessed, updated, and shared across the organization and will comply with one or more interoperability standards, which permit sharing, such as HL7.

From that basic definition, the required attributes of a fully functioning EMR quickly proliferate. According to the Healthcare Information and Management Systems Society (2003), the EMR must possess the following qualities:

- The EMR must provide secure, reliable, real-time access to patient health record information where and when it is needed to support care.
- The EMR must capture and manage episodic and longitudinal health information. Significantly, the EMR must include time stamps, mark information sources, and record amendments to create a secure audit trail.
- The EMR must function as clinicians' primary information resource during the provision of patient care. The provider organization must establish a policy that the EMR is the source of patient information to be used in care delivery. It should be the official medical record under local and state statutes.
- The EMR should facilitate delivery of evidence-based care to patients. This includes everything from simple planning tools that help the physician to organize his work shift to more advanced decision support tools. The latter may include software that guides and critiques medication decisions and decision-support tools, such as care pathways that standardize care among physicians.

- The EMR must capture data to be used for utilization review, risk management, resource planning, and performance management. These include tools to gauge patient case intensity and severity, which can help in resource planning. The data become the basis for the healthcare organization to assess, measure, and manage quality.
- The EMR should capture patient health-related information necessary for reimbursement. This includes verification of coverage, transmission of chargeable transactions to billing, and provision of data to support accurate coding.
- The EMR must generate longitudinal information that can be used in clinical research, public health reporting, and population health management. Such information must be suitably masked to conform to HIPAA (Health Insurance Portability and Accountability Act) requirements. It must also support ongoing evidence-based research and clinical trials.

Clearly, the EMR is a powerful, wide-ranging tool that should be the foundation of any provider's HIT strategy. Numerous industry vendors offer competing tools, including Epic, Ingenix, Athena Health, and Allscripts. Many provide specialized versions for specific practice types.

Nevertheless, relatively few healthcare providers in the United States have fully embraced the EMR. A recent survey by the Centers for Disease Control and Prevention's National Center for Health Statistics showed that fewer than half of the nation's physicians use EMRs, with many using just partial systems and just 10 percent using fully functioning systems (see Exhibit 6.1).

Clearly, the daunting cost of implementing EMRs is a big part of the low implementation. Starter systems can cost from $25,000 to $50,000 for one physician and her assistants. But there are many other factors. As discussed earlier, physicians don't like ceding control to anyone outside of their line of sight, and for many, computerized systems, no matter how sophisticated, are not in the line of sight. For older physicians, working at a computer may never feel comfortable. And older physicians who own their practices may not be comfortable with the investment required to set up an EMR. Some healthcare

Exhibit 6.1 Percentage of Office-Based Physicians with EMRs/EHRs: United States, 2001–2009 and Preliminary 2010

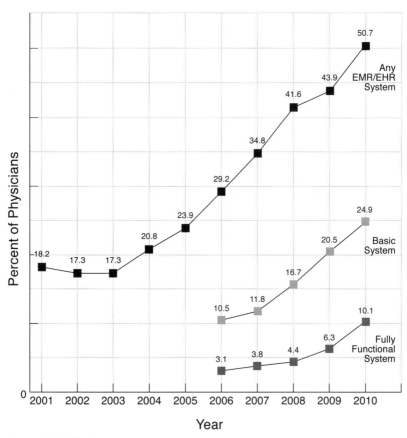

Source: CDC (2010).

systems force the issue by making the EMR a precondition of joining their physician organization.

The numerous benefits offered by the EMR will enable providers who adopt the EMR to generate many quick savings. First movers in their markets will gain key advantages, and the incentives of the American Recovery and Reinvestment Act of 2009 (ARRA) are expected to speed adoption of the EMR. At the same time, it's important to keep in mind that the EMR is just the first step.

"The EMR is the starting point," says Dr. C. Martin Harris, chief information officer of Cleveland Clinic and prime mover of the renowned provider's impressive HIT initiatives (see the sidebar "Peeling the Onion"). According to Dr. Harris (2010), "When you're starting out, the functionality you need is transactional information that will help you understand what you're utilizing and how. This includes electronic ordering, so you can see how much medication, labs, consults, and procedures you are using. Next up should be an electronic documentation system, which replaces physicians' hand-written notes on the paper chart with computerized records. You can't deduce everything from ordering behavior; you have to be able to decode what the physician is thinking. Electronic documentation enables you to count, sort, and draw conclusions from many physicians' documents. And moving up from there, you can add clinical decision support, alerting and notifying, and prompting caregivers to a set of guidelines. You can write rules that would prompt someone under certain conditions to think about a diagnostic test or a medication, or the need to avoid a medication."

Taking Action

Ultimately, adopting the EMR and other HIT tools is a requirement for the ACO. It is impossible to think of a fully functioning ACO that is not supported by a full suite of electronic tools, including the EMR. For instance, most ACO pilots will only treat subsets of larger patient populations from the anchor hospital or physician organization. Primary care physicians will have to start by answering a basic question: Is this patient in the ACO or not?

From a Data Registry to an Integrated Clinical Data Source

Describe a hypothetical clinical information tool to a physician, and he may jump to a conclusion: "This is nothing but a registry." There's some truth to this assessment. The best tools resemble registries in appearance, but they go far beyond registries in functionality. Say you're building a modern registry for an independent practice association (IPA) that is

Peeling the Onion: The Many Layers of Cleveland Clinic's HIT Strategy

For those just starting to think of their HIT needs as they implement an ACO strategy, it is easy to feel overwhelmed by the achievements of Cleveland Clinic. The not-for-profit multispecialty academic medical center has spent hundreds of millions of dollars on HIT over more than a decade. In the process, it has piloted healthcare products from industry leaders, such as Google and Microsoft, and has become an acknowledged leader in developing and implementing new technology-based products and services. Here is an overview of the many elements of Cleveland Clinics' HIT strategy, starting with the first and ending with the most recent:

- The core EMR at Cleveland Clinic is called *MyPractice.* It was launched in 2001 and now connects 6,000 physicians (2,200 employed) at 11 hospitals and 20 health clinics. The vendor is Epic Systems Corporation of Verona, Wisconsin.
- In 2005, the clinic introduced *MyChart,* a Web portal that gives patients access to their medical records. The system is regularly used by about 280,000 of the 750,000 people the clinic treats on a regular basis.
- *MyConsult* is a Web-based service for patients anywhere who want a second opinion or a consult with a Cleveland Clinic physician. It is aimed at a set of 250 diagnoses. The tool gets a patient who is not affiliated with the clinic started on the path toward getting a physician and a second opinion.
- Many doctors send patients to Cleveland Clinic for episodic or specialized care. For those physicians, the clinic launched *DrConnect.* This gives the referring physician access to the full EMR within the system, just as the Cleveland Clinic physician would. It is intended to keep the physician fully informed about the patient's treatment, with the understanding that the patient will return to that physician after treatment at the clinic.
- Cleveland Clinic focused on the 4,000 or so physicians who are not employed or working at the clinic but who admit to the hospital.

> *MyPractice Community* is an attempt to distribute the Cleveland Clinic HIT tools to those physicians at a relatively low cost. For a base fee of about $450 a month for a single physician, a practice can have everything it needs to connect to the same system as Cleveland Clinic physicians. "They just have to buy computers and printers," says Dr. C. Martin Harris (2010), chief information officer of the clinic. "It relieves the physician of the burden of having to be an IT expert."
>
> - Recently, Cleveland Clinic has partnered with Google and Microsoft on two additional services that spread an even wider net. Google Health and Microsoft HealthVault are online personal health records for patients anywhere. Individuals can store clinical, lab, pharmacy, and hospital data in their own account. For patients who ultimately travel to Cleveland for specialized treatment, the personal record can be accessed before they arrive. With up-to-date medical information at the ready, the clinic doesn't need to spend as much time getting a patient workup before surgery or another procedure can begin. Patients move more quickly through the process, and the clinic uses its operating rooms and beds more efficiently.

affiliating as part of a hospital-anchored ACO. Here are the four attributes the "registry" needs to have:

1. *It must integrate multiple sources of data.* Data come from everything from claims to physician documentation. Even the most prosaic data from patients and doctors have value when combined through powerful analytics.
2. *It must be easy to read and understand.* Doctors spend a lot of time looking at computers these days. They don't want a program that is going to require them to spend any more time looking at a screen. They want a tool that enables them to get away from the screen and treat patients.
3. *It must appeal to physicians at all age levels and all degrees of computer literacy.* Older physicians, like many older people, may never feel completely comfortable at the computer. Newly

minted physicians may feel ready to run their practice from their smart phones. The desktop tool has to accommodate both extremes and everyone in between.

4. *It must have real-time interactivity.* Something that updates at midnight every night is no longer adequate. A physician who looks at a patient chart has to be able to see the current view to assess the patient's health and compliance. Any orders the physician enters need to show up at all other points in the ACO. Integration of data leads to integration of care.

From Data Source to Business Analytics

In the rapidly evolving world of HIT, the data generated by myriad software tools such as the ones we've listed are just the beginning. A new product sector within the HIT industry is focused on gathering data from disparate sources and analyzing them. This generates new, more fully developed information that can better support physician and management decision making.

A simple example begins to show the power of analytics. A primary care physician (PCP) sees a patient with a running injury. An MRI (magnetic resonance imaging) shows torn cartilage in the knee. The PCP refers the patient to an orthopedist for a surgical evaluation. The orthopod, upon seeing the patient, orders another MRI. An analytic engine spots this duplication and prompts the physician with a pop-up window to advise against the additional imaging diagnostic. The analytic engine sees across multiple programs (see Exhibit 6.2). Moreover, the reminder comes from the system, which ACO physicians presumably support. Had the message cancelling the additional image come from a colleague who is not a peer (an administrative assistant or a patient care coordinator), the physician might have ignored the reminder. Physicians prefer line-of-sight relationships, and they don't like taking direction from nonphysicians.

Exhibit 6.2 shows how an analytics engine can take multiple data streams and process them into useful insights that drive physician actions. According to Dr. Todd Rothenhaus (2010), chief information officer for Caritas Christi Health Care, a six-hospital Catholic health system in Boston, "There is a widespread notion that getting everybody on an electronic health record is the only thing we need to do to

Exhibit 6.2 Function of an Analytics Engine

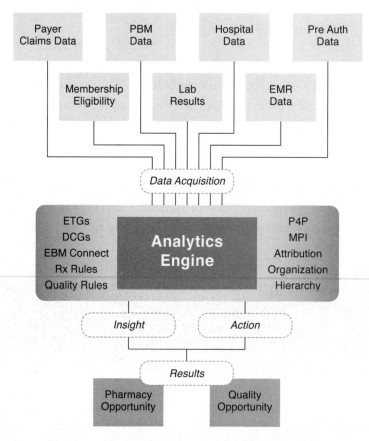

get at all the data we need to deliver better care. That's just not true. It's an oversimplification. There's an enormous amount of analytical work that needs to happen." (See "A Bold HIT Initative" sidebar.)

Understand Meaningful-Use Standards: A Potential Funding Source and More

As part of the ARRA, the federal government is investing some $30 billion into EMRs. The law provides for substantial grants for individual physicians and for hospitals that buy EMR hardware and software and

A Bold HIT Initiative at Caritas Christi Health Care

Caritas Christi Health Care, a six-hospital Catholic healthcare chain located in and around Boston, has gone through a dramatic transformation in a few years. It struggled through most of the 2000s, saddled with financially strapped hospitals with poor payer mixes in low-income communities. It was composed of community hospitals and a second-tier academic medical center in a city dominated by Partners HealthCare and world-famous hospitals, such as Massachusetts General.

Meantime, Caritas's sponsor, the Archdiocese of Boston, was itself coping with the aftermath of the Catholic priest sex scandals, which had been uncovered in 2001. Enormous settlements to victims left it short of cash and having to close churches and consolidate parishes. It had little time and no resources to devote to healthcare.

Two attempts to sell the chain to other Catholic healthcare providers fell through. Then, in May 2008, the chain hired Dr. Ralph de la Torre, a cardiologist from neighboring Beth Israel Deaconess Medical Center, as chief executive officer. De la Torre's style was a big change, and presaged larger changes at the system. In 2010, the system was purchased by Cerberus Capital, a New York private equity firm.

The system has also been shaking up its clinical operations. It is aggressively pursuing an ACO strategy and has ruffled feathers in the marketplace by actively pursuing physician groups to join its IPA. And it has launched a cutting-edge HIT overhaul, through which it intends to become a regional HIT leader in just seven years. These principles underlie the new system:

- *Ubiquitous information systems:* Wire every transaction
- *Advanced interoperability:* Seamlessly integrate all clinical and administrative systems
- *Data reuse and rapid learning:* Deploy data tools to make use of every piece of information gathered during clinical and administrative activities
- *Patient relationship management:* Attract patients through technology, including secure portals, social networking sites, and innovative telehealth applications

It has been installing EMRs in its physicians' offices, starting as part of a statewide pilot, offering solutions from eClinicalWorks or Athenahealth. By fall of 2010, it had about half of its employed and affiliated physicians hooked up and was deploying two new systems a week, at a cost of $20,000 to $45,000 per physician.

According to Dr. Todd Rothenhaus (2010), chief information officer, some of the findings midway through the HIT project have been surprising:

- A single EMR is an "imperfect strategy." It's better to offer different choices for small and large practices.
- Not all independent physicians are sold on the need for shared medical records.
- Small practices are keen to exploit the connection between EMR and practice management integration.

Through 2011, Caritas will be focused on breaking down internal silos and fully leveraging data. It plans to use Microsoft Amalga and Microsoft HealthVault Community Connect to construct a clinical "data mart" for use by clinical, administrative, and financial functions. The goal is real-time detection of patterns and outliers.

Dr. Rothenhaus is sometimes reluctant to put too much trust in HIT as a tool to transform care. But he says this about the Caritas effort: "A high-functioning electronic health record becomes a power driver of financial performance, helping to eliminate network leakage. It supports the cultural mission of the ACO by breaking down the silos that exist between various clinical specialties and among the practices and partnerships that [compose] the organization. But ultimately, as the ACO becomes more adept at processing and sharing information, the EHR becomes a tool for driving care decisions from a population level. The healthcare information technology system will provide real-time detection of patterns, enabling providers to respond more quickly to health trends and identify the outliers that drive costs."

then put it to work to improve outcomes. Under rules set out by the Centers for Medicare & Medicaid Services (CMS), only those who demonstrate "meaningful use" of the technology qualify for the incentives.

For providers—hospitals, physician groups, and individual practices—considering an ACO strategy, the appeal is twofold. First, free money is a good thing, especially when the provider is faced with the daunting investment of setting up an EMR. Second, the rules that define *meaningful use* provide a good, basic road map for those first implementing HIT. Meeting the government's definition of meaningful use doesn't ensure that an organization's HIT will ultimately support its ACO goals. But if the organization's HIT doesn't meet meaningful use, it is likely the technology won't support the larger ACO goals.

The three main components of meaningful use were set out by CMS in July 2010. Technology from a government-certified vendor must be

- used in a "meaningful manner," such as for e-prescribing of medications,
- used to support electronic exchange of health information in a way that improves quality of care, and
- used to submit measures of clinical quality.

The specifics of the meaningful use rule are spelled out in the sidebar "Make It Meaningful."

The money available depends on the program. Physicians who demonstrate meaningful use under traditional fee-for-service Medicare can qualify for federal payments of $44,000 over five years, starting in the first quarter of 2011. Also starting in 2011, hospitals can get base federal payments of $2 million plus additional incentives. Physicians who demonstrate meaningful use for Medicaid can qualify for state payments of $63,750 over six years, and hospitals can also get state base payments of $2 million; state payments are expected to begin in the summer of 2011. The basic plan is for physicians and hospitals to adopt technology, prove that it is being put to meaningful use, and then start receiving payments over time.

Make It Meaningful

As CMS (2010) states, the adoption of electronic health records is not a goal in itself. It is the use of EHRs to achieve health and efficiency goals that matters. CMS spells out five goals of the program:

1. To improve the quality, safety, and efficiency of care while reducing disparities
2. To engage patients and families in their care
3. To promote public and population health
4. To improve care coordination
5. To promote the privacy and security of EMRs

These are all laudable goals, and some seem to closely mirror the goals of the ACO strategy. To achieve these goals, CMS takes a "one from column A, two from column B" approach. To receive payments in 2011 and 2012—what CMS calls Stage 1—physicians must first demonstrate the following 15 capabilities:

1. Use of computerized physician-order entry for prescriptions directly entered by any licensed healthcare professional
2. Implement drug–drug and drug–allergy interaction checks
3. Generate and transmit prescriptions electronically
4. Record patient demographics, including language, gender, race, ethnicity, and date of birth
5. Maintain an up-to-date problem list of current and active diagnoses for at least 80 percent of patients
6. Maintain active medication list for more than 80 percent of patients
7. Maintain an active medication allergy list for more than 80 percent of patients
8. Record and chart vital signs, including height, weight, and blood pressure for more than 50 percent of all patients
9. Record smoking status for at least 50 percent of patients 13 years or older
10. Implement one clinical decision–support rule, and show ability to track compliance with the rule
11. Report clinical quality measures to CMS or the state

12. Provide patients with an electronic copy of the health information upon request
13. Provide patients with an electronic copy of discharge instructions upon request (hospitals only), or provide clinical summaries for each office visit (physicians only)
14. Show capability to exchange clinical information electronically with other providers
15. Protect electronic health information from security risks

These are the basics. Physicians must also choose five of ten additional objectives from a menu (e.g., implement drug formulary checks, incorporate clinical laboratory test results into the EMR, generate lists of patients by specific conditions) and submit six clinical quality measures (many of them related to the initial 15 requirements). Hospitals must also choose five of ten additional objectives from a separate menu, and they must submit 15 clinical quality measures.

The meaningful-use standards promulgated by CMS in the summer of 2010 were just the beginning. Additional standards for judging and categorizing ACOs all take the organization's HIT capabilities into account. In October 2010, the National Committee for Quality Assurance (2010) published a draft set of standards for ACOs. (The final rules will be published in 2011.) When adopted, the final standards will be used to rank ACOs according to their ability to generate better clinical outcomes, increased patient satisfaction, and lower per capita costs.

The following shows that each level of the meaningful-use standards has an implicit or explicit expectation of HIT adoption and mastery (boldface added for emphasis):

- *Level 1.* Meet core qualifying criteria, which include standards for infrastructure (e.g., legal entity, leadership team, available primary care and specialty providers) and processes that promote good patient care and **quality improvement** (e.g., care coordination, managing patient transitions)

- *Level 2*. Meet core qualifying criteria and have some advanced features, which may include **integration of electronic clinical systems** and the ability to integrate data for reporting and quality improvement
- *Level 3*. Meet core qualifying criteria; possess advanced features; and **can report standardized, nationally-accepted clinical quality measures, patient experience, and cost measures**
- *Level 4*. Meet core and advanced criteria, and demonstrate excellence or **improvement in the metrics**

A summary of the full set of requirements, and other EMR fact sheets, is available at www.cms.gov/EHRIncentivePrograms/30_ Meaningful_Use.asp#.

Plot the HIT Plan

The key to a successful IT strategy for an ACO is having a strong vision for the ACO and its business model. Kenneth Barrette (2010), a HIT consultant with Optimity Advisors, says, "We don't do any IT road mapping without a strong business case attached to that. New ACOs have a hard enough time projecting their revenue stream for the next few years, let alone determining what capital assets they need. You've got to project a business case for making the IT investment."

Categorizing Technology Capabilities

For those just starting out, the vast range of electronic tools can be overwhelming. One way of looking at them is to identify which are the basics and which are required to reach a "best practices" or state-of-the-art level. Some tools will differentiate the healthcare organization and make it stand out from its peers (see Exhibit 6.3). Choosing from the latter category, of course, is predicated on having a clear vision of the organization as an ACO and a well-defined strategy of how to achieve that vision. Exhibit 6.3 divides the tools we discussed into three categories.

Developing the Road Map

With all the choices and all the fancy chrome on the showroom floor, selecting and implementing a HIT strategy is not a job for amateurs,

Exhibit 6.3 Three Categories of HIT Tools

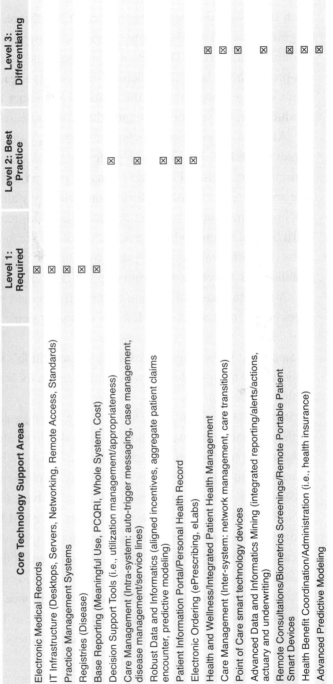

Technology Capability Assessment

Core Technology Support Areas	Level 1: Required	Level 2: Best Practice	Level 3: Differentiating
Electronic Medical Records	☒		
IT Infrastructure (Desktops, Servers, Networking, Remote Access, Standards)	☒		
Practice Management Systems	☒		
Registries (Disease)	☒		
Base Reporting (Meaningful Use, PCQRI, Whole System, Cost)		☒	
Decision Support Tools (i.e., utilization management/appropriateness)		☒	
Care Management (Intra-system: auto-trigger messaging, case management, disease management/service lines)		☒	
Robust Data and Informatics (aligned incentives, aggregate patient claims encounter, predictive modeling)		☒	
Patient Information Portal/Personal Health Record		☒	
Electronic Ordering (ePrescribing; eLabs)		☒	
Health and Wellness/Integrated Patient Health Management			☒
Care Management (Inter-system: network management, care transitions)			☒
Point of Care smart technology devices			☒
Advanced Data and Informatics Mining (integrated reporting/alerts/actions, actuary and underwriting)			☒
Remote Consultations/Biometrics Screenings/Remote Portable Patient Smart Devices			☒
Health Benefit Coordination/Administration (i.e., health insurance)			☒
Advanced Predictive Modeling			☒

Source: Optimity Advisors, used with permission.

even those with decades of experience in healthcare. Except for the largest and best-funded systems, an outside consultant or other expert partner is mandatory. "Don't do it alone," says the head of a large not-for-profit who is helping implement HIT across several states. "You don't stand a chance against the vendors. No matter how good their products are, the vendors have only their own interests at heart."

After the organization has clarified its strategy and what it wants to achieve with HIT, it's time for a professional technology assessment. This analysis is crucial because no matter how primitive, every practice and hospital has some information technology already deployed. It's important to build on what's already there. Moreover, operations must be kept running while the new technology is adopted. And questions of interoperability and system overlap are best left to someone familiar with the entire spectrum of product offerings.

A hospital, hospital system, or large IPA should plan on 8 to 12 weeks for a full assessment. Here are the major steps:

- *Step One: Vision quest*. Finalize the organization's vision and business strategy. Identify which information tools might support that business model.
- *Step Two: Check under the hood*. Take a full inventory of the equipment, software, and processes that have already been adopted. Which were developed in-house? Which were outsourced? How old are they? Can they be modernized?
- *Step Three: Standard equipment*. What are the basic tools, as outlined in Exhibit 6.3, necessary to achieve the provider's ACO strategy?
- *Step Four: Engineering*. Business process design and integration of care must proceed hand-in-hand with the design of the HIT system.
- *Step Five: Scan the options list*. Which tools and capabilities could help the organization differentiate itself once it is treating a patient population as an ACO? Think of these as bells and whistles that can also serve an underlying business strategy.

"If you're headed for an ACO, having an IT assessment is one of the first things you should do," says Dr. Harris (2010) of Cleveland Clinic. "The goal is to map what data you currently have against what data you need to drive your analytics. That is going to be a function of who you are and what you intend to do." Dr. Harris, as mentioned earlier, has been in charge of one of the largest HIT initiatives in the country for 14 years. He suggests that organizations not try to implement everything at once. "Don't boil the ocean," he says. "You have to be very careful not to attack on all fronts and wind up not really being successful at any of them, versus making a decision to cover those disorders or episodes of care that represent the large majority of what you do. You need to capture that information and get really good at it."

Exhibit 6.4 shows one firm's multifaceted approach when helping a provider with the assessment of existing information technology and when evaluating the purchase of a new product or service.

Build It or Buy It?

Veteran industry watchers know the healthcare field is littered with the wrecks of IT projects gone awry. Many of these software disasters—for example, claims systems and coding systems—were tied to payers. But providers are not immune. It just seems that large, widespread programs intended to "revolutionize" work processes have a tendency to get out of control. (This is not limited to healthcare, as anyone who has lived through the implementation of an enterprise software program can attest.)

The challenges are, of course, tougher in healthcare, where records and ordering cannot just disappear for a few days without dire consequences. One challenge for providers is deciding whether to design and implement a program in-house (build it) or buy a program or module from a vendor (buy it). A third option is to have a vendor custom-design a turnkey system. Each approach has its own difficulties. Exhibit 6.5 presents a rough guide to which types of HIT programs are best suited to the various approaches. These are not hard and fast rules; depending on budget and time constraints, almost any approach *could* work for a given tool. So exceptions are to be expected.

Avoid Pitfalls: Don't Get Lost in the Supermarket

Completing a technology assessment and having a sense of build versus buy is just the beginning. Sorting through the expansive list of solution vendors is a logical next step. Vendors from coast to coast

Exhibit 6.4 A Multifaceted Approach to Evaluating Existing Information Technology and Purchasing IT Products

Parameters When Assessing In-House Current State IT Capabilities	Parameters When Assessing Potential Purchase of IT Products
Ability to support evolving business needs	Ability to meet business requirements
Interoperability with data and other systems	Market penetration and reputation of product
Alignment with existing IT architecture	Alignment with existing IT architecture
Security	Ease of use
Applicability to workflow in terms of service vs. post-service	Ability of tool to be customized
Ability to integrate multiple constituent stakeholders (physicians, administrators, patients)	Flexibility of IT infrastructure and/or hosting services required
Data export/import flexibility and adaptability	Data and interface integration capability
Reporting capabilities	Human investment required for initial setup and learning curve
Costs (dollars and resources)	Costs (dollars and resources)
Ability to scale up	Ability to scale up

Source: Optimity Advisors, reprinted with permission.

and overseas are busy dreaming up new software tools that can have a profound impact on medical practice and can help providers reach many goals. What follows is a selective survey of the core technology support areas for which providers can choose products to support their goals (and quickly rack up bills in the millions of dollars):

- *Disease registries.* The monitoring systems track specific categories of medical conditions or diseases for a specific population of the ACO. They track trends in occurrence, patient compliance, and outcomes. These are crucial among providers

Exhibit 6.5 A Guide to HIT Programs

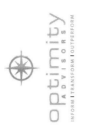

Core Competencies Required by Health System Structure Type

With the vast array of hospital and practice management and care guidelines determined at the specialty level, investing in the proper care management and collaboration systems (and determining in-house vs. outsourcing) is critical.

Accountable Care System Model	IT In-source	IT Outsource	Business Process Outsource
Multi-Specialty Group Practice	Do Not Recommend	Evaluate	Evaluate
Hospital Medical Staff Organization	Recommend	Evaluate	Do Not Recommend
Physician Hospital Organization	Recommend	Evaluate	Do Not Recommend
Interdependent Provider Organization	Do Not Recommend	Recommend	Recommend
Health Plan Provider Organization	Do Not Recommend	Recommend	Recommend

Source: Optimity Advisors, reprinted with permission.

seeking to better manage patients with chronic diseases such as diabetes and congestive heart failure. The best provide proactive case management so that the system automatically communicates with providers and patients to ensure a high level of compliance and proactive management of the disease.

- *Practice management systems.* These are information technology applications that automate daily activities in the medical office, including collecting patient demographic data, scheduling, appointments, billing, reporting, and updating medical records. More than 50 systems are currently on the market, some specializing in specific functions such as scheduling and billing.

- *Meaningful use.* Always-helpful vendors have created tools to monitor and track compliance with CMS's meaningful-use standards discussed earlier. There are also tools to track other reporting measures established by the Institute for Healthcare Improvement and cross-industry committees.

- *Decision support tools.* These are systems that align physician prognosis with medical standards and the latest evidence-based data and provide supporting information to improve health outcomes.

- *Care management systems.* Care management programs apply systems, science, incentives, and information to improve medical practice. They also assist patients and their support system to become engaged in a collaborative process designed to manage medical, social, and mental health conditions more effectively. They seek to improve coordination of care and eliminate duplicative services.

- *Robust data and informatics.* The data captured in the EMR is just the beginning. A growing number of programs mine the data in EMRs and other sources, such as disease registries, to generate reports and other tools for management decision making. Other reporting measures include CMS core measures, readmissions, whole systems measures, and per capita metrics. These metrics are critical in the transitions from a fee-for-service/volume world to a wellness/population management world.

- *Electronic ordering.* At a basic level, these systems replace the traditional physician's scrawled, often-illegible medication prescriptions. They are intended to increase accuracy, cut patient waiting time, and reduce prescription fraud. They are being further applied to lab orders and diagnostic imaging and can be used to track status, results, and history.

- *Patient information portals.* A big goal in the ACO is to engage the patient in her own treatment. These tools provide health records and other information on demand to patients and can be leveraged by individuals and providers to improve outcomes. They have proven helpful in making patients more active shepherds of their own medical records. This is useful when the patient is traveling to a distant clinic for specialized treatment. At a crass level, they are also used as marketing tools by payers and providers.

- *Health and wellness and integrated patient health management tools.* As discussed in Chapter 4, ACOs must look at all patients, not just the sick ones. These tools are aimed at the well cohort of patients and promote behaviors that can improve health outcomes. In the ACO, keeping healthy patients healthy is just as important as helping sick patients get well.

- *Care management.* These tools help support care across the entire spectrum of providers, including those that are affiliated but not economically linked to the ACO. They aim to close the gaps that can occur during care transitions, such as when a patient is discharged with follow-up instructions to go to a physical therapist.

As long as it is, this list is far from comprehensive. Vendors are continually thinking up new tools, creating new categories, and creating compelling pitches for adoption of their products and services. It cannot be overemphasized that ACO leaders, both professional and physician, need to clarify their immediate and long-term goals before letting a sales team anywhere near. Overall business strategy defines the electronic tools required by the ACO. Choosing a set of tools will not help clarify the right direction for the ACO or its components.

Don't Be a "Brochure Buyer"

Everybody loves going to the auto show. All those shiny new models. All those fancy displays. You can touch the new cars. You can sit in them. You can even smell the new car smell. The dreams promised by the automakers—whether it's power, sex appeal, luxury, or virtuous high mileage—seem real. But, of course, if you run out and buy a new car, all you really have is a vehicle that gets you from Point A to Point B. The dream used to pitch the car isn't a reality.

Unfortunately, many buyers of healthcare information technology fall into the same marketing trap. They want what is promised by the technology—whether it's control over doctors, power to bend the cost trend, ways to improve quality metrics, or a secret tool to gain advantages over payers. Some vendors call these providers "brochure buyers," because they believe everything that's in the sales brochures and they seem overeager to start shelling out millions of dollars.

A word of advice: Don't fall into this trap. However appealing, spending willy-nilly on information technology isn't likely to have the profound effect on operations that you are seeking. One scrupulous vendor says, "They get blinded by the sales brochure. They're often buying technology for a very specific function, but the software has lots of other functions. They don't differentiate. They just go ahead and buy the kitchen sink, and half the items they paid money for have no place in their strategy."

This behavior is also known as "buying the black box." The black box—whether it's hardware, software, or some mix—will solve your problems. This, of course, is just magical thinking.

Move from Analysis to Work Flow

Getting the Information Where It Needs to Be

For HIT to promote meaningful behavioral change among physicians and other caregivers (changes that will support higher quality and lower cost outcomes), the knowledge needs to be in the right form at the right place. The right place, clearly, is the physician's or caregiver's computer at the time of care. The right form means a pop-up window or other reminder that can gently steer the caregiver to the optimal action. One vendor, Athenahealth Inc. of Watertown, Massachusetts, calls this "Situational Awareness at the Point of Care." It's a fancy marketing phrase, but it underscores a basic concept: All the IT spending in the world won't do any good if it doesn't influence provider actions.

Many analytic engines and EMRs generate reports. Reports can be useful for physician leaders and professional managers charting medium- and long-term changes in clinical policy and organizational direction. Reports are great, but for most caregivers, they are useless. Physicians and physician extenders have neither the time nor the inclination to read another report. Derek Hedges (2010), senior vice president of product strategy at Athenahealth, says, "What doctors are going to look at the reports? All this information and data and insight are irrelevant if it doesn't surface to impact change at the point of care. If the result of your health information technology is a report that someone has to look at, you're dead. It has to be put into the workflow in a way that's not disruptive."

Take pharmacy management for example. Using tiered formularies to encourage patients to switch from name-brand drugs to clinically equivalent generics is one of the few cost-control success stories of the past few decades (more on this in Chapter 7). Still, compliance with generics isn't complete. Can the HIT system facilitate this to generate savings?

Just flagging that a patient is on a name-brand drug in the physician's online chart isn't adequate. Here are the steps needed to bring about compliance:

- A letter needs to be sent to the patient.
- A letter needs to be entered into the EMR.
- A new prescription needs to be written and forwarded to the pharmacy.
- Someone must follow up to ensure the patient complies with the new medication.

A system that can flag the high-cost drug and automatically follow through with these four actions is one that helps the provider move to accountable care and lower costs.

Using IT to Find Early Wins

Your hospital system or physician organization has just implemented a powerful HIT system. Now what? Start looking for ways to save money.

One early win that several experts have highlighted is reducing system leakage—referrals to specialists outside the ACO. When the ACO assumes risk, fees paid to outside physicians are lost dollars. The solution is a real-time online tool that blocks physicians from referring outside the system. An audit trail ensures that physician leaders and managers can see exactly who writes an order. "It's absurd when you realize we're dealing with a lot of physician groups that are contemplating going to an ACO that only know that a referral went outside of their network because they got a claim from a payer who covered the consult," says Hedges (2010).

The tool will also direct the physician to the approved care pathway, which is likely designed by peer physicians. Standardizing care to approved paths is one of the key guidelines for improving outcomes and efficiency within the ACO.

Want to make the ACO perform even better? Use the online tools to establish a hierarchy for internal referrals. Physicians with the best outcomes and efficiency are at the top of the list and will get the lion's share of referrals. This could potentially create competition among physicians, helping to raise performance among the laggards. Hedges (2010) says, "Physicians who have a more active panel with more patients and are more productive are going to make more money. It will create a free market within the walls of the ACO."

The Limits of Technology

Popular culture is rife with images of technology run amok. From the Disneyfied pathos of *WALL-E* to the dystopian future of *Battlestar Galactica*, science fiction warns us of technology that goes too far and tragically turns on its creators. Happily, this is not a problem with HIT (at least not that we know of yet).

Instead, healthcare leaders who implement HIT and those who help create it warn that technology does not go far enough. It will not solve the problems of an ACO with a fundamentally flawed governance structure or an overly optimistic business plan. It will not magically change physicians' behavior and attitudes. It cannot, by itself, make an ACO successful. The danger, of course, is that we have become so reliant on technology in all aspects of our lives that it's tempting to see HIT as the *deus ex machina* of healthcare.

"I get worried when people think technology is the answer," says Micky Tripathi (2010), president and chief executive officer of the Massachusetts eHealth Collaborative. Tripathi pointed to a CMS study publicized in October 2010 by Anthony Rodgers, deputy administrator for the CMS Center for Strategic Planning. Rodgers said the study, which had yet to be peer-reviewed, showed that advanced HIT contributed to the success of five of the ten ACO pilots funded by CMS. "If that's not a business case [for health information technology], I don't know what is," said Rodgers (*Healthcare Finance News* 2010).

Organizational Questions

The organizational questions raised in this chapter include the following:

- Do we have a HIT strategy? Is it supported by clear management goals?
- How far along are we to meeting CMS's definition of "meaningful use"?
- Have we implemented HIT in a way that empowers physicians and boosts use of new tools?
- Does our HIT strategy improve the patient experience?
- Will our HIT implementation qualify for government reimbursement from the Medicare and Medicaid EHR incentive programs?

Category of Readers	Key Concepts	Actions to Consider
Category A (interested)	• Basic EMR functionality	• Attend educational forums on CMS's meaningful-use standards for physicians and managers
	• Meaningful use as a potential capital source	• Plan physician meetings to discuss use of EMR going forward
		• Encourage physician leaders and department chairs to attend seminars or trade shows to review the current environment
Category B (engaged)	• Commission an IT assessment	• Convene information officers from member and affiliated organizations to choose a vendor
	• Beware of pitfalls	• Initiate market/Web research project to learn patients' usage patterns
Category C (committed)	• How can HIT help us differentiate ourselves in the market?	• Retreat to discuss IT strategy
		• Direct physicians leaders and managers to craft a five-year HIT plan showing costs and anticipated savings
	• Early wins	• Convene meetings between CIO and chairs to identify early win potential

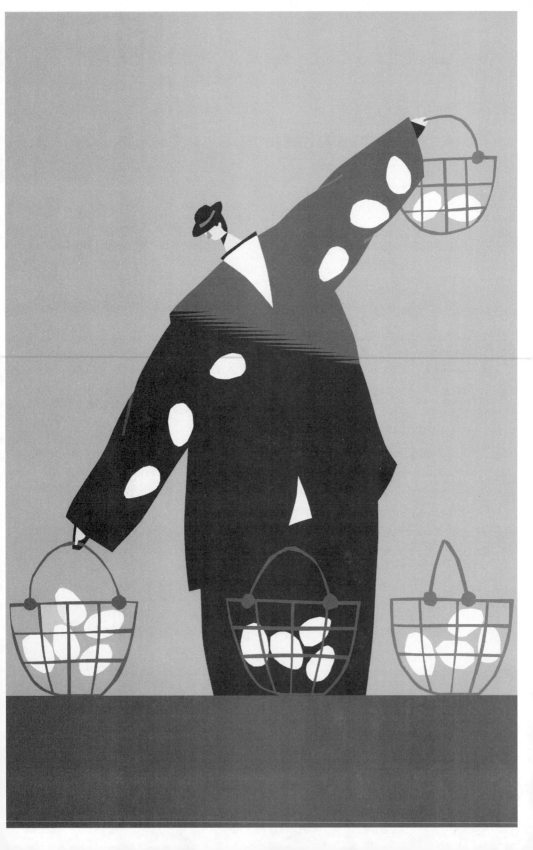

7

Accountable Care Organization Economics

ACOs won't reach their full potential unless purchasers, patients, payers, and providers work together to transition the delivery system to a lower cost, higher quality chassis.

—Anonymous Senior Vice President, Network Contracting
BCBS Plan

Accountable care organizations (ACOs) were created by the Patient Protection and Affordable Care Act of 2010 (PPACA). That word *affordable* in the PPACA means that economics are central to the ACO concept. Yet the need for ACOs to stem healthcare cost increases seems to be escaping many early ACO adopters. That is, many ACO early adopters are thinking of the ACO as simply a managed care vehicle or shared-savings arrangement to maximize reimbursement, rather than as a new approach to expense management, capital investment, funds flow, and incentive alignment necessary to manage margins in a soft unit reimbursement and volume environment.

If ACOs are to be more than aggregators of market power, it is imperative that ACO leaders engage internal finance and clinical leadership, as well as payers, purchasers, and patients, to design an economic model that directs incremental dollars to activities that don't just improve quality but also lower costs. This is no short order given the industry's 25-year track record of robust top-line increases.

This chapter is intended to show payers and providers how their historical economic models need to evolve under an ACO model to improve quality and bend the trend. Here are the topics we cover:

1. Defining the components of the ACO economic model
2. Defining what really needs to be different this time
3. Designing your ACO economic model and strategic margin transition plan to help fund your ACO
4. Defining how payers, policymakers, and purchasers need to support the economic transition
5. Reviewing case studies that illustrate early ACO successes and challenges

Defining the Components of the ACO Economic Model

The ACO economic model starts with the basic functions referred to in healthcare financial management textbooks and certification courses. Following is what is included in the textbook *The Financial Management of Hospitals and Healthcare Organizations* (Nowicki 2007):

- *Revenue and expense management functions.* These include traditional revenue cycle functions such as charge practices, the charge master, charge master prices, coding, billing, collections, and denial management. These functions also include variable and fixed cost savings practices such as supply chain standardization, reduced use of agency labor, leases, and outsourcing. These tactics generate capital for ACO startup activities.
- *Operating, cash, and capital budget function.* This includes annual operating and cash flow budgets and long-term strategic capital planning budgets.

- *Managed care contracting function.* This includes traditional contract analysis, design and negotiations, and day-to-day collections and denial management issues. This domain also includes the design of shared savings, partial capitation, and other payment models specified under Section 1899 of PPACA.
- *Rewards, penalties, and incentives.* These include compensation, incentives, and benefits plans, as well as information about how rewards and penalties are used to motivate shared accountabilities and results.
- *Funds flow and risk management.* This includes the internal pricing principles that underlie the flow of funds among facilities, physicians, school of medicine, and other parties.
- *Treasury functions*

The main difference between the providers' traditional economic model and future ACOs is the fuel the ACO will need to run on. For the past 25 years, the provider's economic model has run on a 4 to 6 percent operating margin built on remarkable 7 to 8 percent annual revenue growth, which is defined as unit reimbursement times volume growth (Carlson 2010). Expense increases have mirrored revenue increases, growing more than 7 percent annually for the past 25 years. Moving forward though, most agree that the economy, competition, and reform will put significant pressure on providers to reduce the 7-plus percent annual growth in revenue and costs. Pressure is also coming from Medicare, Medicaid, commercial payers, and the millions of patients who each year are forced to share a much larger portion of healthcare costs.

Medicare, Medicaid, and Commercial Rate Increases

The PPACA stipulates fundamental changes to provider reimbursement starting with market-based adjustments in 2010. Although Medicaid increases vary significantly by state, most expect Medicaid increases to be flat at best over the long term. Commercial payers are following public payers, generally offering 0 to 2 percent annual increases, down from 6 to 10 percent annual increases just a few years ago. Yet many providers' long-term financial plans still assume 3 percent Medicare increases and 5 to 10 percent commercial rate increases well into the future. The disconnect is striking.

Increased Patient Cost Shifting

Downward pressure on provider revenue is also coming from patient cost shifting. According to the Kaiser Family Foundation's 2010 survey, patient cost shifting has increased substantially among commercially insured members since 2006, with family deductibles almost doubling from $750 to $1,500 for an HMO (health maintenance organization) and from $1,200 to $2,300 for a POS (point of service) plan (see Exhibit 7.1).

A separate report from Hewitt Associates points out that employees' share of medical costs, including employee contributions and out-of-pocket costs, tripled from $1,229 in 2001 to $4,386 in 2011 (projected) (Aon 2010). At some point, this cost-increase trend becomes untenable, which is prompting providers and payers to review the very economic principles their businesses are founded on.

Guiding Principles of the ACO Economic Model

An increasing number of providers are beginning to take a fresh look at how their entire economic model will need to evolve to maintain historical margins required to maintain bond ratings, let alone fund their ACO. Both payer and provider CFOs are re-casting their long-term revenue, expense, and investment forecasts to account for major top-line cuts, as described below.

Revenue and Expense Management

The economic downturn and healthcare reform mean that providers' days of passing 7-plus percent annual cost increases to purchasers and patients are numbered. For many systems, we project 2015 revenue could be 1 to 5 percent *less* than what they assumed before the anticipated disproportionate-share payment cuts and other payment reductions. And assuming the typical hospital needs to reduce variable cost by 5 percent for every 1 percent reduction in revenue to maintain margin, providers would need to trim variable costs up to 25 percent to maintain margin (Nugent 2004).

Exhibit 7.1 Individuals with Deductibles of $1,000 or More

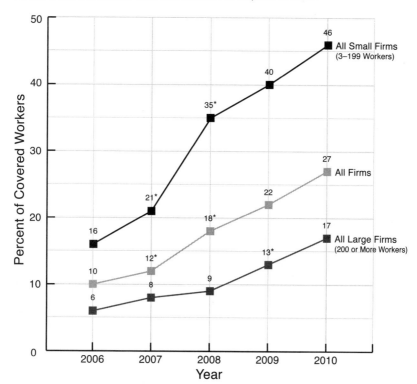

*Estimate is statistically different from estimate for the previous year shown ($p < 0.05$).

Source: This information was reprinted with permission from the Henry J. Kaiser Family Foundation. The Kaiser Family Foundation is a non-profit private operating foundation, based in Menlo Park, California, dedicated to producing and communicating the best possible analysis and information on health issues.

To maintain current margins in a soft reimbursement and volume environment, providers will need to redouble their expense-management efforts. This entails looking beyond traditional variable cost-reduction opportunities (e.g., supply chain, pharmacy, overtime, agency staff) to fixed and variable cost and avoidable utilization opportunities, including salary and benefits, staffing levels and mix, divestitures, and throughput/productivity improvements. Ultimately, expense management and revenue management will need to

Exhibit 7.2 The Three Levels of Expense Management

Type of Expense	Examples	Potential Savings/Increases
1. Traditional variable unit cost and utilization savings	Supplies, pharmacy, overtime, agency staffing, and LOS reduction	~5+% expense savings
2. Next-level variable and semi-fixed cost and utilization savings, including divestitures	Salary, benefits, staffing levels, and mix Requires some process reengineering, space reconfiguration, and exiting underperforming businesses	Additional ~5+% total expense savings
3. Reduction in readmissions, complications, and ambulatory sensitive care utilization across the care continuum, including chronic care	Avoidable readmissions, procedures, complications, etc. Requires significant process reengineering, space reconfiguration, and incentive alignment initiatives	~5+% expense reduction equivalent + opportunity to backfill with profitable patients and share savings, and hence increased revenue and margin

be integrated into a *strategic margin plan*, which divides the initiatives into three levels as shown in Exhibit 7.2.

What's striking is that during the Great Recession of 2008–2009, most providers did not have to execute on all three levels. Only 20 percent report reducing costs by more than 5 percent, and only 16 percent exited unprofitable businesses and only 9 percent monetized assets (HFMA n.d.). But with significantly smaller reimbursement increases going forward, we expect providers will need to take a much more deliberate approach to manage their margins.

Capital Planning

Revenue and expense management aren't the only finance functions that will have to change under the ACO strategy. Chief financial officers (CFOs) will need to revisit their long-term capital plans in search of unrealistically high future volume, cost, and unit reimbursement assumptions in order to eliminate unrealistic assumptions. CFOs will need to rebalance their existing portfolio of potential revenue-enhancing capital investments (e.g., new high-tech service, new tower, regional expansion) with new cost-reducing capital investments (e.g., nurse practitioners, physician assistants, investments that increase scale and reduce costs). CFOs may also need to work with the capital markets to reevaluate how the markets look at hospital capital investment. For example, some assert the markets currently grant higher ratings to facilities that invest greater than 1.5 times the annual depreciation expense, invest in quaternary capacity, and have a lower age of plant. Reform, let alone ACOs, will have some bearing on these rating dynamics in the future.

Managed Care Contracting and Pricing

The CFO will need to oversee the managed care team's transition from unit reimbursement "maximizers" to strategic negotiators who find new ways to maximize the revenue—and over time margin (a.k.a. yield)—per available unit of capacity (e.g., staffed bed, clinic appointment slot) while maintaining quality and access. As one health system executive shares, "I'm realizing I cannot automatically get more unit reimbursement out of undifferentiated services to make up for an ever-increasing cost shift like I did in the past. I've got to manage my margin differently." Internally, the transition will need to start with simply benchmarking your commercial contract's margins, rates, and administrative costs to the market by hospital, physician, and service using publicly available benchmark data. The second step is to draft a credible business case with your hospital and physician leaders to your top commercial payers that describes areas where increases are justified on the basis of performance and patient unmet needs. In some instances, this business case has evolved into clinically integrated joint ventures between providers and employers or trusts to manage total cost of specific populations of chronically ill patients at $5 to $50 per member per month (PMPM). Providers that make their case early will be more likely to get funds than those that wait.

But we also observe that providers who desire to "go ACO" will need to invest considerable time with their top payers to move beyond their historic cat-and-mouse games that cost both sides considerable resources but do not benefit patients. (See sidebar.)

For years, payers and providers have played a series of these cat-and-mouse games. They take place at the negotiating table, in between negotiations, and in many other areas regarding payments, denials, and collections. Many (but not all) relationships are based on tactics by providers to optimize revenue and on efforts by payers to take revenue back. To put it mildly, this is not a patient- (or customer)-centric relationship based on shared vision, trust, and accountability.

Consider some of the revenue-optimization tactics providers engage in:

- Use of sophisticated revenue-maximization software that bills an inpatient case rate versus an observation day rate with unbundled ancillary tests
- Use of a different tax-identification number to maximize reimbursement under site-of-service contract terms
- Increasing gross charge amounts to hit inpatient outlier payment clauses, with limited attention to the defensibility of those gross charges or the medical necessity of an extra day of care
- Extra tests, procedures
- Creative assignment of "billing units" in lab, pharmacy, minute charges, and so forth to maximize revenue

On the flip side, consider some of the tactics payers engage in:

- Unilateral payment policy changes, including no or significantly reduced payment for multiple procedures and unilateral bundling logic changes that unexpectedly reduce unit reimbursement
- Unilateral medical necessity policy changes for new types of procedures and tests, such as genetic testing, for which limited data exist
- Delays in sharing or refusal to share data

Cat and Mouse Games: The Tom and Jerry Show

The following script represents a fictitious, but directionally accurate, dialogue between a typical payer and provider. This points out how the dialogue between payer and provider needs to move beyond "I win/you lose."

Tom (provider): So here we are once again. Time for our annual rate increase.

Jerry (payer): Stop there, Tom. Who said anything about an increase? Times are changing, Tom.

Tom: But your premiums went up 20 percent this year. What do you mean, "No increase?" We're one of the biggest players in the market—and you can't afford to exclude us from your network!

Jerry: Think again, Tom. Average family out-of-pockets increased to $3,500 this past year. Didn't you notice your outpatient ancillary volume that you generate your margins from *decreased* last year for the first time ever? Patients are steering away from your facilities because your prices are two or three times those of your competitors!

Tom (to himself): How does Jerry know this? I'm toast if my CEO finds out. I really need to buy some time here!

Tom: Well, we've got to get a bigger increase on inpatient rates if our outpatient rates are higher than market.

Jerry: Well, Tom, our economics team looked at your inpatient costs, including cost/adjusted discharge, staffing ratios, length of stay, supply costs, and so on. Our customers simply can't afford to buoy your margins on their backs anymore.

Tom: Our margins? What about *your* margins?!? Not to mention all those administrative games you play?! I have five FTEs [full-time equivalents] dedicated to all those prior authorizations you make me do. You've even begun to deny a whole range of readmission DRGs [diagnosis-related groups]. You can't do that according to our contract! And where is this magic data you have, Jerry?

Jerry: We think those readmissions are the results of substandard care. Would you pay for the following readmissions if it were your money? *(Jerry hands Tom a list of readmissions)*. And don't think about telling your doctors to make up for fewer admissions by upcoding or doing extra tests. Your use rates *and* unit reimbursements are well above our overall book of business. You're pricing and utilizing yourself out of the market, Tom.

Tom (to himself): Thankfully we're about to announce a big acquisition that will force all our payers to ante up this time. And I have a 3 percent guaranteed increase if I simply let this contract evergreen.

Jerry *(interrupting)*: Despite all these cost, utilization, and pricing issues, you are an important member of our network, Tom. We also acknowledge the potential acquisition you are considering. My health plan is not leaving this market, nor are you. So if you're willing to engage in a new dialogue about how you manage margin and improve quality under a lower unit-reimbursement trend, let's move ahead. If not, I'll come back and do our dance next year—*after* I steer even more business to your biggest competitors. So what's your response?

Tom (to himself): How did I miss that this was coming? Time to talk to my CFO and CEO before our competitors pull a fast one on us.

Tom: Jerry, you're setting yourself up for a fall! You can expect a call in the not-too-distant future from me and our attorney.

Extrapolate these costly cat-and-mouse games out a few years, and it becomes clear that payers and providers are stuck in a zero-sum game mentality. The outcome has been lose–lose for both parties. As the game becomes better known, patients, purchasers, and policymakers are showing less tolerance for the complexity and expense of paying for care.

Another way of looking at payers' and providers' mutually self-destructive behavior is through the Prisoner's Dilemma, a classic problem in game theory that is used to explain economic behavior.

The Prisoner's Dilemma

The Prisoner's Dilemma is typically presented as follows:

Two suspects are arrested by the police. The police have insufficient evidence for a conviction, but having separated the prisoners, they visit each prisoner to offer the same deal. If one testifies for the prosecution against the other (*defects*) and the other remains silent (*cooperates*), the defector goes free and the silent accomplice receives the full 10-year sentence. If both remain silent, both prisoners are sentenced to only six months in jail for a minor charge. If each betrays the other, each receives a five-year sentence. Each prisoner must choose to betray the other or to remain silent. Each one is assured that the other would not know about the betrayal before the end of the investigation. How should the prisoners act?

We assume that each player is motivated only by self-interest—to minimize his own jail time. As a result, cooperating is strictly dominated by defecting, and the only possible equilibrium for the game is for both players to defect. No matter what the other player does, one player will always gain a greater payoff by playing defect. Because in any situation playing defect is more beneficial than cooperating, all rational players will play defect, all things being equal. Thus, both parties end up with the five-year jail sentence, when if they cooperated, they each would have received only six months.

It's not hard to see the parallels between the prisoners in the sidebar and the payers and providers. Payers and providers, playing hardball and seeking their own self-interest, inevitably "defect"— try to get a worse outcome for the other party. As a result, negotiations create suboptimal outcomes in which the system as a whole loses. It's useful to look at the dilemma using a two-by-two grid (see Exhibit 7.3) that shows the four possible outcomes.

In scenario 1, payers and providers continue to play the traditional game, which costs the system valuable resources in the form of audits, legal and consulting fees, contract revisions, and constant development of software to "catch the other guy in the act." At an extreme, this scenario is exemplified by the hypothetical community where most

Exhibit 7.3 The Prisoner's Dilemma Applied to Healthcare

		Provider	
		Stands Firm	**Collaborates**
Payer	**Stands Firm**	**Scenario 1:** Stalemate—cat & mouse games continue to reduce customer value rather than create it; odds of rate regulation increase	**Scenario 2:** Provider develops programs to reduce excessive readmissions, ED visits, etc.—and loses margins that fund other services in the process
	Collaborates	**Scenario 3:** Payer loses because its investments (IT, new programs, etc.) may not go to initiatives that ultimately improve quality or save its customers money	**Scenario 4:** Each party coordinates delivery and payment over a multiyear transition period (e.g., 2011–15) using reform & CMS "Value Based Purchasing" policies as guideposts

of the citizens work for large, self-insured health systems that spend hundreds of millions of administrative dollars more than necessary to deliver high-quality, efficient, and accessible care. It is just a matter of time until the community catches on to the costly administrative and delivery activities, and the state or federal government legislates premium rate caps or even cost-plus-reimbursement rates because the market could not agree to a more enlightened value-based approach. Given the public's growing awareness of the cat-and-mouse games and the public's general mistrust of insurance companies, this may be where we are headed right now in America.

Two of the three remaining scenarios are unlikely to emerge in this version of the Prisoner's Dilemma, because each party will be worse off if it decides to cooperate but the other party does not. For example, assume the community-based provider extends an olive branch to implement a medical home initiative with its top payers to improve access, quality, and efficiency. To its dismay, the provider loses a sizable amount of margin-generating inpatient admissions and emergency department (ED) utilization because of improvements in primary care access and coordination. The provider did the "right thing" and wound up worse off. On the flip side, imagine the payer agrees to contribute funding to the provider to support a major electronic medical record project. Only in this case, the provider turns around and fails to generate a clear return on investment.

Place these fears and endless tugs of war within the context of the current payer–provider relationship, and no wonder both sides are reluctant to cooperate in shared savings, partial capitation, or other ACO-related arrangements, and skeptical of working with the other party to manage total cost of care. Consequently, payers and providers need to step back; establish new rules of the road for their relationship; and use a transparent, data-driven approach to negotiations that must underlie the ACO. The focus must shift beyond unit-reimbursement increases to tactics to lower underlying costs while allowing the hospital to earn the margin required to maintain its day-to-day operations.

Funds Flow and Incentives

One of the most important changes, from a funds flow and incentive perspective, will be to expose the fundamental disconnect between increasing physician compensation levels and declining third-party reimbursement. The large systems that compensate employed physicians at two or three times the market reimbursement rates know they cannot sustain these internal cross-subsidies as Medicare and other payers scrutinize certain highly reimbursed and/or highly used services. Radiology, urology, and cardiology have already begun to feel the scrutiny and subsequent unit-reimbursement cuts, with more specialties and service lines to follow. Is your organization prepared?

To get out of this squeeze, providers will ultimately have to align compensation and reimbursement with managed care and Medicare, thus aligning their internal funds flow principles with what the market is willing to pay. This includes linking physician bonuses with the base fee schedules and performance-based payments for reducing avoidable costs and complications that providers negotiate with third-party payers.

Risk Management

The final component of the ACO economic model that will require a new, more coordinated approach is risk management. Historically, finance's risk-management strategy focused on negotiating lower malpractice and other insurance rates. In a separate silo, clinical operations were reacting to adverse events and complaints, mitigating and, at times, hiding them. The finance and delivery silos were rarely integrated to eliminate systemic patient-safety risks that resulted in adverse patient and financial events.

The new clinical and financial risk-management approach is more proactive and involves identifying potential financial, operational, and event risks by patient cohort and function and taking action to eliminate them, then demonstrating results to insurance carriers to get lower rates for malpractice, liability, errors, and omissions of insurance premiums.

Summary of ACO Economic Principles

Taken in its entirety, this section underscores the need for ACO architects to consider the entire economic model when designing the ACO. ACOs that are designed merely as a small-scale pilot project in a managed care vacuum where cat-and-mouse games abound are more likely to fail, because, as we've already seen, they don't generate sustainable savings to self-fund future tactics that will sustainably bend the trend.

For example, take a large provider system that was interested in pursuing an ACO. As part of its ACO endeavor, the system sanctioned the creation of a congestive heart failure disease management "ACO pilot" in partnership with a payer. The payer and provider spent considerable time outlining various risk-adjusted methods, but the program began to blow up when hospital and specialist volumes began to decline precipitously, seriously hurting the provider's top line. In retrospect, the parties failed to completely analyze the intended and unintended consequences of their effort. Both parties viewed the ACO simply as a payer–provider "feel-good" relationship builder, rather than positioning the pilot as a longer term commitment to design a new economic and delivery model to improve quality and efficiency.

In particular, the payer and provider failed to fully consider the following questions:

- Where specifically are our best opportunities to improve quality, efficiency, and margins over the next several years as payers/purchasers reduce rate increases and expose pockets of high cost and utilization?
- How will we optimize existing productivity and scale, and even exit certain lines of service, so that we can make more with less? What are the barriers (e.g., cat-and-mouse games)?
- How could an ACO or risk-sharing pilot help us do all this over the next five years?

Organizations that overlook these big-picture questions will tend to get caught up in the mechanics of the deal too early (e.g., who will receive the ACO payment, how will it be distributed, how will claims be handled, what patients should be enrolled, who will sign the contracts?) and ignore the ACO's end goals. As one finance executive shares, "Until our organization is ready to talk about how clinical delivery and economics need to evolve together, we're destined to make the same mistakes we made in the past. I can't let that happen."

Defining What Really Needs to Be Different This Time

This is by no means the first time payers, purchasers, providers, and consultants have proclaimed the need to bend the cost curve and manage the margin. So what needs to be different this time if the industry is to truly and sustainably bend the curve? Exhibit 7.4 summarizes a few of the key differences required of ACOs if they are to sustainably bend the trend. We discuss each past attempt in this section.

Capitation

Capitation represented only a small component of many providers' books of business in the 1990s. Consequently, most providers were able to make up for reduced utilization on its capitated business with increased utilization on other books of business. In other instances, the

Exhibit 7.4 Summary of Gaps in Payment Schemes

Past Attempts	Provider, Patient, Payer, Regulatory Gaps
Capitation	Capitation rates were often set too high, so they did not "incentivize" change; even where they were appropriately set, providers lacked either the information required to improve access, quality, and efficiency or enough capitated patients to warrant changes in the delivery of care. In other instances, many providers signed percentage of premium arrangements with certain payers, who passed the risk to providers, sold products to employers at below-market premium rates, and left providers with multimillion dollar losses.
Unit reimbursement caps	This short-term strategy focused on limiting unit-reimbursement increases and did not address providers' capital investment decisions and high cost chassis that drove costs up in the first place.
DRG and prospective payment	Arguably the most successful program of all in terms of length of stay and productivity improvements; this payment innovation was based on core, evidence-based costs and let hospitals "share in"/retain the substantial length-of-stay savings that ensued.
Balanced Budget Act of 1997	Effectively reduced hospital Medicare reimbursement by more than $100 billion in the late 1990s and early 2000s.
Acute care episode bundles and physician group practice demonstrations	Insufficient revenue to change underlying delivery and efficiency, although most argue it was a step in the right direction.
Market-based prescription drug payment changes	Arguably the most successful market-based bend-the-trend example; several demand and supply forces interacted to improve quality and efficiency.

actual capitation rates were lucrative and did not create incentives to change delivery. In many instances, providers agreed to take a percentage of the premium from the payer in return for managing total risk, but the premiums were set low, leaving providers with the losses. Yet where capitation took root, integrated delivery models have generated demonstrable savings in the form of lower prescription drug spending and lower lengths of stay. So by no means is capitation dead on arrival.

Rate Caps of the 1970s

Several states implemented reimbursement rate caps in the 1970s to contain costs. Researchers report mixed results. For example, Feldstein (1988) reported that mandatory rate regulation held down hospital underlying cost increases when a majority of payers were indexed, but it took several years for these programs to take effect.

DRG Prospective Payment System Versus the Balanced Budget Act of 1997

The implementation of both prospective, case-based DRG reimbursement in the early 1980s and the Balanced Budget Act of 1997 (BBA) reduced Medicare reimbursement increases by billions of dollars. Yet there was a major difference between the two approaches to reducing spending growth.

The BBA simply cut the unit reimbursement by more than $100 billion in the late 1990s and early 2000s but did not significantly change the way care was delivered. On the other hand, DRG prospective payment did not simply reduce annual spending increases (from 15 percent to 8 percent); it also reduced the average length of stay by several days per admission and resulted in a major decrease in inpatient capacity within a few years. Furthermore, the Centers for Medicare & Medicaid Services (CMS) allowed hospitals to keep the savings resulting from the length-of-stay cost reductions, which consequently increased hospitals' profitability despite lower inpatient utilization (Bazzoli et al. 2004). We view bundling readmissions into case rates as the next generation of prospective payment, with hospital/physician bundling to follow. ACOs need to start exploring *now* how these future reimbursement methods fit into their broader economic models.

Recent Lessons on Reimbursement Practices: Acute Care Episode Bundles Versus Physician Group Practice Demonstrations

Our clients' experiences with the acute care episode (ACE) bundles and physician group practice (PGP) demonstrations are relatively positive. In several instances, they have generated reductions in total cost of delivering care (e.g., lower supply costs) and higher clinical quality. However, many, but not all, participants cite some frustration with the relatively low bonuses these programs generated for providers, which limited their influence in overall day-to-day operations.

Prescription Drug Spending: Perhaps a Best-Case Scenario for ACOs?

Exhibit 7.5 shows how market forces interacted with public policy to significantly lower one key cost driver for more than 10 years. Between 1995 and 2006, innovative, tiered pricing systems significantly reduced (and for one year, even reversed) the rate of increase in spending on prescription drugs.

By tiering prescription drug prices so that patients paid significantly lower co-pays for generics and higher co-pays for name-brand drugs, annual spending increases fell precipitously. Patient education further reinforced the effectiveness of the pricing incentives. For providers, stricter formularies forced doctors to prescribe generics where supported by evidence-based cost-effectiveness research. In addition, computer-based tools, including electronic medical records, e-prescribing, and drug reminders, lowered administrative costs.

Large employers and benefits consultants led the charge, followed by pharmacy benefit management companies that took advantage of scale economies and purchasing power. Providers who saw the patient safety and margin opportunities before others benefitted financially.

Two Alternate Visions of the Future

Using these historical examples, we can create two hypothetical scenarios that payers, purchasers, and providers should consider as they plan for their ACO.

Failure Scenario: ACOs Consolidate the Market and Drive Costs Up More

ACOs consolidate the provider market and drive costs up. These actions set the industry up for a sudden shift to all-payer rate regulation before the end of the decade. Here's how it happens:

Demand increases modestly. Aging baby boomers and new insured lives (enrolled via insurance exchanges) generate increased demand, albeit at relatively low reimbursement points, which do

Exhibit 7.5 Growth of Prescription Drug Benefit Costs, Private Insurance
1995–2006

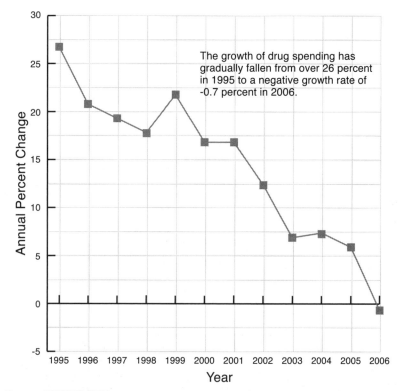

The growth of drug spending has gradually fallen from over 26 percent in 1995 to a negative growth rate of -0.7 percent in 2006.

Source: USDHHS 2010

not help providers' margins. Patient cost shifting continues to rise rapidly, resulting in lower-than-expected volumes of discretionary and nonemergent services on which providers currently earn significant margin. Tepid volume and unit reimbursement increases put considerable pressure on provider margins.

Supply decreases. Providers consolidate to primarily achieve higher reimbursement rates from payers. Input costs continue to rise faster than revenue. Certain ACOs cherry pick only healthy members of the health insurance exchange to fill their margin gap, to the detriment of other ACOs.

Consider the Impact of Patient's Skin in the Game

Payers and providers have limited information on patient willingness to comparison shop on the basis of quality, price, access, and so forth. However, WellPoint, one of the nation's largest insurance carriers, conducts extensive research on this topic. Research shows patients are becoming increasingly willing to comparison shop as out-of-pocket expenses continue to increase. Payers and providers can achieve a competitive advantage by integrating these insights into the products and services they offer to help steer patients to high-quality, low-cost sites of care.

Willingness to Use a Select Set of Providers If Resulted in Premium Savings
Consumers

	Willing to Select If Savings Was 10–15%	Likely (rated 4 or 5)	Unlikely (rated 1 or 2)
Provider relationships	Primary doctor visits	41%	41%
	Specialist visits	41%	38%
Non-serious test	Blood work	69%	14%
	MRI or other high level scans	65%	16%
	X-rays	67%	14%
More serious procedures	Minor outpatient surgery	42%	37%
	Inpatient surgery with overnight stay	34%	46%

Steerage opportunities exist

	Willing to Select If Savings Was	Won't Use Restrictive Network or Would Need at Least 50% Savings
Provider relationships	Primary doctor visits	87%
	Specialist visits	85%
Non-serious test	Blood work	77%
	MRI or other high level scans	84%
	X-rays	77%
More serious procedures	Minor outpatient surgery	84%
	Inpatient surgery with overnight stay	87%

Result. Short term, providers offset weak reimbursement increases from Medicare and Medicaid by increasing utilization. Medium term, costs continue to increase rapidly. By 2019,

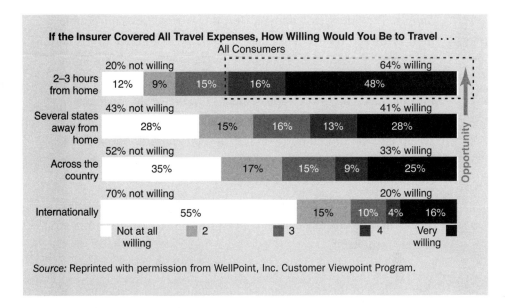

If the Insurer Covered All Travel Expenses, How Willing Would You Be to Travel . . .
All Consumers

2–3 hours from home	20% not willing				64% willing
	12%	9%	15%	16%	48%
Several states away from home	43% not willing				41% willing
	28%	15%	16%	13%	28%
Across the country	52% not willing				33% willing
	35%	17%	15%	9%	25%
Internationally	70% not willing				20% willing
	55%	15%	10%	4%	16%

Not at all willing   2   3   4   Very willing

Opportunity

Source: Reprinted with permission from WellPoint, Inc. Customer Viewpoint Program.

simple economics overwhelm political opposition to all-payer setting and multiple states adopt 1970s-era all-payer reimbursement caps to control costs.

Success Scenario: A Sustainable Bend-the-Trend Model

Under this scenario, market and regulatory forces come together to lower underlying input costs and prices. Here's how it happens:

Demand stays flat. The slow economy and ever-increasing patient cost sharing means inpatient and outpatient volume growth is flat despite newly insured lives. Employers discover and become much more vocal about the inefficiencies within the delivery system's cost structure and force payers to pursue shared-savings arrangements (e.g., 30-day readmission bundling, hospital–physician bundling) with ACO and non-ACO providers. Government restricts increases in annual health insurance premiums and aggressively invests in bundled reimbursement for readmissions and other cost-saving initiatives and allows providers to keep most of the savings (similar to the DRG prospective payment changes in the 1980s).

Supply. Providers exit underperforming businesses and double their efforts to reduce fixed and variable costs to break even on Medicare. Providers reevaluate how delivery and economics need to evolve before they pull the trigger on the next new $100 million medical tower replacement. Primary care, specialists, and post-acute services achieve new utilization and cost targets set up and monitored by Medicare and purchasers. The medical home model takes off, targeted at members with multiple chronic conditions.

Result. Annual cost trend increases go from 8 percent to just under 5 percent, and this buys the industry a few more years to continue to transform itself.

Regardless of the exact scenario that emerges, the probability of lower unit-reimbursement increase and volume growth going forward is significantly greater than in the past. At least for the next five years, this behooves financial leaders of ACOs and non-ACOs to formulate their ACO economic playbook and strategic margin transition plan.

Designing Your ACO Economic Model and Strategic Margin Transition Plan

So how can your ACO begin to design its economic model? We recommend following four steps:

1. Project your revenue gap in light of likely reform and market scenarios; establish a sense of urgency.
2. Benchmark unit cost and utilization savings opportunities.
3. Develop a strategic margin transition plan, consisting of short- and long-term delivery and financial tactics to close the margin gap over time.
4. Integrate the strategic margin transition plan into the care transformation plan to ensure patient benefits.

Step 1: Project Your Revenue Gap

Unlike past reforms, PPACA lays out a series of revenue hits that will affect all providers over the next several years, including cuts in reimbursement to disproportionate-share hospitals, market basket adjustments, and value-based purchasing. Using historical financial statements and cost and volume data, it is easy to plot multiple reform-induced revenue shortfall scenarios, as illustrated in Exhibit 7.6.

Key assumptions include the following:

- Expected increases in bad debt, charity care, and write-offs as a function of projected payer mix and demographic changes.
- Expected Medicare cuts associated with
  a. provider-specific hospital-acquired conditions;
  b. avoidable readmissions (and/or days), including admissions for chronic and ambulatory-sensitive conditions;
  c. disproportionate share and uncompensated care scenarios; and
  d. wage index reclassifications.
- Hospitals and specialists with excess capacity and no backfill opportunities will be especially hit hard by reimbursement cuts, as will integrated delivery systems that are employing physicians at salary ranges at a considerable markup over future reimbursement rates.

Based on our analysis of several systems to date, 1 to 5 percent of many systems' top-line revenue may be in jeopardy over the next five to seven years. One of the largest health systems estimates it would experience over $600 million in cumulative cuts between 2010 and 2019. This revenue shortfall will require health systems to rethink their traditional cost-management tactics: A 1 percent top-line reduction requires providers to reduce variable costs by 5 percent or more to maintain their historical 4 percent margin, depending on their mix of fixed and variable costs.

Exhibit 7.6 Quantify Providers' Anticipated Revenue Shortfalls

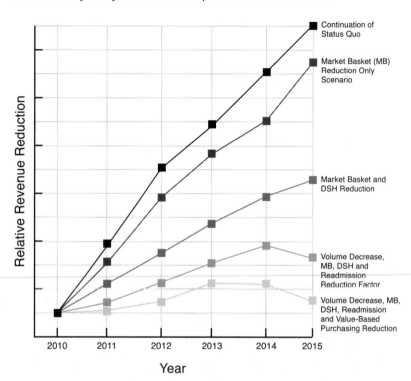

Step 2: Benchmark Unit Cost and Utilization Savings Opportunities

The second step is for providers to benchmark unit cost and savings opportunities relative to competitors and best practices. This starts by putting avoidable costs and complications into three categories:

1. Traditional variable unit cost and utilization savings, which can amount to ~5 percent cost-savings opportunity. The savings come from reducing unit cost and overuse of certain supplies, drugs, and agency staffing, for example.
2. Next-level variable and semi-fixed cost and utilization savings, including divestitures, which can be an additional ~5 percent of

cost savings. These savings are achieved by reducing excessive bed days, unnecessary ambulatory procedures, and ICU utilization. Nursing and physician support is required to achieve these savings.

3. Reduction in readmissions, complications, and ambulatory-sensitive care utilization across the care continuum, which can be an additional 5-plus percent cost savings. Achieving these reductions requires new levels of clinical, financial, and organizational integration among hospitals, post-acute providers, primary care providers, and specialists.

To quantify these opportunities, in the hospital for example, organizations should consider using DRG and APG (ambulatory patient group)–level analysis of cost and utilization variance. Using cost-report data and Medicare claims data, it is possible to quantify total cost variance versus benchmark by DRG and drill into cost drivers (e.g., ICU/CCU [intensive care unit/critical care unit] cost variance versus peers, clinical productivity variance, length-of-stay and readmission variance, drug and supply chain costs). Payers and providers are increasingly using these episode-based analyses to tier comparable providers and set mutual performance improvement targets and tactics that go well beyond traditional analysis of potential supply and labor savings. See Exhibit 7.7 for a summary of common cost drivers or savings areas.

We urge payers and providers to look beyond DRG and APG cost and utilization variance opportunities to uncover *additional* avoidable cost and utilization opportunities across the care continuum. Three additional methods are summarized below:

1. *PMPM population–based unit cost, utilization, and mix analytics.* Where payers are willing to share, we highly recommend that your organization assesses its track record in managing population utilization, quality, and cost trends. This entails obtaining payer reports for patients associated

Exhibit 7.7 Major Diagnostic Category (MDC) and Service Line Based on Author Research of Hundreds of Providers

Operational Areas \ Service Lines	MDC 05 Circulatory	MDC 08 Orthopedic	MDC 04 Respiratory	MDC 06 Digestive	MDC 19 Psychiatry	MDC 23 Rehabilitation	Surgical Services
Surgical Supplies and Implantables Devices	√	√		√			√
General Drugs and Supplies			√				
Operating Room and Anesthesia Costs	√	√		√			√
Length of Stay	√	√	√			√	√
Routine Room and Board Costs	√	√	√	√	√	√	
ICU/CCU Utilization Rates	√		√	√			
Outlier Management					√	√	√
Physical, Speech, and Occupational Therapies						√	

with your physician practice to assess their unit cost and utilization patterns versus those of fellow providers and national benchmarks. These PMPM analytics help organizations find additional deep-drill analyses, such as detailed analysis of pharmacy costs, diabetic and cancer patients, care transitions, and inpatient use rates. Some of the nation's top-performing systems have used these analytics to facilitate 10 to 30 percent reductions in unnecessary emergency room visits, bed days, and referrals.

2. *Analysis of ambulatory-sensitive inpatient admissions.* The Agency for Healthcare Research and Quality published a list of these admissions by DRG, along with other adverse event indicators based on claims data; this list is available at www.qualityindicators.ahrq.gov/pqi_overview.htm. The Commonwealth Fund provides state-specific reports on these metrics as well. Payers and providers are increasingly incorporating these metrics into both provider profiling tools for patients and their contract negotiations. We even know of

one national carrier that is withholding payment on potentially avoidable readmissions.

3. *Advanced avoidable cost/use methods.* Methodologies such as Prometheus focus on avoidable costs across the inpatient–outpatient–post-acute care continuum by disease.

Take a diabetic patient for example. The logic identifies patients using specific triggers in the claims data, such as ICD-9 codes. A series of co-morbidities and risk factors can be defined as well to further segment these patients. Then with input from clinicians, a series of potentially avoidable complications and costs can be defined (e.g., in the case of diabetics, specific wound care, readmissions, ED utilization). Although claims data are typically used to do the preliminary quantification, follow-up observational data (collected, for example, at the bedside or through electronic medical record data) are used to further refine the analysis so that it is clinician ready. Exhibit 7.8 shows a sample analysis.

In general, we find that the advanced cost and utilization analyses tend to uncover additional savings (over and above traditional functional analysis) in the realm of 5 to 10 percent of the total costs of a population if physicians participate with hospitals in the process.

Step 3: Develop a Strategic Margin Transition Plan

The next step is to combine the revenue projections with the cost benchmarking/opportunity analysis to draft what we call the *strategic margin transition plan*. The strategic margin transition plan contains a set of sequenced strategies, tactics, and financial pro forma that outlines how payer, hospital, and physician margins will transition over three to five years to bend the trend and improve quality.

The strategic margin transition planning process includes a plot of your organization's offerings from the *market's* perspective of differentiated, proprietary commodity services versus undifferentiated commodity services and from an overall cost–value perspective, using the four-quadrant graphing method in Exhibit 7.9.

Exhibit 7.8 Sample Cost and Utilization Analysis

Prometheus ECRs	Episode Window (days)	Number of Eligible Patients	Total Allowed Amount	Total PAC Amount	Average Episode Cost IP, OP, Rx, and Professional	PAC as Percent of Average Episode Cost
Diabetes	365	1,173	$6M	$2M	$5,500	30%
Hypertension	365	1,697	$4M	$900k	$2,100	25%
GERD	365	843	$4M	$700k	$4,200	20%
Asthma	365	647	$2M	$575k	$2,700	33%
CAD	365	224	$2M	$250k	$7,300	15%
COPD	365	292	$1M	$500k	$4,100	42%
Other	Etc.	Etc.	Etc.	Etc.	Etc.	Etc.
Totals and Weighted Averages:	333	5,488	$25M	$7M	$9,596	29%

Note: PAC = potentially avoidable complication/cost; CAD = coronary artery disease; COPD = chronic obstructive pulmonary disease; GERD = gastroesophageal reflux disease; IP = inpatient; OP = outpatient; ECR = evidence-informed case rates

Ironically, payers are ahead of providers in beginning to plot these dynamics for providers in their network, albeit with limited data that require more attention. In fact, this new way of looking at margin management represents a new compact between payers and providers under reform. This framework also provides a fresh starting point for payers and providers to begin negotiations from a common set of principles that give both sides a framework to optimize their margins and quality in an environment of lower premiums and unit reimbursements.

Here's a breakdown of the graph in Exhibit 7.9:

- *Quadrant A margin optimization tactics.* This upper-left quadrant represents high-cost, proprietary services. Classic examples include transplant services at smaller geographically isolated academic medical centers, where much larger programs exist

Exhibit 7.9 Margin Optimization Discussion

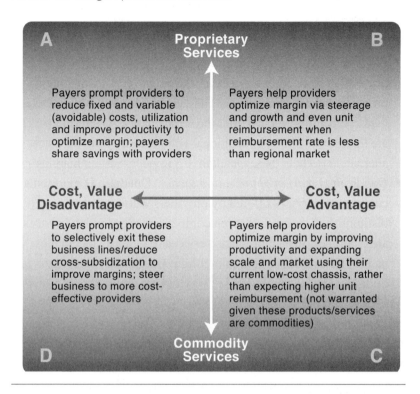

within a three-to-four-hour drive. Employers are increasingly demonstrating less willingness to grant these providers historical rate increases to buoy margins, particularly when lower-cost substitutes (even a few hundred miles away) exist. One such employer is Lowe's, the home improvement chain, which incentivizes its employees to get heart surgery at Cleveland Clinic rather than at local higher-cost care sites.

- *Quadrant B margin optimization tactics.* This upper-right quadrant represents specific proprietary products and services that providers offer in a cost-effective manner. High-volume, advanced proton beam therapy is one example of such a service; in markets where only a handful of institutions offer the service, we observe that purchasers are willing to pay a premium price for a premium service. This premium price, in turn, generates higher margins, which can be used to fund other mission-oriented services.

- *Quadrant C margin optimization tactics.* In the lower-right quadrant are commodity services that providers can offer at lower prices than competing services. For example, certain imaging providers have lower costs per FTE, equipment, and square footage than competitors, yet can offer the same quality. As a result, payers are finding ways to steer additional volume away from high-cost alternatives to help these Quadrant C providers sustain margins.

- *Quadrant D margin optimization tactics.* Quadrant D represents commodity services offered by providers who have not distinguished themselves from competitors. Several lab services are examples of such products/services (e.g., basic metabolic panel). Payers are starting to highlight Quadrant D performers and finding ways to steer business away from these underperformers.

Quadrant A Case Study

Consider, for example, the case of a community hospital's lab that had high costs (and high prices) on its sophisticated cytology services (Quadrant A, upper left). On the surface, the services appeared to be generating a positive contribution margin, so the hospital was not inclined to change its behavior, until a large payer shared some price and cost benchmarking results that forced the hospital to consider whether it should offer those services.

As it turned out, the lab director's "maximize prices to maximize margin" strategy came under attack because of a number of internal operational and competitive issues. First, the underlying productivity of the lab equipment was low. Furthermore, the hospital had costly technology that ordinarily would be found only in large academic medical centers. The lease terms for the equipment were poor. Furthermore, market research showed the hospital was losing market share to lower-priced competitors.

Upon further discussion with the lab director and pathologists, the hospital leadership team agreed to improve margin by lowering prices and decreasing their costs. They hoped to increase volume and market

Finding New Sources of Capital for ACOs

The Healthcare Financial Management Association reported (www.hfma.org/pulse) that even during the recent economic downturn, only 9 percent of surveyed systems reported they would consider monetizing assets in response to capital needs; see Exhibit 7.10.

Exhibit 7.10

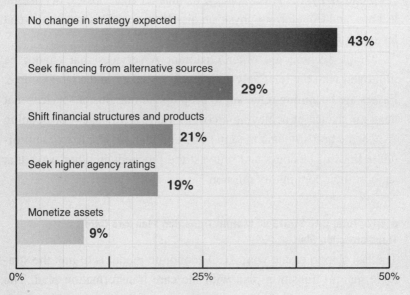

What steps are you taking in response to higher cost of capital?

No change in strategy expected — **43%**

Seek financing from alternative sources — **29%**

Shift financial structures and products — **21%**

Seek higher agency ratings — **19%**

Monetize assets — **9%**

0%   25%   50%

Source: Healthcare Financial Management Association (www.hfma.org/pulse). Used with permission.

When assessing your service portfolio, consider these telltale signs of opportunities to generate cash to fund cost-saving innovations:

- No divestiture or closure of any of your hospital's services in the last five years
- Lack of analysis of new business opportunities based on mission, margin, and capital requirements
- Little confidence in product-line strategies and financial analysis
- Difficulty prioritizing capital investment items
- A pattern of budget shortfalls followed by urgent cost-reduction mandates

share that had been lost over the past two years, in part because of the hospital's high prices. The hospital renegotiated its equipment's lease terms and told referring physicians about its new prices. Ultimately, volume, market share, and net margin rebounded, even as price and patient out-of-pocket amounts decreased. This illustrates that high prices do not automatically optimize margins. By analyzing the lab prices relative to cost and market and rebalancing the product portfolio, the chief operating officer (COO) and chief financial officer (CFO) resolved five issues: (1) productivity, (2) price strategy, (3) market share losses, (4) margin leakage, and (5) referring-physician dissatisfaction. This is an important lesson for ACOs.

Granted, there are other Quadrant A services that cannot be improved with the relatively simple actions taken in the lab example. Payers are becoming reluctant to prop up the margins of services that have no chance of achieving a cost or value advantage. For budding ACOs, the best strategic margin transition plan may be to exit unprofitable lines of business and reinvest the proceeds in other ways that support their community mission.

Step 4: Integrate Strategic Margin Transition Plan into Care Transformation Plan

The last step to create your ACO economic model is to link the strategic margin transition plan with the care transformation plan. The process begins with the five patient cohorts discussed in Chapter 4: well patients, minor episodic illness patients, major episodic illness patients, chronic patients, and catastrophic patients. Next, array cost avoidance, outcomes improvements, and patient incentive opportunities by cohort (columns) and by service line or grouping of clinical resources (rows); see Exhibit 7.11.

Here's an explanation of how to do this:

- *Well-patient cohort.* Avoidable cost-savings opportunities include decreasing unnecessary tests and steering patients to lower cost sites of care. Opportunities also exist to monitor health via annual checkups; telehealth; and cost-saving, patient

Exhibit 7.11 Array of Five Patient Cohorts

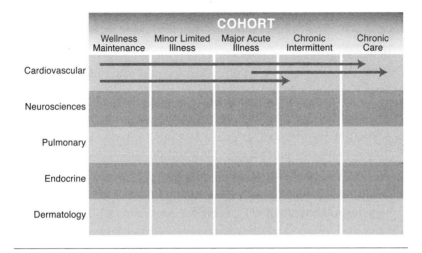

self-education tools the ACO invests in with payers to keep the trend low on this group.

- *Minor/major illness cohort.* Bend the ACO trend within this cohort by early identification and active management of co-morbidities. Adopt protocols for high-dollar procedures, including robust ICU resource management. Embed order sets, prompts, and triggers in delivery of care. Focus on transitions to post-acute sites via pre-discharge planning.

- *Chronic-patient cohort.* Avoid complications and cost by adopting protocols around the use of specialists versus primary care and the use of interventions (medications, procedures, and testing). Select testing and procedure sites on the basis of cost, quality, and clinical efficiency. Conduct active outreach and surveillance of care using telemedicine, home care, and so forth.

The strategic margin transition plan and care transformation plan become aligned when the CFO, COO, nursing, and physician leadership sit down to profile (and track) how these delivery and incentive changes will improve a specific patient cohort's outcomes, service, and cost.

Micro Case Study: 30–40-Year-Old Diabetic Cohort

In this case, we worked with finance and delivery leadership to quantify avoidable costs and complications and to map the clinical pathways necessary to improve quality and efficiency within a particular patient cohort.

Avoidable costs within this cohort included the following:

- Avoidable ICU utilization
- Excessive readmissions
- Brand-name and unnecessary prescription utilization
- Unnecessary ED visits
- Multiple physician touch points—the number of different physicians the patient was seeing for conditions related to diabetes

The economic and delivery model implications for the ACO included the following:

- Expense management: standardize formulary usage
- Capital investment: invest in a diabetic educator for the sickest patients to prevent downstream admissions
- Managed care contracting: modify benefit design to favor generic utilization; negotiate bonus for specific process and outcomes measures, new reimbursement arrangement for home care and telemedicine, and shared-savings arrangement for keeping patients out of hospital; provide patient-education materials and incentives for members to self-steer toward lower-cost sites of care

This exercise was run across a dozen conditions to vet and integrate the strategic margin transition plan and care transformation plan.

Summary of the Design of the ACO Economic Model

In summary, this four-step process to design your ACO economic model reinforces that the ACO economic model is much more than a managed care contract. To bend the curve, let alone maintain financial viability, ACOs must coordinate multiple initiatives, including revenue and expenses, management, capital investment, acquisitions, divestitures, and funds flow/incentive design. But, as the next section covers, providers cannot do all this on their own. They need external parties—payers, policymakers, and purchasers—to change some perverse incentives if the ACO model is to thrive.

Defining How Payers, Policymakers, and Purchasers Need to Support the Transition

Payers, policymakers, and purchasers need to do their part to improve quality and help bend the trend. Two items warrant attention in this regard:

1. Payers and purchasers need to share population data with providers to set targets and prioritize tactics.
2. Payers, policymakers, and providers need to adopt simplified, standardized, value-based payment approaches, which include payment off of core evidence-based costs, a separate performance-based bonus, and even direct investment.

Share Population Data to Set Targets and Prioritize Tactics

Like providers, payers can be siloed organizations that do not share data internally, let alone externally. Network contracting staff are often in a separate division from sales and marketing staff, who are in charge of benefit design and incentives. Sales and marketing staff, in turn, are separate from underwriting, finance, and actuarial staffs.

This fragmentation results in a lack of coordinated strategy between sales, underwriting, and contracting to bend the trend. One way to begin to align is for purchasers to insist that payers partner with providers to integrate population-based claims data with registry and electronic health data to quantify key cost drivers by patient segment; set performance targets; and formulate product and benefit design, reimbursement, and medical management tactics to bend the trend.

Exhibit 7.12 summarizes how payers and providers can work together to manage key trend drivers, using a combination of product

Exhibit 7.12 How Payers and Providers Can Jointly Bend the Trend

Trend Driver/ Segment	How Services Are Priced	How Care Is Managed	How Incentives Are Set
Emergent, major acute, differentiated care services	Increase reimbursement for differentiated outcomes as long as underlying costs are competitive	Since unit reimbursement would increase commensurate with value, be vigilant at measuring/monitoring outcomes, value	Cover these services with a deductible similar to what competitors charge
Nonemergent, discretionary, elective, nondifferentiated care services (Savings = $x)	Set reimbursement of core, evidence-based costs for these services. Don't pay extra for nondifferentiated care	Employ rigorous prior authorization; monitor provider-specific overuse or misuse	Employ high patient cost sharing to discourage unnecessary utilization; create patient incentives to steer to most cost effective/high quality providers
Preventive care services (Savings = $x)	Set reimbursement off of core, evidence-based costs and a bonus if provider hits particular targets	Promote utilization practices in accordance with national guidelines, medical home programs, etc.	Promote appropriate use through benefit design
Chronic disease(s) requiring ongoing management and occasional flare-ups (Savings = $x)	Pay for care transitions, telemedicine, etc.; pay a bonus for reduced readmissions, avoidable ED use targets, etc.	Promote utilization and compliance in accordance with national guidelines, medical home programs, etc.	Promote appropriate use through benefit design
Undifferentiated ancillary services (Savings = $x)	Set reimbursement off of core, evidence-based costs	Employ prior authorization; incentivize providers to steer patients to low-cost providers; monitor abuse	Employ high patient co-pay to discourage unnecessary utilization

and benefit design, medical management strategy, and unit-reimbursement and direct-investment tactics.

Adopt Value-Based Payment or Pricing

Payers and providers also need to help design and implement simple, value-based payment schedules that promote behavior for both underperformers and superstars that will actually bend the trend. That is, the trend will not bend unless purchasers insist that fee schedules (1) pay for services that add value, (2) reward results, and (3) reduce administrative cost. A simple example brings this to life.

Take the case of a CT (computed tomography) of the abdomen, which can easily be reimbursed off of hundreds of different fee schedules for any particular provider in America. We observe that a single provider may get reimbursed between $200 and $2,000 for the exact same service, which ranges from well under cost to a significant multiple of cost. This may create incentives to do additional services, particularly on highly reimbursed commercial patients, even if it adds significant cost over what we call core evidence-based, best-practice, or Medicare breakeven costs. At least some of that additional utilization arguably does not add value. Yet the patient, purchaser, and payer foot the bill.

Alternatively, consider how payers and providers are coming together on behalf of patients/members to explore, at a service level, (1) core, evidence-based costs, (2) avoidable costs, and (3) a bonus or shared-savings arrangement—all three of which can be rolled into a value-based fee schedule as illustrated in Exhibit 7.13.

We are working with various payers and providers to initiate a process that defines core, evidence-based, efficient-care costs (dotted line) for common resources used in the delivery of care (e.g., guide wires, operating room [OR] minutes). As part of the process, we work with payers and providers to analyze how these resources are combined to deliver value-added products and services patients and purchasers actually buy. As part of this process, we work with both parties to quantify potentially avoidable costs (gray bar) and design a direct investment or value-based bonus that shares some of those savings with high-performing providers (black bar).

Using this collaborative process, we see an opportunity for the industry to rally around a common set of resource and product definitions, tools, and metrics to perform this work, such that the administrative burden is reduced. In time, this approach has the potential to replace the hundreds (and even thousands) of traditional charge masters and fee schedules the typical managed care plan and provider

Exhibit 7.13 Value-Based Fee Schedule

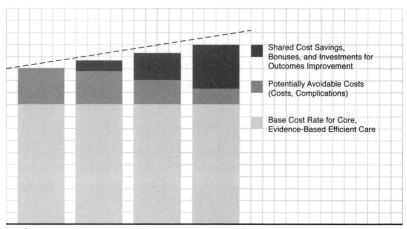

Shared Cost Savings,
Bonuses, and Investments for
Outcomes Improvement

Potentially Avoidable Costs
(Costs, Complications)

Base Cost Rate for Core,
Evidence-Based Efficient Care

Current

Payer Perspectives

1. Set fair base rate without automatic yearly increases
2. Reduce payment fo avoidable costs
3. Share cost savings for better outcomes

Result: lower yearly cost increases

have to track (e.g., by product, provider type, site of service, geography). The traditional schedules would be replaced with a simplified base-fee schedule table for individual clinical resources *and* a table of specialty-specific, value-based multipliers by provider. The multipliers would specify bonuses for various access, efficiency, quality, and satisfaction results that demonstrably bend the trend and improve quality.

Over time, this approach will prompt the industry to greatly simplify and standardize hospitals' charging practices across the industry. After all, patients do not derive "value" by the guide wire or by the OR minute. Nor do patients derive "value" based on whether a provider bills a service as a facility-based or office-based service. Providers spend considerable sums finding new items or ways to charge for services that may enhance margins but do not create patient value. This would be equivalent to a hotel starting to charge guests for the ounces of shampoo, number of sheets, and minutes of television consumed.

Over time, the ACO needs to create a new line of sight between cost, price, and value for patients, payers, and providers. This way, providers will earn profit on things patients value. Pricers in other industries, like airlines, hotels, and rental cars, have long created lines of sight by linking units of resource capacity (e.g., a seat, bed day) to products or packages of resources people buy (e.g., Flight 102 from Chicago to Los Angeles). For "elective" flights, customers know that if they book in advance, travel at off-peak times, and are willing to make a connection, the flight will cost less. As the following case study exhibits, though, this is *not* the case for most healthcare services.

Case Study: The Price Is "Wrong"

The following case study is indicative of how the lines of sight between cost, price, and value remain blurred in a rush to "go ACO."

In a hurry to satisfy internal pressures, a large system pieced together various facility, ancillary, and professional resources into an acute episode "bundle" to attract specific employers and payers to use its new facility. The problem was that underlying lab resource prices were completely out of line with market, cost, and Medicare; the basic lab resource alone was priced at 800 percent of Medicare. To make matters worse, the team included low-revenue-producing supplies in the bundle (e.g., $1 toothbrushes), which actually cost more to track than they generate in revenue. The result wasn't just an outrageously priced "bundle" composed of mispriced resources. The result was a convoluted, administratively burdensome fee schedule and funds flow problem. Not to mention, time would be wasted severity adjusting the bundles, which eventually patients with increasing out-of-pocket obligations would have no interest in buying.

Here's a better way to design a value-based bundle:

- *Step 1.* Update variable and fixed cost allocations for associated resources across the hospital.

- *Step 2*. Rebase charge master prices on underlying costs, market, and Medicare norms.
- *Step 3*. Understand the need to maintain margin on a softer top line, and quantify avoidable resource utilization and how to price that into packages (e.g., build a case rate that assumes a 30-day readmission is included).
- *Step 4*. Market-test the concept with key patients, payers, and purchasers to assess volume-growth potential and the potential for the payer to steer new volume to your facility.
- *Step 5*. Approach specific payer/purchaser channels with special pricing in return for real, sustainable, and exclusive volume steerage.
- *Step 6*. Negotiate a bonus system or direct investment for exceeding specific quality and service metrics in which the bonuses would flow directly to the provider.

Summary of Value-Based Payment

In summary, healthcare payment is especially complex because there is no line of sight between price, cost, and value. (See Exhibit 7.14 for creating a line of sight.) This is exacerbated when parties do not share common views about how value is created and distributed, and it is made even worse when they don't share data. But until payers and providers establish standardized payment approaches that acknowledge core, evidence-based costs and what patients value, the ACO's ability to improve quality and reduce cost is limited. So payers and providers need to start with administrative simplification and proceed to quantifying the value for every resource or unit of capacity, based on underlying cost, market comparisons, Medicare, and work effort. Once resources are valued and captured in a standardized, cost-effective manner, payers and providers will find new and innovative ways of packaging resources to reward reductions in avoidable costs and complications. This will give ACOs a clear pathway to earning premium prices rather than being commoditized to death.

Exhibit 7.14 Creating the Line of Sight and the Evolution of Healthcare Payment Model

Current System	Cost-Based, Market-Based System Milestones	Value-Based Payment, Incentive Principles
• "Pay me more" versus "pay you less" rhetoric at the negotiation table • Major cross-subsidies and cost shifts—internally and externally to the provider • Success = contractual loopholes + negotiation power • Limited (if any) relationship among price, cost, quality, and value and the prices, rewards, and compensation systems	• Awareness of cross-subsidies, irrational unit reimbursement, over/mis/underuse of resources • Establishment of a method that bases prices on incremental costs and market competitors and on qualitative indicators of value	• Customer first • New payment and patient and provider incentive mechanisms, such as hospital/physician bundling, 30-day episodic payments, guarantees, and peak pricing that clarify mutual accountability to maximize patient value for the incremental dollar

Reviewing Case Studies That Illustrate Early Successes and Challenges

The following case studies are intended to bring the aforementioned economic principles, analytics, and tactics to life for your ACO.

Case Study 1: Large Payer's Journey Toward Value-Based Contracting and Benefit Design

Like other multimillion-member, not-for-profit health plans, this payer's (a composite of several large payers) historical strategy was to maintain high market share and low administrative costs. But faced with declining margins and increased employer and regulatory scrutiny, the payer proactively set up a process and an integrated internal team to manage both insurance premium and medical cost trend in tandem, in anticipation of not being able to pass large PMPM increases onto customers in the future.

Value-Based Funds Flow Design and the ACO

Resource-based *internal* pricing is at the heart of any funds flow exercise. Navigant Consulting's CARTS funds flow methodology is effectively a resource classification system, in which resources are classified into C(linical resources), A(dministrative resources), R(esearch resources), T(eaching resources), and S(trategic resources). Each of these resources/units of capacity entails its own unit of analysis, such as a work relative value unit (RVU) for clinical production or a research unit for research. These resource units can be costed and compared with national norms to generate an internal cost (or price) point (or range thereof). The key that most funds flow and compensation models miss, though, is that the external unit reimbursement/price on the resource (as determined by, say, managed care contracts) needs to be in synch with the internal price for that same resource so that the sources of funds match the uses of funds and cross-subsidization is minimized.

That is, the root of funds-flow evil is when internal cost and prices do not match external market reimbursement rates. The most common example is when payers reimburse $50/work RVU, but physicians are paid twice that amount under an employment contract. This disconnect can easily deteriorate into a lack of trust and accountability within the organization—ACO or not.

So the payer set off to explore a bend-the-medical-cost-trend strategy. Using some of the provider profiling analytics noted earlier in the chapter, the payer analyzed its network's cost drivers, including unit reimbursement, utilization, and mix, relative to competitors and found some interesting results:

- Hospital unit reimbursement was spread across 100 fee schedules, with a 400 percent variance between the highest and lowest reimbursed providers. Physician reimbursement was considerably lower than that of competitors, and several commodity services that could be contracted for nationally were over-reimbursed (e.g., reference labs at a significant markup over Medicare).

- Inpatient and outpatient utilization was largely unmanaged. The plan did not delegate any medical management to the network. Limited staff and loose interpretation of various medical guidelines, such as InterQual, yielded relatively high utilization rates across the board.
- There was significant provider-specific unit reimbursement and utilization variation (similar to that seen in *Dartmouth Health Atlas*), with particularly high variation in use rates and practice patterns among procedural specialists.
- There were up to 20 percent avoidable savings opportunities (readmissions, high-cost outliers, skilled nursing facility days, brand-name utilization, avoidable utilization in the ED, and other high-cost sites of care despite alternatives) in particular regions.
- A major disconnect existed between what was in the contracts and how claims were actually paid, resulting in pockets of substantial overpayment rather than underpayment.
- There was a 10 percent reduction opportunity in administrative costs.

With this fact base in place, the payer embarked on a strategy to do the following:

- Build internal and external awareness around bend-the-trend and value-based purchasing—why and why now.
- Establish value-based reimbursement "rules of the road" with providers over a five-plus-year time frame to bend the trend.
- Plot strategic margin transition plans with specific providers, which include performance target setting, value-based fee schedules, shared savings, and direct investments in cost-saving technology.

The payer did not begin by diving into an ACO pilot. The payer began by engaging individual specialties in conversations about insurance premium, utilization, administrative cost, and reimbursement trends. The analytics helped to address the what, why, and how for providers and customers:

1. What is the objective: Maximize value for our customers—our patients.

2. Why: Future premium and reimbursement increases will be lower than in the past. The medical cost trend curve will need to bend downward without jeopardizing quality, access, and affordability.
3. Why now:
    - Employer/customer demand for lower costs
    - Increased patient cost sharing
    - Unemployment and increase in uninsured
    - Today's price increases are tomorrow's bad debt
    - Provider access gaps
4. How:
    - Need to *do this together*, rather than apart; move beyond pay more/pay less rhetoric.
    - Highest and best use of the incremental dollar: Dedicate incremental reimbursement and capital dollars to the highest and best use of those dollars to improve health, which will include cost saving and quality-improving technology, facilities, and so forth. Likewise, exit businesses others can do better.
    - Core, evidence-based costs and savings targets: Set reimbursement based on core, evidence-based reimbursement rate plus a value-based multiplier for unique cost savings and/or quality your organization can achieve that others cannot. The value-based multipliers are based in part on the provider's ability to reduce avoidable costs and medical cost trend, relative to the do-nothing scenario.
    - All this under the guise of shared accountability to our customers

With those key messages in place, the next step was for the payer to establish a set of rules of the road with its provider network. The payer extended the following to cooperating providers:

1. Voice at the table for purposes of planning and operating in an accountable care model
2. Financial resources in the form of bonuses and direct investments to improve quality and efficiency

3. Clinical resources in the form of case managers, physician extenders, and others to manage transitions of care and special populations
4. Administrative simplicity in the form of less paperwork, faster payment, lower administrative costs, and so forth
5. Volume growth potential in the form of a new product that could steer patients to highest-performing providers
6. Data analytics to identify high-risk patients, practice variation, daily census and referral reports, shared medical management guidelines, and target setting

In return, the payer expected the following from its provider network:

1. Accountable provider's willingness to manage "total cost" of care over time
2. Commitment to achieving specific access, quality, affordability, and productivity metrics across all components of their practice and across all sites of care
3. Provide clinical leadership to advance the development of multidisciplinary, evidence-based, team-based approaches to care delivery and patient engagement, including structure (staffing, scheduling) and process (protocol development, medical management activities)

With the rules of the road in place, the next step was to plot the multiyear transition plan, provider by provider.

The payer engaged specific high-cost provider groups (including the hospital association) to plot out a series of tactics to deliver value—by reducing cost and improving access, service, and quality. Provider-specific initiatives to bend the trend included the following:

- Hospital- and physician-tiered networks with differential patient cost sharing or waived co-pays
- Nonemergent ED utilization control

- Durable medical equipment purchase versus lease
- No payments for never events or certain avoidable complications
- Domestic medical tourism
- Development of narrow network
- Generic substitution
- Supply standardization and gainsharing
- Money-back guarantees
- 340b pharmacy pricing
- New payment for case management
- Bundling for orthopedic and cardiac surgery

Next, the payer and provider network translated these shared-savings opportunities into a value-based fee schedule that consists of a base rate for evidence-based costs without guaranteed annual increases. This became the base fee schedule amount. They next estimated the avoidable cost by provider and took a percentage of that amount and allocated it to a shared savings/performance bonus factor added to the base fee schedule to be paid to providers that exceeded their expected performance on a quarterly basis. Aside from the implementation of the value-based fee schedule changes, they also provided some direct investment dollars to fund medical home and on-site case-management pilots throughout the region.

A year into the initiative, progress is deliberately slow but steady. The level of provider communication and support is quite significant and appears to be yielding cost savings and health improvements. Providers have broadly supported the millions of dollars of extra reimbursement in the form of primary care multipliers and payment for certain telemedicine and case management services. This has created momentum and enthusiasm for additional value-based fee schedule multipliers and direct investments in coming years.

Case Study 2: A Failed ACO Initiative

Sometimes, failures provide more useful insights into future improvements.

In this instance, the CEOs of an independent payer, a large multispecialty physician group, and a hospital system came together to explore their ACO possibilities. From a process perspective, all three CEOs had concluded that their individual destinies rested in the success of each other. They then set off to explore how the economics and delivery could work. Ultimately, their efforts failed on two accounts: (1) the analytics were not rich enough to generate the urgency necessary to sanction even a pilot, and (2) one of the three parties used the initiative as a platform to negotiate immediate savings with another party, rather than look at the longer-term merits of the arrangement for all three parties.

Specifically, the analytic focused exclusively on PMPM benchmarks of unit reimbursement, utilization, and mix and did not quickly identify early wins (e.g., specific expense reductions, growth opportunities) that could help fund future ACO initiatives. One of the three parties was also extremely insistent on fully capitating the entire arrangement, rather than easing into an arrangement with a shared-savings or value-based fee schedule approach, which would have created immediate traction and financial rewards for all parties.

As the initiative progressed, that same party used the PMPM analytic against the other two, threatening to reduce unit reimbursement immediately if no deal were done, as one of the two ran into roadblocks with union renegotiations. The other two parties became frustrated with the third, and the potential arrangement died a quick death less than eight weeks into the initiative (despite the long-term strategic merits and codependencies among the three parties). Clearly, all parties failed to lay out the rules of the road from the beginning, let alone the early wins that could have at least improved the working relationship in a manner that could open up subsequent partnership opportunities.

Case Study 3: Using the ACO to Energize Service Lines

This was a classic case of a struggling cancer service line that was losing margin and competitive positioning in its market, despite new facilities, technologies, and some advanced medical techniques. Like most cancer programs, it lacked adequate coordination among independent subspecialists and had gone through a series of medical leaders who could not get adequate cooperation/coordination to design and implement standard care paths, supply use, and so forth.

Service line leadership embarked on a data-driven approach to quantify go-forward vulnerabilities and opportunities in light of reform. The leaders laid out a compelling set of problems:

- Future Medicare cuts put 5 percent of the net revenue in jeopardy
- Avoidable costs and complications represented another potential 5 percent cut in future revenue, not to mention the unnecessary testing and (at times) surgical procedures based on independent medical review.

At one level, the analytics opened up the proverbial can of worms. But under hospital executive leadership, a series of focused, quality improvement sessions occurred, including finance and the physician hospital organization leader, with the explicit goal to define (1) an economic model and (2) a delivery model required to improve quality. Up to that point, meetings had simply focused on incremental delivery improvements and patient chart reviews (and they were poorly attended). But when the CEO put the delivery *and* economic models on the table for debate and joint design, key stakeholders lined up outside the door.

Key payers were also invited to participate in the data-driven initiative. They provided key hospital, physician, drug, and other claims data to the effort, which allowed all parties to uncover some immediate opportunities, and a few surprises, as follows:

- Some patients saw literally dozens of doctors over the course of their treatment.
- Significant ancillary overutilization (e.g., labs, radiology, pharmacy) was occurring as compared with well-established clinical best practices.

- Incentives were completely misaligned to coordinate care (e.g., payer did not pay for care coordinators, payers paid terribly high rates for certain services that had created a glut of capacity in region).

Physicians, the hospital, and payers took a step back and plotted care paths for the top-four cancer diagnoses in the region. They used this exercise to drive (1) clinical reconfiguration priorities and (2) new payment models, direct investments, and incentives required to get to a lower-cost, higher-quality outcome (see Exhibit 7.15).

Predictions for the Future

A sustainable economic model is critical to the success of ACOs and the US delivery system in general. As such, ACO economics are not simply managed care arrangements between payer and provider; rather, they are the revenue and expense management, capital, risk, and funds flow tactics required to improve quality and bend the trend. Unlike past attempts at reform, payers, providers, patients, and purchasers need to achieve a new level of coordination to manage the transition from the current system to the future system. This requires all parties to focus efforts on how their economic and delivery models need to evolve together, in a manner that maintains margins and quality. It also requires all parties to create a clear line of sight between the cost, price, and value of items they are buying so that all payers, providers, patients, and purchasers can be held accountable to improving access, service, and efficiency. Fortunately, many providers and payers are not waiting for reform to make this happen.

For these organizations, we recommend the following:

1. *Immediate term.* ACOs should focus on "early savings" that will help self-fund future investments in efficiency and quality improvements.
   a. Create a sense of urgency by quantifying your top-line *vulnerabilities* (e.g., Medicare payment changes, unsustainable cross-subsidization) under reform.

Exhibit 7.15 One Size Does Not Fit All: Oncology Contracting

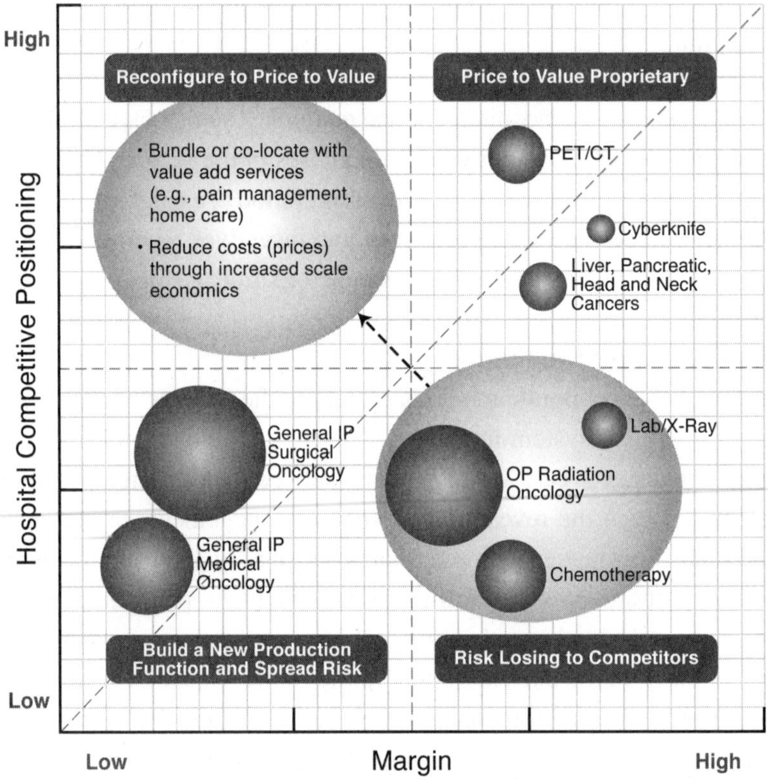

Note: Bubble size reflects relative market size based on current experience.

    b. Quantify short-term and long-term savings *opportunities* (e.g., avoidable costs, monetization of assets) across different services and populations.

    c. Beyond the analytics, sketch a picture of "what will be different this time" and how to close the margin gap.

2. *Long term*. Manage the transition to a new payment and delivery model. Coordinate economic and delivery model changes to sustain improvements over a multiyear period.

    a. Establish with key stakeholders (e.g., CFOs, payers, physicians) the rules of the road, including a core set of principles that underlies revenue and expense management, capital planning/allocation, acquisitions and divestitures, pricing and managed care contracts, risk management, and funds flow and incentives.

b. Eliminate misalignment.

- Stop the cat-and-mouse games between payers and providers.
- Rebase pricing, managed care contracts, compensation and incentives, capital priorities, and internal funds flow consistent with cost, market, and value.
- Integrate your strategic margin transition plan and care transformation plan, including primary care model changes and post-acute care readmissions and care transitions.

Organizational Questions

The organizational questions raised in this chapter include the following:

- By how much may reform trim our revenue over the next decade?
- How will we sustain our margins, considering that our options are volume growth, unit-reimbursement increases, and cost reduction?
- Where are the greatest opportunities to reduce avoidable costs and complications, and with whom?
- How do we tie our financial plan to our clinical improvement plans?
- How do we work with our top payers to manage the transition?

Category of Readers	Key Concepts	Actions to Consider
Category A (interested)	• ACO economics is more than a managed care deal • Your organization needs to consider its entire economic model if it is to sustainably bend the trend and improve quality	• Size your margin gap under future reimbursement environment
Category B (engaged)	• Strategic margin transition plan to optimize margin under a soft reimbursement and volume environment • Payer–provider "Prisoner's Dilemma"	• Develop your strategic margin transition plan with physicians and payers • Confront the cat-and-mouse games
Category C (committed)	• Clear line of sight between price, cost, and value for the things customers buy • Explicit linkages between economic transformation and delivery transformation	• Adopt new metrics/scorecard that includes revenue per available bed day and cost per available bed day • Adopt value-based fee schedules and align with internal funds flow

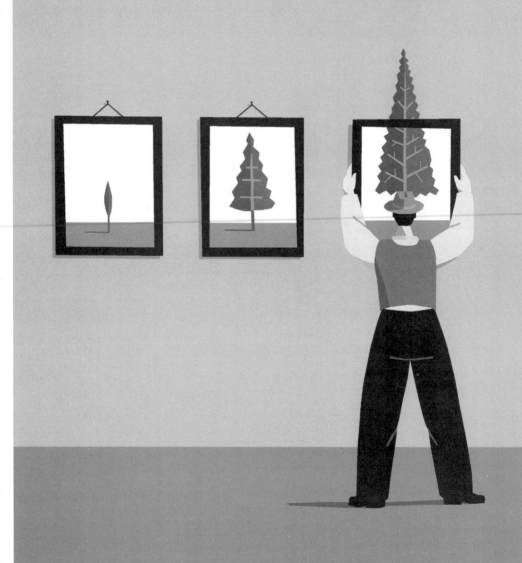

8

Assessing Your Organization's ACO Readiness

Becoming an ACO is a daunting task at the same time that it is a compelling strategy. How do we know where to start our journey?

—Executive, Baystate Health

███████████████████

Running a hospital isn't like performing a total hip replacement. The hip replacement, if done correctly, is a standardized procedure: Perform a preoperative assessment, explain to the patient what to expect, perform the procedure using a standard protocol, administer postoperative care, and discharge the patient to physical therapy or a rehab center. Simple, ready or not.

The performance of a complex organization such as a hospital or a physician practice doesn't lend itself to such linear predictability or assessment of readiness. Nevertheless, most complex, adaptive organizations (such as hospitals, seaports, or cities) engage in a set of activities that tend to follow each other in a somewhat predictable order, like shown in Exhibit 8.1.

Exhibit 8.1 Organizational Activities

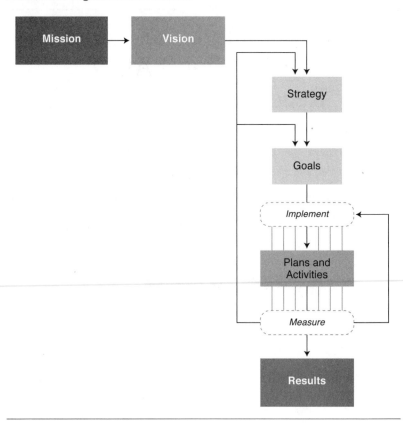

It works something like this: Organizations clarify their missions, thereby defining their reasons for being—missions are enduring and change only in response to significant internal or external discontinuities (such as *healthcare reform*). Once clear about the mission, the organization crafts a vision, or picture, that describes what it intends to look, feel, and operate like when fulfilling the mission in its preferred way. The vision generally includes the core values that drive and measure performance.

That picture, in turn, invites the selection of a strategy that describes precisely *how* the organization intends to achieve its vision in the service of its mission. All of this is then translated into a budget and a set of well-defined, sequenced, and measurable goals. The strategy and the goals in turn cascade into a portfolio of coordinated plans and activities that get implemented across the enterprise. The results are measured, and feedback loops support ongoing performance improvement.

While the real world is seldom this simple and things rarely progress in quite so orderly a fashion, most successful organizations follow some adaptation of this sequence. Problems arise, however, when organizations plan their ACO in a strategic vacuum.

After all, all healthcare delivery organizations, by design or default, have strategies. The success or failure of each strategy can only be evaluated against the organization's broader goals and intentions. Strategies, such as ACOs, are always a means to a higher end.

The ACO represents one of several potential reform and market-facing strategies. As stated, all the other potential strategies and tactics (e.g., Medicare breakeven, build scale) that existed before the Patient Protection and Affordable Care Act (PPACA) became law are still available. Yet ACO *strategy* has captured many providers' attention because independent tactics (e.g., divest underperformers) simply fail to inspire a critical mass of providers, payers, and policymakers to expend the effort required to transform delivery and payment simultaneously. The "accountability" concept also resonates with many providers at the end of the day, as does the threats (e.g., regulatory rate setting) inherent within the do-nothing scenario.

Five Questions When Considering the ACO Strategy

Ultimately, it is up to each organization to determine whether pursuit of an ACO is the right competitive strategy to help it reach its goals. So to inform whether the ACO is the right strategy, we recommend healthcare leaders across America to ask five fundamental questions:

1. *What is it?* What is an ACO, and what does it take to become one?
2. *Could it be good for us?* Is it a strategy that could help us achieve our goals and fulfill our mission?
3. *Should we do it?* What will it take for us to become a successful ACO?

4. *Can we do it?* What would the investment and the potential yield be to pursue this strategy?
5. *How do we do it?* What's our business plan for becoming an ACO?

We explore each of these questions.

What Is It?

The ACO is new. As stated above, it is really a work in progress. We don't yet know what the first functioning ACOs will look like. Moreover, the ACO is an abstraction. There really isn't an ACO that exists separately from the healthcare delivery system. Rather, the ACO is a strategy or road map for achieving certain ends—in particular, clinically superior integrated care that helps bend the cost curve to a lower, more sustainable trajectory.

So it's important to start educating your organization about this emerging model, regardless of whether or not you've made a firm decision to pursue it. Translated into action, a hospital CEO considering the ACO might say to her staff, "Given that healthcare reform is already being implemented, it is up to us, as leaders, to make certain that we are fully educated about the facts, the implications, and the options that we need to consider in order to continue to carry out our mission in a changing environment."

This education process is valuable, regardless of the outcome. It's a litmus test of the readiness of the organization to embrace the disruptive change required to adopt the ACO strategy. Many organizations are using this time to educate their boards, management teams, medical executive committees and medical staffs, community-based physicians, and external community groups that participate in patient care. Responses to the educational process provide important information for many healthcare executives as they reflect on the five questions related to the ACO. Astute healthcare leaders gain insight into the level of concern, fear, opportunity, or enthusiasm expressed by different stakeholders. These stakeholders' reactions will be useful for those organizations interested in further exploring how an ACO could be good for them.

Could It Be Good for Us?

This question can only be answered if the organization has well-defined goals. The answer can be discovered using a "shallow dive"—consulting industry jargon for a research exercise that, over the course of a few days, can assess local market conditions, internal interest, and organizational commitment and capabilities. Section 3022 of the PPACA makes *only one* new strategy available to healthcare organizations to achieve their goals: the ACO. All previous strategies are still available. At the end of this shallow dive, an organization is able to determine whether pursuit of the ACO strategy (versus others) could be helpful in achieving its goals. It will also be able to assess the magnitude of effort and investment required.

Additional innovative strategies can be expected to be introduced over the next few years. Separately from the ACO effort, the CMS (Centers for Medicare & Medicaid Services) Innovation Center, established in May 2010, will be working with private healthcare organizations to identify new ways to improve Medicare and Medicaid. The center will be establishing pilot programs to test emerging delivery, financing, and organizational innovations.

But the shallow dive may be more than a planning tool. Some organizations will use the tool to simply establish their *goals* in light of healthcare reform. For these organizations, the shallow dive is a useful tool for clarifying or reformulating goals and then communicating them clearly throughout the organization as an initial step in considering a potential ACO strategy. The shallow dive assessment explores (at minimal depth) the five organizational core competencies and the external environment (see the discussion later). It focuses primarily on the organization's expressed goals, commitment, interest, and high-level competencies to answer the question, "Could it be good for us?"

The shallow dive assessment and its cousin the deep dive assessment differ in both purpose and detail. The shallow dive answers whether the ACO is a reasonable option for an organization to consider for achieving its strategic goals. The deep dive is designed to answer the question "Should we do it?"—that is, "What will it take for us to become a successful ACO?"

Should We Do It?

Answering this question requires an in-depth assessment or a "deep dive" that evaluates all five core competencies along with an evaluation of local competitive-market conditions, including the payer market. Details of each component of this assessment are described later.

The answer to "Should we do it?" is partially supported by analytics, but ultimately it is a leadership decision. Because the ACO strategy requires significant redesign and creates many discontinuities in organizational anatomy, physiology, sociology, and economics, the decision to move forward should not be taken lightly. The ACO is not a strategy that can be approached tentatively. It requires deep commitment from the CEO on down, and it demands true leadership passion.

To repeat from Chapter 2, Judy Rich (2010), CEO of Tucson Medical Center (TMC), one of three ACO pilot projects, notes:

> At TMC we have embraced the ACO as an alignment strategy with our physicians and as a means to improve the health of our community through coordinated care. Unlike models in the past, this one is not designed to produce volume for the hospital. This model keeps patients out of the hospital. We have learned that our physicians value a partnership that is focused on the patient and "doing the right thing." It has been a journey that has required an "all in" leadership commitment. No dabbling in an ACO...this model fundamentally changes the way we do business. The ACO put us into a partnership with our medical staff that is supporting their autonomy and expertise as managers of patient care. It lowers the costs of care by reducing repetitive, unnecessary care and lowering length of stay and utilization of expensive resources. TMC's ACO is a model for the future of healthcare in Southern Arizona, which I am sure will evolve in its appearance and makeup over the next few years. This journey is not for the timid, it is full of risk and potential obstacles, but it is the necessary path for us at TMC to fulfill our core mission of providing exemplary healthcare with access for all in our community.

Can We Do It?

For those who have studied ACO strategy, decided that it could be helpful for them to pursue their organizational goals, and agreed to pursue it, there's another hurdle: "Can we do it?" This question warrants the development of a detailed business plan. Conversations with local payers, patients, purchasers, other healthcare resources, and community-based independent and employed physicians are likely required to truly understand the unmet needs and the gaps that create them.

Preparing a detailed ACO business plan follows the same steps as standard business planning processes. It uses reasonable assumptions, business analytics, business modeling, and careful planning. While there are no benchmarks for comparison, much of the gap analysis and benchmarking can be based on organizations inside and outside of healthcare that operate at higher levels of quality and efficiency.

Beyond the analytics, three additional factors are prerequisites for any organization that wants to answer this question:

1. *Leadership passion*. As Rich observes, it will take a dedicated CEO ready to move mountains to guide the organization through a candid "Can we do it?" discussion because this isn't for the lukewarm or casually interested.
2. *Active management*. Does the organization simply drift onward in response to stimuli from the market? An organization needs to be actively and professionally managed to handle the tests of the ACO.
3. *Physician organization and interest*. Hospitals without well-developed physician organizations will be at a loss when they implement the ACO strategy. A well-functioning physician organization cannot be created overnight, and without it, the ACO effort is doomed to failure.

How Do We Do It?

Organizations that thoroughly address the first four questions realize by the end that there is no silver bullet, blueprint, script, or recipe for building an ACO. Like any change, it begins with a clear picture of what is desired, an honest assessment of the current state, a rigorous business planning process, and an operating plan for closing the gaps between the current and the desired state. The process for answering "How do we do it?" warrants a separate chapter—see Chapter 9.

ACO Education: Coming Soon to a Theater Near You

Educating your organization about the ACO will include many of the topics covered in this book. They include the evolution of the US healthcare market; PPACA reforms; the advent of the ACO; definitions; requirements; ACO models and core building blocks; CMS's goals for the ACO; core ACO competencies; ACO structure and operations; payment options; assessments of organizational readiness; and evaluation of what it will take to build a real, functioning ACO.

We strongly recommend that leadership follow up all presentations to employees, medical staff, governing bodies, and others with facilitated conversations. In many ways, these conversations will be more illuminating than the presentation itself. It is in the conversation that the staff's hopes, fears, excitement, and concerns get revealed. These conversations have enabled organizations to accurately assess the level of interest and enthusiasm among critical stakeholders, such as members of the governing body, senior management, middle management, medical staff, community-based primary care physicians, hospital-dependent specialists, and leaders of other community institutions. These conversations will reveal crucial data that may not surface in either the shallow or deep dive assessment.

Assessing Readiness: Many Shades of Gray

Organizational readiness cannot be assessed as a simple yes or no. Instead, there are many shades of gray that must be evaluated. Readiness is a relative assessment and must be considered inside a rational cost versus benefit framework. More precisely, the question the organization needs to answer is, "Do we choose to make the effort and investments necessary to close the gaps between where we are and where we need to be to become an ACO?" A useful tool—an effort/yield model for weighing the options—is presented in the 2 × 2 grid in Exhibit 8.2.

Business Plan ABCs for ACOs

At a high level, an ACO business plan should be thought of as a business plan designed to interest a local payer or self-insured group to contract with a delivery system in a manner similar to an ACO. While the ACO business plan will probably be used primarily internally to secure resources (e.g., capital, personnel, systems), writing it as an externally focused document will ensure appropriate comprehensiveness and discipline. In some cases, it will serve as a business plan to enlist some investment capital from a local payer as well. Either way, the business plan should include, at a minimum, the following ten components:

1. Description of the ACO division's business purpose—reorganizing to support ACO goals of improving outcomes, efficiency, and care experience in return for shared savings; includes why, why now, and why the organization believes it can be successful

2. Explanation of how the ACO strategy integrates with other competitive and organizational strategies

3. Description of the market that will be served and how that market will be accessed

4. Assessment of the local market and competitor positions

5. Description of organizational assets and investments that will contribute to success in the ACO

6. Description of the organizational design to deliver the services and outcomes

7. Anticipated organizational structure—partnerships, governance, and executive leadership team

8. Operating plan—the physiology of how this model will operate

9. Business model for this product, including
   a. Revenue, including payment model
   b. Estimated membership
   c. Funds flow
   d. Opportunity assessment for achieving operating efficiencies along with strategy

The most favorable quadrant is the one in which the investment is relatively modest and the yield is relatively robust (lower right). An organization in this position has an easy decision to make. The inverse is the least favorable quadrant (upper left), where the investment is relatively high and the yield is relatively modest. This represents an organization with a more daunting decision.

Both deep and shallow assessments use a common framework that analyzes five core competencies (first discussed in Chapter 2) in addition to the external environment:

1. Leadership and culture
2. Operational excellence
3. Care integration
4. Physician alignment
5. Technology enablement
6. External environment

Each assessment category is evaluated against similar organizations or markets, and each category can be evaluated using a combination of objective and subjective data. The results for each category can be represented with a score from one to five (see Exhibit 8.3). One reflects low readiness, and five represents an organization that, for all practical purposes, is already organized as an ACO and merely needs to develop alternative payer strategies to function as an ACO. While

Exhibit 8.2 Effort/Yield Model for Weighing Options

High
Low
Effort / Investment
Least Favorable
Most Favorable
Low
Yield / Benefit
High

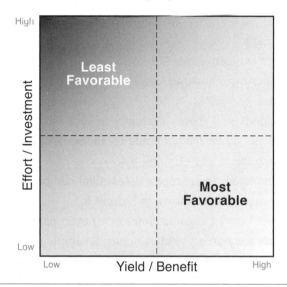

Exhibit 8.3 Levels of ACO Readiness

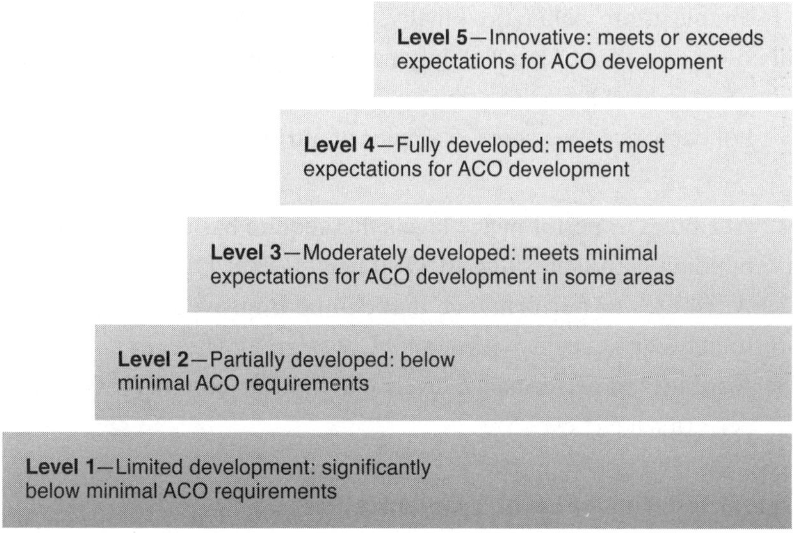

Level 5—Innovative: meets or exceeds expectations for ACO development
Level 4—Fully developed: meets most expectations for ACO development
Level 3—Moderately developed: meets minimal expectations for ACO development in some areas
Level 2—Partially developed: below minimal ACO requirements
Level 1—Limited development: significantly below minimal ACO requirements

physicians are scientists and tend to value objective data exclusively in clinical decisions, we consider subjective data just as important in organizational assessments. An objective measure such as "cost per adjusted discharge" can say a lot about the operational readiness of an organization; a subjective measure such as "staff's level of confidence in current leadership," however, can say even more about the organization's readiness.

Organizations will score differently in each category. An aggregate assessment can be made by adding the scores. The full assessment looks like the chart in Exhibit 8.4.

Once completed, an aggregate assessment can be mapped on the 2×2 effort/yield grid, as shown in Exhibit 8.5.

Notice that Level 1 organizations aren't even plotted on the grid. That's because they aren't ready to consider implementing an ACO strategy. In particular, they don't have the required leadership, management skills, or physician organization—the core building blocks. Moving forward with an ACO strategy at Level 1 would be an unwise decision. Level 2, 3, and 4 organizations are ready to pursue the ACO strategy—beginning at different levels, focusing on different areas, and proceeding at different rates as long as their assessments suggest a favorable effort/yield ratio. Finally, those at Level 5 essentially meet all criteria for an ACO and simply need to focus on their payer strategy. (See Exhibit 8.6.)

For each level, we share examples of attributes or performance:

1. Attributes or performance levels that require basic foundation building before pursuing ACO strategy (Level 1)
2. Attributes or performance that can be improved or expanded to achieve success within an ACO strategy (Levels 2, 3, 4)
3. Attributes or performance levels that indicate current ACO-level performance (Level 5)

Characteristics of Level 1 Organizations

This level consists of those that require some foundation-building work before considering the ACO strategy.

Exhibit 8.4 ACO Readiness Assessment Chart

	Level 1	Level 2	Level 3	Level 4	Level 5
Leadership and Culture					
Operational Excellence					
Care Integration					
Physician Alignment					
Technology Enablement					
External Environment					
Recommendation					

Exhibit 8.5 Completed Effort/Yield Model

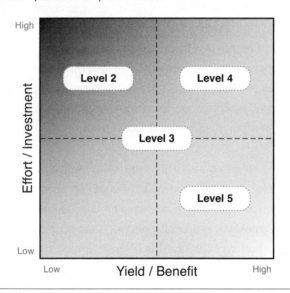

Leadership Commitment and Culture

Level 1 organizations tend to have underdeveloped strategies and short-term goals. They are focused as freestanding or holding company–type hospitals or hospital systems, not *healthcare* systems. There is little

Exhibit 8.6 Considerations for Each Readiness Level

Level	Consideration
1	Foundational work is strongly advised before pursuing the ACO strategy
2, 3, 4	Ready to pursue the ACO strategy; use assessment to guide design and implementation efforts
5	Already organized as an ACO in all but name and may already operate as an ACO with a captive MCO; ready to negotiate payer strategy

emphasis on the ambulatory components of delivery and the integration of care between the ambulatory and inpatient environments. These organizations place a priority on revenue, occupancy, volume, and market share as primary drivers of success. They see physician engagement, care integration, and margin enhancement through operating efficiencies as secondary or even tertiary drivers of success. Finally, these organizations tend to see physician integration in terms of practice acquisition or employment rather than in terms of shared leadership and partnership.

Generally, hospitals and healthcare systems in this category suffer low trust among the physicians and between physicians and the hospital. There is evidence of physician–hospital tension and competition for patients in diagnostic and specialty services and hospitals. Primary care physicians are no longer involved in hospital affairs, and specialists tend to leave the hospital or build their own competing facilities. Medical staff meetings are often poorly attended. If other hospitals are active in the same market, many members of the medical staff split allegiance among the hospitals, pitting one against the other for "benefits," such as technology investments, medical directorships, or favorable call compensation.

Finally, these organizations tend to exhibit a culture of "working alone together" among the medical staff and between physicians and the hospital. There is no common vision, no collective goals, and no sense of shared destiny.

Operational Excellence

As noted, achieving operational excellence is often subordinated to goals such as maximizing revenue, occupancy, and market share. This approach is often reflected in higher-than-average operating costs; high cost per discharge; low productivity; higher lengths of stay; and less focus on internal measures of operating performance such as waiting times, discharge time of day, utilization of scarce resources, and clinical throughput measures. The organization's average or substandard performance outcomes generally reflect its lack of commitment to operational excellence.

Care Integration

Level 1 organizations show little evidence of effective care integration. These organizations tend to operate more as silos than as systems of care. Measures that reflect a low priority for care integration often include high readmission rates and case mix–adjusted length of stay, low referral capture among employed or affiliated physician practices, and below-average core measures performance. Other notable performance observations include high use of emergency services for low-acuity care, high one-day admission rates, and little or no use of clinical pathways to integrate multiple disciplines of care beyond those used—for example, in the emergency department (ED) or the neonatal intensive care unit (NICU). In these environments, hospitalists are poorly utilized, and standardized specialist-driven critical care oversight is frequently resisted. This often indicates distrust or self-interested unwillingness to participate in programs designed to better integrate care. Finally, lack of an electronic health record (EHR), while possibly the result of other factors, often indicates of lack of emphasis on care integration.

Physician Alignment

Physician alignment in Level 1 organizations is often tribal. Doctor allegiance is limited to their specialties, ethnic groups, medical training sites, board certification, and so forth, setting up competitive factions that protect each "tribe's" members and compete with others. Even when there is civility among the physicians, integrated service lines rarely exist and tensions between competing specialties abound (e.g., orthopedics and neurosurgery compete for spine procedures; cardiology, interventional radiology, and vascular surgery all compete for patients with peripheral vascular disease; general surgery and specialty surgery compete for breast, oncology, or colorectal surgery). In these organizations, the medical executive committee is frequently reactionary and oppositional, seeing its role as that of protecting physicians from the hospital. Bad behavior and inferior performance by physicians are inadequately addressed by peer-review processes. These problems show up in daily behavior and are reflected in core indicators or pay-for-performance contracts.

Physician leadership tends to be weak, political, and disengaged in Level 1 organizations. Clinical department leadership is elected. Often, the job goes to someone merely because "it's her turn" to assume the role. Finally, in these systems the chief medical officer or vice president of medical affairs is frequently perceived as a physician who has "gone over to the dark side" rather than a physician who is actively involved in executive decisions to the benefit of everyone on the medical staff.

Technology Enablement

Not surprisingly, the lack of cohesion and commitment to a shared agenda delays the investment in technology. In other cases acquisition of technology has been a reactionary response to strong lobbying or threats by key ("royalty") physicians. Too often, unfortunately, the acquired equipment (e.g., gamma knife, da Vinci surgical robot, computer software) is significantly underutilized. The adoption of an EHR tends to be highly politicized in these environments. Design and implementation of the EHR are difficult; physicians don't give enough input, and thus the systems that result are not user-friendly or accessible to some physicians. Other well-functioning technology supports, such as a clinical decision support system, are underutilized because of lack of physician buy-in, training, or commitment.

External Environment

Level 1 organizations tend to have less competitive urgency to pursue an ACO strategy. Any glimmer of interest in the ACO is associated with "locking up the physicians" rather than pursuing outcomes. Consequently, unlike the other levels, the external environment plays little role in determining readiness because the real challenges lie within the organization rather than outside of it.

Characteristics of Levels 2, 3, and 4 Organizations

These levels consist of those ready to pursue an ACO strategy.

Leadership and Culture

Organizations in Levels 2, 3, and 4 each start from a different place and will likely proceed at a different pace. Level 2 requires foundational work. Level 3 must close identified gaps. Level 4 needs to refine structures, systems, and practices.

These organizations tend to have emerging (Level 2) or well-developed and well-communicated (Levels 3 and 4) market differentiation strategies; those strategies and goals reflect a focus on clinical quality and operational efficiency. The goals reflect an appreciation of the continuum of health delivery from the ambulatory to the inpatient and back to the ambulatory environment. Level 2 organizations are aware of the need for integration, while Level 3 and 4 organizations are designing and implementing systems to address that need. Performance dashboards—computer screens that show real-time performance measurements intended to assist management decision making—emphasize components of quality, patient satisfaction, employee and physician satisfaction (Level 2), integration of the components (levels 3 and 4), and efforts to manage resources.

These hospitals and systems tend to have physicians in leadership and management positions who are involved in decision making at both the strategic and operational levels of the hospital. This is reflected in organizational structure and mechanisms for direct feedback from physicians. As with all attributes in this category, Level 3 and 4 organizations tend to be more advanced than Level 2 organizations.

The most significant cultural attribute of Level 2, 3, and 4 hospitals is that they are beginning to operate or already operate as systems of care. Turf issues, tribal issues, departmental issues, specialty issues, nursing issues, physician issues, and so forth are subordinated to "system" issues. Increasingly, the focus is on the patient. Tensions among the medical staff are less evident, and tensions between physicians and the hospital are either minimized or relatively isolated. Physicians manage themselves as a more tightly coupled system, which is a critical attribute for ACO success (see sidebar on page 77).

Distrust among physicians and between physicians and the hospital has lessened or is absent. Physicians are actively involved in strategic and operational decisions through formal and informal shared leadership. The insidious, creeping cynicism that often pervades hospital culture has been replaced by growing trust among employees throughout the organization.

The system of care is united around a common vision of the future, and most caregivers who operate in the system have at least a rudimentary understanding of the system's vision and goals. Incentives are well aligned with goals, minimizing cynicism and resignation. Staff turnover is below industry standards and staff satisfaction is higher than average.

Medical staff meetings are well attended and substantive, and there is little sense that some participants are being treated differently from others; when they are, leadership transparency explains why and makes a rational case for the treatment. Physician and staff pride is growing or high. When they have a choice, doctors prefer to work in the hospital over alternatives. Teamwork is apparent in work processes and results.

Operational Excellence

Performance dashboards, committee structures, incentives and rewards, and performance outcome measures in Level 3 and 4 organizations reflect a commitment to and focus on operational excellence. Outcomes often include above-average or even market-leading performance on core measures, safety measures, revenue per available bed day, length of stay, throughput and productivity measures, and cost per discharge or overall care process. Cross-subsidization is deliberate and based on an intentional strategy rooted in the organization's mission. Physicians and hospital managers work together to optimize hospital or system efficiency from emergency services to bed utilization, operating room management, ICU utilization, discharge, and follow-up.

Hospitals in these three levels tend to have the financial resources to invest in cost-savings technology and understand they cannot exclusively cut or grow their way to profitability; they realize a balanced approach is warranted. They are apt to have a balanced fiscal strategy focusing on revenue, cost, and margin per unit of available capacity. That lets them see the merits of shared-savings payments in return for reduced readmissions as an opportunity to reduce suboptimal utilization or to reduce fixed costs rather than as a threat to their bottom line. As a result, these organizations, particularly in Levels 3 and 4, are beginning to view their role in the full continuum of care.

Care Integration

Level 2 organizations are experimenting with cross-functional teams to design and manage care integration processes; Level 3 and 4 organizations use them heavily. Clinical protocols, pathways, and care plans are embraced and widely used to integrate care and optimize clinical outcomes. Hospitalist programs are widely and effectively used to manage inpatient care, and, particularly in Level 3 and 4 organizations, they focus on operational excellence. The hospitalist programs and emergency and urgent care services communicate effectively with affiliated community-based physicians. Referrals for specialty care are generally captured within the overall system; more so as the organization moves up the performance ladder.

Hospitals in Levels 3 and 4 are more likely to have functionally integrated service lines, fully qualified centers of excellence, and functioning institutes, and most operate using a combination of physician leadership and professional management. Level 2 organizations are just beginning to develop such programs. They have not just attacked pockets of clinical waste but, in anticipation of the future, also have begun to actively consolidate and automate various functions to operate at a 5–10 percent lower variable and fixed cost structure than competitors.

Hospitals and systems in these categories also rely heavily on EHRs for clinical management and decision support. The resulting outcomes demonstrate low readmission rates, above-average or market-leading core measures performance, better performance on pay-for-performance contracts, and low utilization of the ED for lesser-acuity care.

Finally, incentives and rewards throughout the organization reflect a genuine commitment to care integration at all levels. Many incentives are team based rather than individual based. The incentives (financial and non financial) are designed to motivate top performers to continue to raise the bar, and underperformers to improve. And, perhaps most important, Level 3 and 4 organizations tend to enjoy measurably higher satisfaction among employees and medical staff than Level 1 and 2 organizations do.

Physician Alignment

While clearly reflecting a continuum, Level 2, 3, and 4 organizations demonstrate greater physician alignment. Physicians actively participate in setting system strategy and designing and managing system operations. The imprimatur of the physicians is no longer solely vested in the medical executive committee: Clinical department leadership, service line leadership, programmatic leadership, and functional leadership are beginning to be shared between physicians and hospital or system leaders. There is minimal evidence of tribal behavior, and while competition among physician groups exists, it is managed in such as way that it is rarely disruptive.

Physician leadership is strong, active, and accepted by both peers and system professional managers. Physicians are beginning to manage the behavior of their peers. There are formal programs and growing participation in physician leadership development, including classes, training, and the pursuit of additional degrees. In Level 3 and 4 organizations, individual report cards are being introduced or are already being used for performance improvement.

It follows that in Level 3 and 4 organizations protocols and care pathways are widely used and great pride is taken in system performance. These hospitals and systems have also begun to develop formal programs to reengage independent, high-performing, community-based physicians who no longer actively participate in hospital activities, further supporting a sense of systemness. Finally, particularly in Level 3 and 4 systems, the chief medical officer (CMO) or vice president of medical affairs is seen by physicians as an important and integral part of the system leadership team, building trust and confidence in the role of physicians within the system.

Many Level 4 organizations are bifurcating the role of the CMO into two roles—the chief medical informatics officer (CMIO) and the chief quality officer. Both are critical roles in the ACO. In organizations that pursue this strategy, the role of the CMO is frequently being absorbed by integrated physician leadership teams composed of physicians and professional managers. Organizations that operate in this manner frequently boast that they "don't need a chief medical officer anymore." Rather, they prefer subject matter experts in informatics and quality.

Technology Enablement

Level 2 organizations are in the throes of introducing EHRs and other technology supports. Level 3 and 4 systems have fully operational EHRs into which they are beginning to integrate employed and independent ambulatory practices so that outside doctors have access to hospital records. Some are experimenting with newer technology that enables information exchange between information technology platforms. In Level 4 organizations, care pathways and protocols are fully integrated into the EHR as its decision support. As noted, many of these systems now have CMIOs to co-manage clinical interfaces with technology.

Investments in technology are integrated into hospital or system strategy to ensure high return on investments, and physician input is actively sought for these strategic capital investments. In Level 3 and 4 systems the physicians actively use technology supports and actively participate in their improvements.

External Environment

Levels 2, 3, and 4 organizations invest time, energy, and resources to engage other providers and payers in ACO tactical design and operations. Currently, Level 3 and 4 organizations are engaging other institutions to contribute to the full continuum of care, including subacute hospitals, rehabilitation hospitals, home health care agencies, dialysis programs, and care management programs. These institutions are actively engaged in conversations to determine their interest and readiness to participate in integrated care programs within the ACO model.

In some advanced markets, assisted living communities are seen as another set of potential ACO partners, as these communities include many residents who have had to endure dislocation with previous healthcare systems when joining the community. Management should consider exploring opportunities with local, regional, or national assisted living programs. In most markets, this is an untapped opportunity.

Level 2 organizations are beginning to consider reaching out to local payer organizations. Levels 3 and 4 are already approaching their payers outside the normal negotiation cycle to think strategically about what changes in market demographics, Medicare and Medicaid products and policies, and technology mean to both sides. They coordinate plans to pay for the data and tools to measure avoidable costs, reduce those avoidable costs, and align incentives to share and ultimately sustain those savings among themselves and even with patients. These providers partner with their payers to help fund the movement to a lower-cost, more competitive business model rather than merely hope that past reimbursement increases can be sustained.

These initial market explorations and conversations with outside institutions can begin with something as simple as the two CEOs meeting for coffee. Even if nothing comes from the meeting, you've gained additional market intelligence that will be useful as your institution becomes more fully integrated.

Characteristics of Level 5 Organizations
This level consists of those already functioning as ACOs.

Chapters 3, 4, and 5 describe the attributes, capabilities, and outcomes required for ACO participation. Generally speaking, hospitals and systems at Level 5 already demonstrate many of the characteristics described in those chapters. Therefore, the characteristics found in the assessment process are reviewed here only briefly.

Leadership and Culture

Level 5 organization leaders are avidly committed to care integration and operational efficiency. This is reflected in the organization's vision, the strategic and performance goals, and the actions and outcomes produced by physicians and staff who actively support these goals. There is no ambiguity about what the leaders or the organization stand for and care about. This is experienced at all levels of the organization by everyone employed by or affiliated with the system.

Perhaps most significant, however, is leadership's acceptance of the paradox described at the end of Chapter 2: Leaders understand and can manage the conflicting realities of the present and future states of healthcare delivery. They are not thrown off balance by having one foot in each world.

Level 5 organizations display many of the cultural attributes described in Chapter 5, as witnessed by the results of their "Changing the Rules®" assessment (see Chapter 9). These organizations have strong cultures, with people who are willing to do whatever is necessary and accept whatever consequences are associated with supporting their culture, because they recognize that culture is the silent driver of organizational performance. In brief, the "simple rules" in Level 5 organizations reflect the wind at their backs with respect to clinical effectiveness and operational efficiency.

Operational Excellence

Commitment to operational excellence is evident in strategy, goals, performance measures, rewards, incentives, and day-to-day operations. Waste, redundancy, unwanted variation, and rework are abhorred and, wherever possible, eliminated. Opportunities to standardize and automate administrative and care processes, consolidate operations, or lease and outsource to more efficient providers are part of the standard operating procedure for these providers. This focus on operational excellence is evidenced in many or all of the performance measures noted above, especially metrics like cost per adjusted available bed day, revenue per adjusted available bed day, length of stay, and other productivity measures.

Care Integration

Level 5 organizations view care integration as a high-order priority, and clinical outcomes reflect that focus. Core measures results and other metrics are market leading. The financial and clinical rewards from pay-for-performance reimbursement strategies are apparent to all who participate.

Above all, however, care integration is apparent to the patients cared for by the system. While they may or may not be able to articulate what accounts for their experience, they feel well cared for by the system and demonstrate preference to receive care within the system. While "patient stickiness" is not a concern for the system, efforts and resources are continually applied to maintaining or improving patient satisfaction. New patient-interfacing systems are constantly being piloted and those that demonstrate value are implemented.

In addition, organizations have moved beyond treating individual patients. They have begun to manage care at the population level. Clinicians are discovering useful causal relationships between treatment and overall population health. They are learning which interventions have the greatest impact on entire cohorts of patients, such as patients with diabetes, cancer, and other chronic diseases.

Physician Alignment

Whether employed or affiliated, physicians in Level 5 organizations are fully supportive and avid proponents of the organization's mission, vision, strategy, and values, because these reflect the physicians' values as well. There is no we/they dynamic. Tensions that develop among the physicians and between the system and the physicians are actively managed and resolved. The popular saying "Stuff happens" still applies, but when it does there are clear structures, processes, and expectations in place to manage the situation. Over time, those who do not share the culture and goals of the organization are weeded out and replaced by individuals who do. They either self-select or are ushered "off the plane," to refer back to the clarity of the flight attendants in Chapter 5.

Technology Enablement

Level 5 organizations don't just *have* the technology and don't just *use* the technology, they also *invent* the technology and innovate using it. While Level 3 and 4 organizations are willing to use the technology to support care, Level 5 organizations use technology to change how care is delivered. They can begin to see health trends in the entire population of people they serve and can move beyond just caring for individual patients into using technology to improve the health of their communities.

External Environment

While Level 5 organizations, with a few notable exceptions, operate in competitive environments, they are the market leaders and set the standards and pace for their markets. Payers compete with other payers to steer business to these high-quality, low-cost providers, instead of the other way around. These providers can even employ peak pricing, charging less at off-peak hours to steer patients to underutilized capacity, much like leaders in other industries do.

After the Assessment: What's Next?

Going forward, organizations evaluated, whether by shallow dive or deep dive assessment, as Level 1 require a fundamentally different approach from those evaluated as Level 2, 3, or 4. Level 5 organizations' strategies reflect their unique positions as well. Because Level 1 organizations are not ready for design or implementation of an ACO model, strategies for them are addressed in this chapter. Suggested strategies for Level 2, 3, 4, and 5 organizations are described in Chapter 9.

Those assessed as Level 1 have one of two profiles: (1) they demonstrate more or less "global" results and have foundational work to accomplish on many dimensions, or (2) they are ready on some dimensions but not ready on a small number of key dimensions, most notably leadership commitment, physician alignment, and operational excellence. Significant deficits in these areas put these organizations in nonstarter status for considering ACO strategies. The deficits must be addressed before proceeding with any further consideration of this strategy.

This chapter concludes with a description of activities and actions that would represent foundational work in each of the five categories, plus market environment, for those organizations deemed not ready for ACO strategies. This work is crucial regardless of whether the organization scored low in all areas or did well overall but fell down in a key area such as leadership and culture.

Leadership and Culture—Foundational Work

The most common and critical readiness gap for organizations assessed as Level 1 on leadership and culture is the absence of a system-of-care perspective on the part of their administrative leaders. Leaders in these "systems" still see their organizations as hospitals and their work as inpatient care. They have invested little in the development of a managed ambulatory component to their care. They generally have vastly underdeveloped primary care programs and relationships.

They focus most heavily on engaging admitting proceduralists, like spine and heart doctors, and the engagement frequently focuses on the acquisition of capital equipment, the selection of medical directorships, and appointment to the hospital board. These institutions have to start at the beginning by educating their boards, senior leaders, and physician leaders (either the medical executive committee or other formal and informal physician leaders) about how healthcare reform is likely to affect their community. The hospital and the physicians need to envision themselves as part of a system of care, and use that as the starting point for recrafting the vision of the hospital.

Leaders need to make the case for why a real disruptive change needs to take place in the organization. Often, this will result in the appointment of a physician advisory group (separate from the medical executive committee) to help the hospital integrate both the ambulatory environment and the inpatient environment. This is an opportunity for hospital leadership to engage ambulatory-based physicians who have drifted away from the hospital over the past decade and use them to advise the hospital on manpower planning, program planning, and quality and safety improvement initiatives. More important, they can engage this estranged collection of physicians around handoffs and care continuity. These are the resources who really understand the need for care coordination and the current deficiencies associated with that need. That's a good place to start the conversation. Despite the fact that physician advisory councils typically focus on small, parochial issues of concern to doctors, over time these councils can be useful in helping hospital leaders make important strategic and operational decisions. At least they can point out the land mines so that they can be avoided and defused.

The next step in the process is to create a strategy and a plan (or revise an existing one) that support the new vision for the healthcare system. Conversion of the vision into a strategic plan reinforces leadership commitment to a new way of being, and if that process is accomplished with the imprimatur of the physicians, its credibility and relevance will be reinforced. The medical executive committee is often too political a forum to be used effectively as the innovative voice of the physicians. Rather, we suggest the physician advisory council be used to give input into this process and enough members of the medical executive committee be included on the council so that endorsement of the strategic plan by the committee can be expected. Innovative tools are available to assist with the envisioning process.

Cultural alignment is one of the most difficult issues to address. As we stated in Chapter 5, simply declaring that a new culture will take effect next Tuesday will not erase the years of policies and actions that produced the current culture. An effective technique to use here is a cultural assessment tool that exposes aspects of the current culture, makes them more manageable, and maps current cultural attributes to the emerging vision and strategy. Assuming physician participation (either an advisory council or the medical executive committee or both) along with participation from board and management, this process is an excellent opportunity to engage all parties in identifying some opportunities to change relationships and build trust. When this process is undertaken, we strongly advise the process include hospital middle management, such as nursing managers and clinical directors, because they are the managers who generally have the most visible and substantial relationship with the physicians.

Building Trust—Foundational Work

Trust is an issue that comes up frequently in healthcare cultures. Here are some ways to deal with a lack of trust. Contrary to common perception, trust represents the ability to accurately predict another individual's behavior. Most relationships begin with no trust but evolve, over time, into either trusting or distrustful ones. The direction of the evolution is the product of explicit or implicit promises made and then either kept or violated. Most of these promises are inferred, primarily on the basis of expediency or the imprecision of the English language.

The process of building trust first requires that participants let go of the past or at least suspend feelings and beliefs rooted in history. The second step requires a set of *explicit* compacts or promises between parties along with identification of "conditions of satisfaction." All parties must agree on what represents the fulfillment of each promise. It is best to start with promises that have little ambiguity and short time spans, and that both parties are highly confident can be delivered. Then, over time, the promises can expand in complexity and impact.

For example, trust is often eroded with such common phrases as, "Let me get back to you on that," uttered in passing in response to an issue that cannot be resolved at the moment. Unfortunately, this phrase creates a commitment on the part of the speaker. When the instigator doesn't circle back, the small interaction creates a withdrawal in the "trust account" with the other individual. Handled properly, such a small interaction can build or reinforce trust. The response is important, regardless of how trivial the issue at hand is. In fact, it is often the most trivial response that is most appreciated. A little effort can make a big deposit in the "social capital account." Such interactions are extremely important when healthcare organizations ask doctors for input into decision making. This issue is discussed further in Chapter 9.

The term *transparency* is often used in discussions of organizational culture and is raised in one of the simple rules suggested in Chapter 5. Unfortunately, it is impossible for executives to be *fully* transparent on all issues of interest to internal stakeholders. It is suggested, rather, that transparency refer to making certain processes (e.g., decision-making rights, responsibilities) transparent. When announcing decisions that affect stakeholders, trust is enhanced by sharing the decision; the rationale for the decision; the likely implications of the decision; and the process, data, and reasoning used to arrive at the decision. Sharing this information "tells the story" about the decision in a way that builds confidence and trust rather than eroding them.

Operational Excellence—Foundational Work

In the new vision and strategy, operating efficiency has to be elevated to the same level of importance previously accorded to revenue, occupancy, and market share. Then, it has to be reflected in the activities, incentives, and rewards that drive performance. Foundational work entails a close look at whether the organization has the financial health (both margin and cash) required to pursue an ACO strategy on its own or in partnership with another organization. Assuming the finances are sufficient, leadership must focus on improving its variable and fixed cost structure (supply chain, bed configuration, staffing levels, capital needs) within a soft reimbursement and volume environment. This focus on financial health requires the hospital, in turn, to improve productivity of current operations (e.g., waiting times, clinical throughput, integration with ambulatory care, bed management, length-of-stay management) to generate the margins required to invest in further improvement efforts.

As throughput is better managed and length of stay shortens, hospitals will have more empty beds. This is part of the paradox that has to be managed as hospitals move from traditional fee-for-service models to the ACO. With the old mind-set, the empty beds are a cause for panic. In the new ACO mind-set, the empty beds represent low-cost expansion of capacity. The hospital can respond by growing clinical service lines to fill the new capacity, or it can consolidate operations to reduce fixed or operating costs. Sometimes a combination of both is best. Systems that fail to capture all referrals within the system are best advised to take a good, hard look at why that is. The simplest way is to ask the referring physicians. Recapturing those referrals is often what fills the beds emptied by greater throughput efficiency.

Care Integration—Foundational Work

Either of the two assessment processes (shallow or deep dive) will usually expose opportunities for improvement in operational efficiencies or clinical outcomes. Level 1 and 2 organizations need to review their anatomy (structures) and physiology (operations) to locate and dismantle the silos that impede care integration. Leaders must pay special attention to the ambulatory environment so that pre- and post-hospital care is integrated as well. Medicare's 30-day readmission reimbursement policy has created a new vulnerability for these institutions. These institutions need to quickly integrate care to reduce avoidable readmissions.

The physician advisory council would be an excellent incubator for initiating or expanding care pathways. These can include high-volume or common clinical conditions, such as total joint replacement, chest pain management, management of congestive heart failure, stroke, or diabetes. Proprietary indexes available from Navigant and other consulting groups can help physicians identify which high-volume diagnoses are good places to start.

The new vision will highlight the hospital as part of the larger continuum of healthcare. Physician leaders will need to look at gaps in the system—areas where care isn't seamless for either the patient or the doctor. Each problem should be assigned a small taskforce of about five hospital managers and five physicians to help craft a solution. The task force builds trust and intimacy among the participants. It also enables all participants to leave behind the obsolete concept that they are solely in the "hospital business." And whenever a doctor comes forward to point out a problem, leaders should see an opportunity to engage that doctor to help craft a solution.

The council would also offer an excellent forum for addressing unresolved issues pertaining to the hospitalist program; emergency services; or communication, including the EHR. Additionally, that body could sponsor a subgroup that focuses on specific service lines, critical care, or perioperative care. Some hospitals have been successful at bringing together subspecialists or subspecialty groups to design and implement care pathways. This has the added benefit of fostering greater cohesion among the physicians, though the competitive nature of the physicians often makes such collaboration difficult.

Physician Alignment—Foundational Work

Establishing a physician advisory council is a good first step in building physician alignment. It is often helpful for that body to work with senior management to establish ground rules to guide hospital–physician relationships in financial agreements, medical directorships, joint ventures, employment, and so forth.

The next level of physician alignment often involves the development of an integrated leadership structure for the hospital or components of the hospital such as a key function (e.g., emergency services) or strategically important service line (e.g., women's health). Such structures reflect needs and capabilities that are unique to each hospital, but all share some common threads: In the case of hospital-level integrated leadership, physicians are appointed by executive management to serve as senior managers of the hospital, along with, for example, the chief nursing officer, chief operating officer, chief financial officer, chief medical officer, and legal counsel. These physicians bring clinical care insights and perspectives to strategic and operational decision making. Those who participate in such a structure must act as fiduciaries rather than as representatives of their specialty, discipline, or practice. This type of structure can be an excellent stepping stone to the integrated leadership, comprising both physicians and professional managers, required for the ACO.

Level 1 organizations are not ready to form a physician organization or physician hospital organization. The trust just isn't high enough among the physicians for them to comfortably surrender independence. For that reason, attention focused on building physician–hospital relationships should be balanced with attention on building intra-medical-staff relationships. Strategies that have worked to improve these relationships include the following:

- Sponsoring specialty-specific educational forums
- Conducting educational workshops on healthcare reform
- Convening committees to aid relationships with common services and emergency services, ambulatory testing, or hospitalists
- Designing referral processes and systems

Much like leadership commitment, physician alignment is one of the two critical core competencies that need to be at sufficiently high levels to support the initiation of the ACO strategy.

Technology Enablement—Foundational Work

In healthcare, nothing represents a shared destiny more than the EHR; no topic produces the same level of interest, concern, and engagement. If technology is at Level 1, you need to assemble a forum of physicians, nurses, and managers to develop attributes and specifications for an EHR. While physicians ought to be included in developing strategic priorities for other technology investments, the EHR is a technology prerequisite for the ACO and should be developed first. Previous limitations on making such technology available to community-based physicians are being reconsidered in light of the ACO. As mentioned in an earlier chapter, avoid the mistake of introducing too sophisticated a medical record. It is too easy for physicians to feel lost in the process. Rather, select an EHR that can be enhanced over time so that the physicians don't need to swallow it all at once.

External Environment Positioning—Foundational Work

Hospitals and healthcare systems assessed as Level 1 are not competitively positioned to succeed. Consequently, an ACO strategy may be a stretch and other alternatives (e.g., affiliation, merger, turnaround) may be in the cards before an ACO strategy can bear fruit.

For these organizations, the first market-facing step is to assess the immediate market's unmet needs. For one safety net hospital in a blighted portion of the Northeast, this meant meeting with local leaders (e.g., schools, city council, county, places of worship, business groups) to inventory the basic health needs of the community and then rallying around a core set of services. From there, the hospital worked on getting the funds, which came from several sources:

- Grant funds aimed at the biggest healthcare cost drivers for the population (including diabetes management, substance abuse, and readmissions)
- Increased collections rates (the hospital partnered with the more prosperous hospitals in the region to share in the cost of the software and processes to improve collections from third-party payers)
- Aggressive negotiation strategy with third-party payers that involved
  - Demonstrating that payment rates had dropped well below market parity
  - Illustrating the recent efforts to reduce waste and unnecessary costs, such as standardizing supply usage, negotiating 20 percent discounts, and pursuing 340(b) status (this helped payers see they were not simply propping up an inefficient, strategically irrelevant player)
  - Board-level conversations with the payers to invest in certain cost-saving technologies (e.g., physician assistants and nurse practitioners, generic versus brand-name drugs, simple diagnostic imaging and lab equipment rather than more expensive equipment a competitor used)

With an influx of cash, the hospital was able to get back on its feet. The partnership with other local hospitals was crucial. It enabled the hospital to meet market needs without unnecessary and costly duplication of technology. Moreover, this "indirect partnering" approach laid the groundwork for a regional ACO strategy.

Organizational Questions

The organizational questions raised in this chapter include the following:

- Is the ACO a rational and reasonable strategy for our organization to pursue?
- What are our gaps, and what will it take to fill them?
- Do we have the resources and leadership commitment to pursue this strategy?
- How should we pursue this strategy?
- How can we fund this pursuit?

Category of Readers	Key Concepts	Actions to Consider
Category A (interested)	• Shallow dive	• Shallow dive assessment to determine whether an ACO strategy could be advantageous for the organization
	• Maturity model	• Educational events to familiarize stakeholders about what an ACO is
	• Deep dive	• Participation in collaborative or other learning options
Category B (engaged)	• Deep dive	• Educational events to build clarity about the organization's ACO model and intentions
	• Contemporary models used by leading organizations today	• Deep-dive assessment to develop a coordinated, integrated ACO road map
	• Funding sources	• Development of a funding plan
Category C (committed)	• Deep dive	• Assessment of current strategy and plan against the elements identified for the deep dive to make sure that all bases are covered
	• Funding sources	• Development of a funding plan
	• Business planning	• Development of a business plan

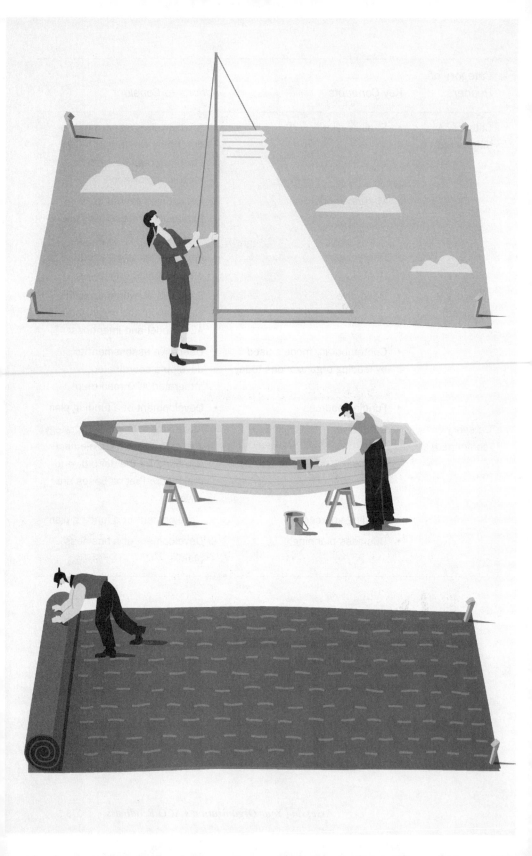

9

Building the ACO

Building an accountable care organization means re-designing and reorganizing care and reprogramming people and systems within a new care model. This is really hard work. But we're going to tackle this because it's the right way to deliver care.

—Ralph de la Torre, MD
CEO, Caritas Christi Healthcare System

Every healthcare payer and provider organization that has been in operation for the past 25 years is already somewhere along the journey to an accountable care organization (ACO); no organization is starting *de novo*. Building an ACO, therefore, is much like changing the tires on the car while it is driving down the highway: Unlike restaurants that can close for business for at least a few hours each night, healthcare organizations cannot shut down during renovation. Each participating entity in the ACO has taken its own course to get to where it is today, and each has envisioned where it wants to be tomorrow. The ACO was not part of any organization's vision or strategic plan back in 2005. Therefore, the chance to create an ACO as an alternative financing and delivery practice model represents a true discontinuity that affords each potential participant with the opportunity to reevaluate its future course. Each must bear in mind that the ACO strategy is but one of a multitude of competing approaches available to healthcare organizations that face the uncertain future under healthcare reform.

Entering After the Movie Has Started

As stated earlier in this book, the ACO is not a model that should be of interest to all payers or providers. Its success is not based on universal acceptance. Yet, improved quality and efficiency are likely to be important goals that every healthcare system must strive for, regardless of whether they choose to operate as an ACO. Without that focus there is little hope that the United States can transform its healthcare ecosystem from its activities-based, transactional market to a value-based system dedicated to improved clinical outcomes and efficiency.

Building an ACO is more like renovating an existing house or building an addition than constructing a home from scratch. Certain components already exist and undoubtedly function well, others exist but need improvement, others need a complete overhaul, and still others do not yet exist and must be created. The purpose of the assessment process is to accurately identify which components fit into each of these categories. The assessment phase is a critical precursor to building the ACO.

Recognizing that each organization that adopts the ACO strategy will be starting from a different baseline, this chapter is organized as if the ACO is starting tabula rasa (a blank slate), even though, as just stated, it is understood that none will be starting without at least some elements already in place. Additionally, the recommendations in this chapter should not give the erroneous impression that we believe that the restructuring process will be linear and orderly. Nothing could be further from the truth. Rather, the goal of this chapter is to be reasonably comprehensive to make certain that important design and implementation elements are not overlooked. Some parts of the chapter will be irrelevant to many organizations that are further along in their ACO implementation.

Organizations that achieved Level 1 ratings (see discussion in Chapter 8) should not embark on the course outlined in this chapter.

They first need to do the foundational work to get ready. Organizations in Level 2 should begin but be prepared for a long and arduous journey that will require significant commitment and resources to attain the full ACO readiness. On the other hand, organizations that have achieved Levels 3 or 4 are in good shape, and those at Level 5 are on the threshold of operating within a fully functioning ACO strategy.

We presuppose a certain level of prior organization, without which it would be difficult to contemplate, let alone design and build, an ACO. For example, it would be completely naïve to think that a hospital system could effectively create a functional ACO with a group of independent physicians who lack any formal organization. Therefore, when we address issues around physician organization, it assumes the preexistence of a reasonable level of physician coalescence that may require some renovation, rather than an unorganized group trying to start from scratch. In similar fashion, many elements addressed in this chapter presuppose a preexisting baseline level of function. As with many processes, the first step focuses on engagement.

Let's Start Talking About the ACO

Any component of a healthcare finance or delivery system could be the convener of a conversation about an ACO. The conversation could be initiated in any number of ways. Many organizations have sponsored informal meetings with local or regional payers and/or provider organizations to initiate a conversation about potential interest in forming an ACO. Some initiate the dialogue with an educational session so that everyone in the conversation begins with a common knowledge base and a set of similar assumptions. Other healthcare leaders have sponsored local or regional symposia about healthcare reform and the ACO, bringing together many payers and providers, followed by a facilitated conversation about the benefits and challenges of such a model in their community. Still others have invited potential partner organizations to accompany them at a regional or national ACO conference and used the down time between presentations to explore interest among the potential partners.

No matter what initial venue is selected, the output of that meeting should be an expression about whether there is sufficient interest in the ACO among the participants to continue the conversation. The participants also need to identify who else should be included in the conversation and create a list of questions to set an agenda. Consistent with the "mall anchor" analogy presented in Chapter 3, we strongly advise that representatives from the hospital or hospital system and physicians from the medical community be included in the conversation from the beginning. This will reinforce the concept that the ACO must include a partnership of two (historically) adversarial groups.

Don't necessarily confuse engagement for antagonism: Animation is often the strongest indicator of engagement. In virtually every change process, four changes are recognized:

- Stage one is characterized by *denial*. While leaders often think the lack of pushback is a positive sign, most often it is denial.
- Stage two exhibits *resistance*—when those asked to change are beginning to recognize that leadership isn't giving up. This is the stage when leaders, often uncomfortable with the antagonism, must recognize that the resistance is actually a demonstration of *engagement*.
- Stage three is exploration.
- Stage four is commitment.

A recent example illustrates this cycle well.

We gave a presentation to a group of IPA (independent practice association) physicians at one community hospital of a six-hospital system in the Northeast that is pursuing an ACO strategy. Two months earlier, we tried to arrange a meeting but no one responded. At this meeting, 70 physicians showed up. There was considerable pushback. Discussion was heated at times. We, as consultants, were repeatedly challenged. But at the end of the evening when we called the question about whether the IPA physicians wanted to endorse moving ahead with this strategy, the vote was nearly unanimously in favor of supporting the strategy. Afterwards, doctors came up and told us they thought it was a great meeting. Said one, "This was a great start to the process. This is the way we're going to have to work if this transformation is going to be a success." Some were beginning to enter the exploration phase of change.

The lesson here is that the emotions surrounding healthcare reform run high. Don't be put off by what appears to be initial resistance. From the outset, it's a good idea to include in the planning those local or regional agencies and service providers that focus on care coordination, particularly those with a historic interest in quality performance. Later in the process, it will be useful to invite local business leaders and patient advocates to join the conversation. Experience has shown us that it is best to invite them only when there is a reasonably strong internal commitment to pursue the ACO strategy. They will be much more valuable in the assessment and design phases of ACO development than in the strategic conversation about whether pursuit of an ACO could be beneficial to the participating organizations or to the community as a whole. At the beginning the hospital could easily represent perspectives and interests of the larger healthcare delivery system as well as those of the business community. As noted in Chapter 2, the hospital is often one of the largest employers in the community.

Each party participating in the initial conversation should be assessing the other participants along several dimensions:

- Do the other parties appear interested and engaged, or are they distracted with other strategic priorities and different time horizons?
- Is the conversation strictly about protecting turf, or do the participants recognize the potential beneficial opportunities and demonstrate enthusiasm?
- How are the other leaders balancing community/population needs with their own organizational needs?
- Are the other leaders focusing on clinical outcomes and efficiency or financial security?
- What windows exist for new, innovative ways of delivering and paying for care?

- Do some of the physicians—particularly community leaders—see potential value in the model?
- Do the participants have the capacity to commit their organization's resources to such an endeavor?
- Are there others at the meeting whom you could see as partners in creating an ACO?
- Do the others sound like people who support a movement, or people with a specific destination in mind? Are the participants setting out on the same journey?

The Shallow Dive Assessment

The initial question posed in Chapter 8 is "Could an ACO be good for us and our patients?" This tests the feasibility of the ACO for each organization and the local community. The shallow dive explores the local marketplace, payer environment, competitive landscape, physician relationships, and high-level clinical and operational performance to answer that question for all potential collaborators, including payers.

The shallow dive can be undertaken in several ways. Ideally, potential partnership organizations would jointly sponsor the shallow dive assessment, involving all the likely partners, or at least the "first round" of identified partners. Reporting the results of the shallow dive transparently could be a good way to build trust among all the participating organizations. It can also serve as an effective "stress test" for future ACO partnership relationships.

The shallow dive can answer questions that aren't threatening to the participants, such as the following:

- Could this be good for the community?
- Are there enough doctors in a physician organization (broadly defined) to make the ACO work?
- Would a more detailed analysis help prepare the organization for the ACO strategy?
- What is the magnitude of effort and investment needed for us to become a successful ACO?

Albert Mehrabian and the Secret to Handling Difficult Conversations

Throughout this book, we have stressed the importance of communication—among healthcare leaders, between various organizations that will compose the ACO, and with the rank-and-file who actually deliver care to patients.

Professor Albert Mehrabian (1971) of the University of California in Los Angeles has conducted groundbreaking research into how communication works between individuals. He hypothesized that any face-to-face communication involves three elements:

1. Words
2. Tone of voice
3. Nonverbal behavior, such as facial expressions and body language

Among Mehrabian's more striking findings is the 7 percent–38 percent–55 percent rule. He looked at situations where individuals expressed messages concerning emotions, and polled listeners whether they *liked* the person who delivered the message. In these situations, the words used by the speaker accounted for only 7 percent of whether the speaker was liked, tone of voice accounted for 38 percent, and nonverbal behavior accounted for 55 percent.

Mehrabian did not say that the words conveyed only 7 percent of *the message* the speaker delivered. But his research underscores how important tone of voice and body language are in charged situations where people are communicating about their feelings.

As they negotiate and implement the ACO strategy, healthcare leaders are likely to find themselves in many situations where they are confronted with angry, frightened, or disengaged listeners. It would serve them well to keep Mehrabian's findings in mind and think about how their *nonverbal* communication affects how their message is received.

Alternatively, one or more of the organizations could sponsor its own assessment process or sponsor the assessment on behalf of others. The shallow dive must end with an appraisal of whether the ACO *could* be good for the community and for the payers and providers within the community. However, it is far too early to determine whether it *would* be good. The decision about whether to proceed to a deep dive assessment should be based on subjective and objective findings rather than on emotion. In either event, the shallow and deep dive assessments have two purposes: The primary purpose is discovery, while the secondary is to offer the opportunity to build relationships among the prospective ACO partners.

The shallow dive process (how it's done) must be transparent to all members of the medical community, even if all the results are not shared openly. The process gets more difficult when there are two aggressive hospitals or provider systems in the community that are competing vigorously for market dominance. But this is a situation where, assuming legal challenges are passed, enlightened self-interest could overcome long-standing rivalries to create collaboration among competitors.

The Deep Dive Assessment

As noted in Chapter 8, the deep dive assessment is much more comprehensive and is used to make the business case for a go/no go decision to pursue the ACO. Because the deep dive requires data and insights from a number of potential participants, it requires full commitment and participation from all parties. It also invites leaders from all participating organizations to make a decision about how they want to pursue an ACO strategy—sequenced through pay for performance, bundled payments, the Medicare program, the second wave of Medicare participants (potentially with Medicaid), their own captive managed care organizations, or negotiations with local commercial payers (as described in Chapter 7).

The deep dive assessment also identifies where the readiness gaps are for the participating organizations. While quantification of the gaps is strongly advised, the strategy for building the ACO should not be based simply on the size of the gap but rather on the order in which to tackle the gaps. For many organizations, it is valuable to narrow a small strategic gap before tackling a larger but less strategic gap. Too many organizations develop strategies based on the size rather than the strategic importance of their real or perceived challenges.

One of the most effective processes for completing the deep dive assessment is a two-day retreat during which the participating organizations review the findings together and make a tentative go/ no go decision for the next step. The participants should identify a steering committee and cross-organizational work groups that can begin to make recommendations about corporate structure, organizational design, governance, management, and so forth. The retreat should end with the development of a timeline for the steering committee to integrate recommendations from the various work groups. The final decision regarding participation will ultimately be made by each participating organization at the end of the design phase.

There is no predictable timetable that will work for all organizations; each will have its own rhythm and pace. If the pace is too aggressive, participants will feel as if decisions are being forced upon them. If it is too slow, the process will exceed the attention span of the participants, and they will begin to lose interest. Eventually, they will stop devoting energy to it. It is best to think of the process as a flywheel that gains acceleration. If it spins fast enough, the flywheel process will reach a self-sustaining speed and will begin to generate trust and confidence on its own.

The Organizational Stress Test: Do We Even Have a Chance Here?

Most organizations that are initially uncertain about whether to adopt the ACO will have performed a shallow dive. If sufficient interest is generated, a targeted deep dive assessment will follow. If, at one extreme, the result of the shallow dive suggests an alternative strategy or, at the other extreme it suggests a high level of readiness, the decision is reasonably easy. The more difficult situation is when the shallow and deep dives do not provide clear direction.

A reasonable strategy for organizations in this ambiguous middle zone would be to designate a pilot area for clinical redesign. On the basis of that trial, they will be able to evaluate whether proceeding to a full ACO model makes sense. Organizations faced with this option might consider the following strategy:

1. Identify the system's highest-volume diagnoses for which care redesign might influence clinical, service, and business performance. Likely candidates include chronic illnesses such as diabetes, congestive heart failure, chronic obstructive pulmonary disease, or chronic renal failure. Alternatives might include high-volume procedures the organization performs, such as total joint replacement or coronary bypass.

2. Compare clinical and operational performance with local, regional, or national benchmarks to determine which of these diagnoses have room for improvement across the entire continuum.

3. Select a small number of these diagnoses—one to three—for redesign.

4. Appoint a small committee of providers, subject matter experts, care coordinators, and others necessary to provide optimal care and service in the ambulatory and inpatient settings for each diagnosis selected: Nonemployed providers might be offered a small stipend to participate. It is best if a highly committed physician leads the committee.

5. Establish a limited set of performance targets.

6. Review currently available protocols or care pathways and select one for modification.

7. Modify the protocol or care pathway to meet the needs and requirements of the system.

8. Redesign the delivery system to support the new pathway as enabled by current technology and provider commitment.

9. Require employed physicians to follow the new pathway; invite any interested voluntary physicians to participate.

10. Measure clinical, service, and business performance against baseline.

11. Tell the story of the successful redesign throughout the organization, and use it as a way of engaging those within or affiliated with the system.
12. Consider a second wave or use the experience to answer the question about whether or not to proceed with a broader ACO initiative.
13. Declare an organizational intention to continue operating using evidence-based best practices as learned from the pilot program.
14. Repeat the procedure as needed.

The above cycle should not exceed six months, or it will exceed the attention span of the organization and fail to serve as a meaningful pilot.

Now You're Committed: Steps After the Deep Dive

If you're committed to the ACO strategy, chances are you've undertaken a deep dive to identify the performance areas that require development or refinement. The steps described in this section are organized around the areas identified during the deep dive. It is important for the organization to recognize and acknowledge that everyone in the organization selected to participate in ACO design already has a fully consuming day job. For that reason the process is best organized like the process of designing a home, where an architect integrates input from the client and then reengages the client to review options and make choices. It is difficult for busy physicians and professional managers to be self-generative, particularly when focusing on innovation.

Form a Steering Committee

The steering committee is the cross-organizational body that guides and integrates the components of the design process. It should consist of senior executives from the "anchor tenants" of the ACO—typically, the hospital, the physician organization, and core participating organizations. While it is politically important to populate the steering committee with leaders authorized to make commitments on behalf of their respective organizations, it is also important to populate the committee with people who understand the core processes involved in clinical integration and operational efficiency, because they must make certain that the structures and functions designed by the subcommittees support clinical integration and operational efficiency.

The steering committee will have five primary functions:

1. Guide and integrate the design process
2. Identify design subcommittees and choose their members
3. Approve the design elements produced by the design subcommittees
4. Select the corporate structure for the ACO with respect to the parent company (discussed in Chapter 3)
5. Choose a strategy for funding the ACO initiative

We discuss each of these functions more fully.

Guide and Integrate the Design Process

The steering committee will approve the overall design process; review the recommendations of the subcommittees; and have the final authority for approving design-element recommendations for the bylaws, initial policies, management structure, and so forth. If external resources are used to assist in the design process, the steering committee will approve the request for proposals, review the applicants, select the partner, provide oversight, and manage the relationship with the consulting partner.

Identify Design Subcommittees and Choose Their Members

A number of subcommittees will be identified throughout the design process. Membership in these subcommittees will be chosen by the steering committee, so care must be taken to ensure that the members of the steering committee have enough familiarity with the participating organizations to make effective appointments and hold subcommittee members accountable for their contributions.

Approve the Design Elements Produced by the Design Subcommittees

The work product of each subcommittee (discussed later) is a set of recommendations about one or more elements of the initial ACO design. It is the responsibility of the steering committee to charter each of the subcommittees and ultimately approve, disapprove, or modify its recommendations.

Select the Corporate Structure for the ACO

Selection of the corporate structure cannot be delegated to a subcommittee. Therefore, it is the responsibility of the steering committee to select the corporate structure of the ACO, as described later.

Choose a Strategy for Funding the ACO Initiative

As noted in Chapter 7, designing and building an ACO requires capital investment. Of the many opportunities to generate new revenues and savings, select two or three and initiate them immediately. We call those "fast lane" activities. They should be initiated without delay. You want to form a work group immediately to design and implement the fast lane activities concurrently with the design of the ACO. Examples of the strategies that organizations are using to fund their ACO development, some of which are in paradoxical conflict with the overall intentions of the ACO, include the following:

- Revenue enhancement
  - Increasing reimbursement rates on services with low reimbursement relative to competitors in the market and the cost of providing the services
  - Improving collection rates via improved coding, billing, documentation, and charge capture
  - Growing profitable service lines
  - Capturing out-of-system leakage
  - Keeping the beds filled with appropriate cases
- Efficiency enhancement
  - Elimination of avoidable costs, such as nonstandardized supply usage

- Steering patients to lower-cost sites of care
- Reducing administrative overhead associated with payer–provider negotiations
- Exiting unprofitable businesses
- Improving throughput and length of stay

Whatever activities are chosen, the final task of the steering committee will be to select the strategy that will be used to fund ACO development, assuming current collective organizational reserves are insufficient or imprudent to use as the ACO financing strategy.

Select a Corporate Structure

With advice from in-house and external counsel, the first step in the design process is to choose a corporate structure, as described in Chapter 3. The benefits and challenges of a range of models should be weighed carefully and the steering committee itself, rather than a subcommittee, should select the preferred corporate model for the ACO. In many cases the structure will be obvious and will require little or no analysis. In other cases it will involve a deeper look at tax implications, corporate liability, physician compliance issues, leadership capabilities, and other issues. No matter what structure is selected, it is strongly advised that the physicians be represented on the committee that selects the corporate structure. At some point in the process the physician participants will need to explain the rationale for the model selected to all the participating physicians. It will be important for participating physicians to know that their physician leaders participated actively in choosing the corporate model.

Charter the First Design Subcommittee: The "Continental Congress"

The First Continental Congress met briefly at Carpenter's Hall in Philadelphia on September 5, 1774. Though many of the delegates from the colonies wanted to amicably resolve grievances against Great Britain, among some attendees there was a growing realization that a rebellion was underway and would be impossible to stop. The delegates organized an economic boycott of Great Britain and petitioned the king for a redress of grievances. By the time the Second Continental Congress met on May 10, 1775, in Philadelphia, fighting had begun in the Revolutionary War. Moderates in the Congress still hoped that the colonies could be reconciled with Great Britain, but a movement toward independence steadily gained ground. Congress established the Continental Army in June 1775; coordinated the war effort; issued the Declaration of Independence in July 1776; and designed a new government in the Articles of Confederation, which were ratified in 1781.

Healthcare organizations must similarly convene a meeting of delegates to determine the course of their undertaking. This is the meeting of the first design subcommittee to establish the ACO's governance and management structure. It must begin with a clear set of goals and principles, which will be translated into operating policies and procedures.

Like the Continental Congress, which was superseded after independence by the Congress of the United States, this design subcommittee will be dissolved when its job is done and the ACO is adopting its formal governance and management structure. And like many members of the Continental Congress, participants on this design subcommittee will logically be leaders of the successor organization.

No Three-Cornered Hats

For our Continental Congress, the governance committee will work with attorneys to establish ACO control and decision-making authority with respect to the parent company and all participating entities. This generally involves the development of a set of rational and fair checks and balances through policies and procedures to ensure appropriate input into decisions and to facilitate efficient and effective decision making. All participating parties will naturally want to retain as much control over the decisions as possible, relinquishing as little authority as possible to the parent corporation or the ACO. This need will abate over time as all parties get comfortable with one another. The design process is, itself, the enabler of the design, as comfort among participants facilitates design. This is what Marshall McLuhan had in mind when he declared this about television in the early 1960s: "The medium is the message."

The "art" in the design is to create a model that optimizes participants' input into decisions while avoiding overly democratic processes that risk stalling or paralyzing decision making. Even though the governing body will be a fiduciary body, it will inevitably be composed of individuals with strong ties to their legacy entities—be they the medical group, the hospital, the home health agency, and so forth. This will inevitably make consensus difficult as a decision-making process. While certainly some decisions will require full consensus, many others can effectively be made by simple or supra-majority of the members of the governing body. When using a parent company model, it is important that the parent company retain the power to authorize decisions when the ACO governing body is functionally deadlocked. In essence, then, the parent company will want to be able to influence decisions but, whenever possible, avoid making them unless the governing board of the ACO is unable to reach a decision. The prevailing subliminal message from the parent company should be "Why would you possibly ever want to abdicate decision making to us? Avoid deadlock and make your best decisions. If you can't, we will."

After designing the governance of the ACO, the same committee should create the executive and senior management structure of the organization. As has been recommended throughout this book, while there is no best model, the executive management team should reflect the principle of "physician led and professionally managed." The governance and management committee can decide between a relatively traditional organizational structure or one of the integrative council structures suggested in chapters 3 and 4. If one of the council structures is selected, the committee should decide which councils to establish during the initial phase of ACO establishment. It should be expected that the initial design will evolve over time.

A simple principle to consider is to use the initial councils first to design the functions for which they are responsible and then to remain in place as the actual councils. For example, a finance council may establish a sense of urgency, by evaluating reform-induced revenue and balance sheet vulnerabilities or by quantifying margin-improvement tactics for key stakeholders. The council would also design a core set of value-based principles that guide managed care rate setting as well as internal funds flow. After the design phase, it would become the ongoing finance council of the ACO that would be charged with creating the strategic margin transition plan defined in Chapter 7. In similar fashion, the initial clinical councils would collectively lay the groundwork for the design of all clinical councils before designing and implementing their identified clinical focus.

Another area of work for the governance and management committee (the Continental Congress) is to define the boundaries and interfaces between executive management and governance. Reviewing medical group operations from chapters 3 and 4, it should be noted that physician groups frequently obfuscate distinctions between governance and management, so great care must be taken to help them understand the distinctions between these two important functions.

The ultimate design must enable the governing body to establish and adjudicate policy; select and manage the executive management team; partner with the management team to establish vision and strategy for the ACO; and provide meaningful oversight for key functions, including the setting of priorities, performance goals, capital investments, operating budget, and key interfaces with the parent company. Management must have clear lines of authority to establish priorities, performance goals, capital investments, and operating budget and to allocate resources subject to the budget oversight approval of the governing body. In addition, executive management must be able to select and manage its senior management team, consistent with the design created by the Continental Congress.

Often, a natural tension exists between strategy and operations: Brilliant strategies that cannot be implemented are as ineffective as brilliant implementation for ill-conceived strategies. The tension between the two functions is healthy and important and will need to be managed by the enterprise. For example, governance may seek to expand the scope or reach of the ACO, and management may feel that its executives are already overwhelmed with other initiatives; they don't feel that the infrastructure exists to support that strategy. Ultimately, the decision for action will be determined by the degree to which they can resolve the tension without compromising on the organization's goals.

When this tension or conflict arises, healthcare professionals often gravitate toward their default operational mode: seek consensus. However, in areas of strategy, consensus may be fatal for the nascent ACO. Difficult as it may be to implement, the governing board's strategy may be the only right one, and compromise may result in a flawed strategy. Moreover, much as in a family, whenever there are situations where opposing points of view are required in order to make the best decision, it's best to have those opposing views expressed by different groups or individuals. When opposing viewpoints are vested in a single individual, there's no platform upon which to make arguments pro and con. Whatever the decision, it's best for the organization to have the debate out in the open and be fully transparent about it. Paradoxically, full transparency usually promotes confidence, not anxiety or unrest.

It should be clear why it is advisable, whenever possible, to make certain that the likely candidates for executive director and medical director are included in the Continental Congress, as it will be best for them to inherit an organizational model within which they are comfortable managing. It will give the two future leaders ownership of the design that emerges. It also provides the likely candidates with an opportunity to test-drive their relationship before actual operations commence.

Tell the Story

Once the governance and management design committee (the Continental Congress) has completed its initial design work, it is time to "tell the story" (at least Chapter One) to leaders in all current and potential participating organizations. The nomenclature of telling the story is recommended for specific purposes. One of the characteristics that differentiates highly successful leaders from those less successful in their leadership positions is their ability to weave messages into a coherent story that not only provides important information but also provides the rationale behind that information. Humans are acclimated to learning through stories during infancy and their capacity to integrate information is greatly enhanced whenever disparate facts, observations, data, events, conditions, and so forth can be woven into a coherent story that has a setting, a journey, a struggle, a climax, and a resolution.

In the case of the ACO, the story is a repeat of the tale already used in the education process followed by the work that has been initiated locally to build an ACO. Care must be taken to craft the story in a way that engages listeners, lets them know what has transpired, what alternatives have been considered, and what results have emerged. The story should always include a section that describes how the listeners are involved, what is or might be expected of them, and what they can expect from others (and these elements should always be customized to the particular audience being addressed).

The most effective leadership stories prompt the listener to ask "why?" and preempt that question with the rationale that explains "why" wherever appropriate. Finally, a successful leadership story ends with an invitation for the listener(s) to participate in some way so that the end of the leaders' story is effectively the beginning of the listeners' story. In some cases, the participation is simply to watch and wait; in other cases, those listening will be invited to participate in leadership or to take some other action. And they always end with firm commitments about what the listeners can expect from leadership during the change process. Most often, this focuses on keeping them informed and involved. It is important to be clear with the listeners about what they can anticipate as the next chapter in *their* story.

Refine the Physician Organization

As has already been noted, the design process is neither linear nor neatly sequenced. Obviously, if some preexisting physician organization does not exist as the nucleus of the physician organization for the ACO, it is highly unlikely that an effective physician organization

Healthcare's Master Storyteller: The New Director of the Centers for Medicare & Medicaid Services

Over the past 25 years, Dr. Donald M. Berwick has made the most consistent and compelling case for improvements in reliability and quality in every facet of healthcare. As head of the nonprofit Institute for Healthcare Improvement, Berwick's work has embedded quality and safety into the lexicon of every facet of healthcare delivery.

In the early days of Harvard Community Health Plan, one of America's leading health maintenance organizations, it was Berwick who recognized the pivotal role of quality in healthcare delivery and introduced that into the design and delivery of every aspect of care. His title, vice president for quality, spoke of his pivotal role. I recall an early management meeting of Harvard Community Health Plan. We were basking in the glory of some early quality performance measures in which we had scored quite well. Everyone was engaged in self-congratulation. It was Don who stood up and said that, while proud of our results, they were "simply not good enough." And everyone in the room realized he was in a different plane than the rest of us. He reminded us that we were the best of healthcare provider organizations, though we held no candle to other industries. Thus began his journey to Bell Laboratories and other organizations to learn about quality and introduce new concepts into healthcare. No one in healthcare matches Donald Berwick's ability to envision and tell the story.

can be created *de novo* at this stage of the process. We assume both the shallow and deep dive assessments have revealed enough physician alignment around a nuclear physician organization to support the development of an ACO. This is the opportunity for the physicians to answer some extremely important questions regarding the development of the ACO. Here is a suggested list:

- Should we expand the number of participating caregivers (primary care, specialists) beyond our nuclear group to achieve the ACO's broader goals?

- If so, how should we expand the practice? Who and where?
- Is our internal structure strong enough for us to be effective partners?
- If so, how do we need to modify our internal governance and management structures and functions to be effective partners in an ACO?
- What principles and priorities are important to us and must be embedded within the ACO?

We address each question individually.

Should We Expand the Number of Participating Caregivers Beyond Our Nuclear Group?

As noted in Chapter 3, we believe that the ACO will evolve over time. The physician organization will also need to evolve over time. It is difficult to envision a high-performing ACO whose physician organization does not make use of the same principles of operation as effective multispecialty group practices do. That does not imply that the group must have the legal or economic structure of a multispecialty group practice, but the group must certainly operate with the ethos of a group practice.

Characteristics of this type of practice include acceptance of a shared (group) destiny; a common mission and vision; embrace of physician management; and adherence to group principles, values, standards, and policies. It also implies that the group members have enough confidence in their colleagues that few patients are referred outside the group. If, on the other hand, attitudes, ethics, or competence inhibit capture of internal referrals, the concerns must be addressed and corrected.

The "nuclear group" must decide whether it has sufficient depth and breadth to provide the full continuum of care to a defined population of patients. Relatively infrequently used services, such as thoracic surgery, deep brain neurosurgery, or transplant surgery, can be acquired through professional service agreements with high-performing local or regional physicians or vendors. More common referral specialties, such as dermatology, endocrinology, and gastroenterology, are less likely to be managed effectively through such vendor relationships. The group should probably consider adding those specialties through an expanded physician organization, IPA, physician hospital organization, foundation, or expanded multispecialty group practice to optimize use of these resources (see discussion later and refer to Chapter 3).

How Should We Expand the Practice?

If the decision is made to expand the practice, the nuclear group must decide on its preferred model, create a legal structure to support its model, and specify governance and management of the expanded entity. If the nuclear group is already a multispecialty group practice, expansion is easier, with the obvious exception of raising capital if practice acquisition is part of the strategy. Once expanded, the group must create policies and procedures so that leadership can hold the expanded group accountable for adhering to standards, values, and policies. Once again, this should be addressed as early as possible in the process. Ideally, it should begin with early informal conversations with potential group members. Don't make the beginner's mistake of starting off talks with negotiations or offers. It's far better to initiate a collaborative conversation than start a negotiation. Negotiation should only begin after a reasonably secure platform of trust is established.

Is Our Internal Structure Strong Enough for Us to Be Effective Partners?

Members of the nuclear physician group should now shore up internal governance, infrastructure, and management to improve the expansion's chances of success. There may be no need for the group to change its economic arrangement with the anchor hospital or healthcare group of the ACO. The nuclear physician group might prefer to maintain its prior economic arrangement with the ACO's anchor hospital. It will, therefore, want to make certain that it has a strong internal management team for addressing and managing internal financial matters. The existing structure can be maintained and added to within the ACO.

If the nuclear group is a wholly owned subsidiary of the anchor healthcare system, it should maintain that relationship. As it potentially expands, the nuclear group might want to consider inviting some of its newer clinicians to participate in clinical leadership and management positions within the expanded practice, to involve them in decision making.

How Do We Need to Modify Our Internal Governance and Management
Structures and Functions to Be Effective Partners in an ACO?

Using the policies and bylaws of the nuclear physician group as a base, the expanded group might want to redesign some elements of governance and management to strengthen both functions moving forward. Depending on the model selected, the newly expanded physician organization might need to revise some internal management structures. Conversely, it could also integrate some of the structures and processes directly into the ACO. Either way, it is important for the physician organization to ensure that it has a strong enough internal management for it to be a full and effective partner in ACO development.

What Principles and Priorities Are Important to Us and Must Be Embedded
Within the ACO?

The final step in preparing the physician organization to participate in designing the ACO is for the physicians to identify their collective priorities and their own design principles so that they can be fully integrated into the governing principles, bylaws, and policies of the ACO. Writing new policies and bylaws is far less onerous than amending previously existing bylaws. Moreover, it is best to introduce the principles during the ACO design phase rather than rewrite them after the ACO is up and running lest any party be accused of deception.

Expand the ACO Clinical and Financial Management Structures

The steering committee is now ready to charter the next two design councils—one that focuses on business and finance and the other that focuses on clinical integration. If the ACO executive director (professional manager) has been selected, it would be ideal for that designee to appoint a design council to identify the issues of the economic model, business strategy, and development that will need to be addressed. At the same time, the council should examine managed care contracting, internal ACO funds flow, and alternative methodologies for the sharing of potential savings.

Consistent with the principle of physician leadership working alongside professional management, the second design council on clinical integration would ideally be chaired by the designated medical director, if he or she is identified at this point. This design council would select the organizing principles for clinical care design and ongoing management, whether a more traditional model or the innovative model (suggested in Chapter 4) is used.

These two councils should meet at least once to share recommendations and to ensure that there are no internal conflicts or incompatibilities in their designs. Then, each should present its design to the steering committee for endorsement and approval. As the process picks up momentum, the steering committee will find that internal modifications will be required to optimally integrate all the functions, much as the design of a house changes from the original architect's drawings as it is built, sometimes turning out much different than the original.

Care Design Modeling: Pedal to the Metal

Managing the full continuum of care eventually requires reevaluation of every facet of care delivery (from outcomes achieved to resources used) and the levels of satisfaction of those who provide and receive care in that process. Once the initial business/finance council and the clinical integration council have been established and chartered, it would be valuable for the two councils to meet. This should be in a retreat-style setting where the councils can share initial activities and initiate or accelerate joint modeling. It is critical for these two groups to see one another as partners, just as their leaders—the executive and medical directors—see themselves as partners. Clearly, some advanced evaluation must precede the retreat.

We suggest one approach to modeling that is based on the clinical delivery model introduced in Chapter 4. In this facilitated process, subgroups are created in each of the delivery categories/patient cohorts (see Exhibit 9.1).

A retreat-style meeting is used to identify opportunities for care redesign and initiate the care/efficiency modeling process. Small integrated teams that consist of operations and finance experts, clinical care professionals, and most important, care coordination specialists are created in advance of the retreat and assigned one care delivery

Exhibit 9.1 ACO Design Subgroups Based on Clinical Delivery Model

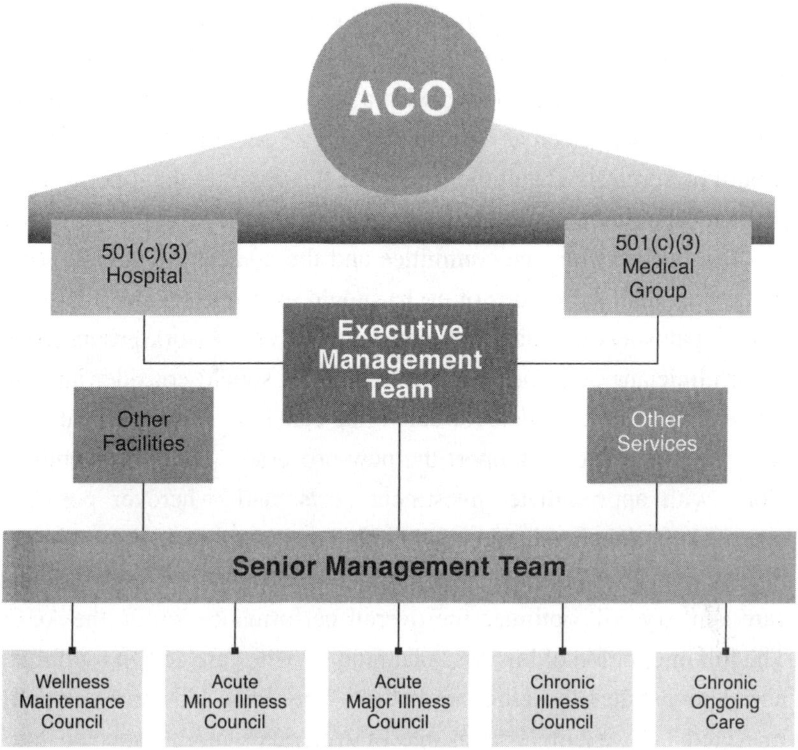

category. One or more relatively common conditions are selected as a model to study in that category. Using internal experience along with available benchmark performance data, processes and outcomes are evaluated along three parameters:

1. *Clinical outcome performance.* Are our clinical outcomes optimized?
2. *Resource utilization performance.* Is our resource utilization optimized?
3. *Patient/provider satisfaction.* Are those who deliver and receive care satisfied?

Using whatever scoring process is selected, specific disease pathways linked to the condition being evaluated are identified for review and redesign. Each selected pathway is viewed as one example of care within its delivery category and is therefore used as an archetype for how care is currently provided within its category. If one current care pathway is recognized as a particularly high performer, that pathway should be scrutinized and the leaders of the program that operates the pathway should be invited to participate in or even lead the process.

The business/finance committee and the clinical integration committee (or small subgroups of each) should then select a small number of care pathways to study and redesign. The initial work group, made up of clinicians and operating professionals, should consider alternative and innovative models for delivering care to the identified patients. Resources required to support the new processes should be identified along with approximate investment costs, and, wherever possible, potential efficiencies should be identified and quantified.

As a general principle, the integration of business modeling and care delivery will optimize the overall performance within the ACO. The full integration of business planning into the care design reinforces and demonstrates the rationale behind "physician led, professionally managed." An example from one of America's most respected integrated delivery systems might reinforce this observation (see sidebar).

Care must be taken to anticipate the resources needed to support the new process and quantify the efficiencies achieved within the new model. The importance of using disciplined business planning processes cannot be overemphasized: The modeling must look at required investment capital and resources, potential lost revenue, and resource savings possible in the alternative care pathway. Discipline in this process will set the standard for ACO-related planning processes that follow.

Models that show particular promise for clinical outcomes improvement, greater efficiencies, and improvement in satisfaction (e.g., 30-day bundled readmission pilot) should be endorsed for pilots. The early results can be shared with the initial retreat participants at the end of three and six months. The expressed goal of the pilot is to initiate innovative care delivery processes and learn from the experiments. The implicit goal of the pilots, however, is to demonstrate that collaboration between clinical design and delivery and business planning is a critical capability for the ACO.

An Approach to Creating a Clinical Pathway Here's one approach to creating a new clinical pathway.

Identify the condition—say, stroke treatment. Then, gather the relevant physician specialists and have them review all the recent literature on "best practice" treatment protocols and pathways. Each physician must sort the articles into those whose recommendations she agrees with and those she doesn't. If 5 of the original 100 peer-reviewed articles are in every specialist's "agree" pile, those treatment recommendations become the core of the new pathway.

Experience teaches us that a core set of standardized activities in a care pathway that is followed regularly will significantly standardize the overall process and improve the outcomes. Generally, the more that can be agreed to, the better, although the improvement curve is asymptotic and does flatten out at some point. Having been critical of consensual decision making, we must point out that this is an example of where consensus can be helpful. It's not important to have all the participants agree on everything, but they need to agree on a small part of the literature, and follow it together, to significantly improve the outcomes of care.

Create the New Dashboard: The Parable of the Lost Balloonist

A man in a hot air balloon realized he was lost. He reduced altitude and spotted a woman below. He descended a bit more and shouted, "Excuse me, can you help me? I promised a friend I would meet him an hour ago, but I don't know where I am." The woman below replied, "You are in a hot air balloon hovering approximately 30 feet above the ground. You are between 40 and 41 degrees north latitude and between 59 and 60 degrees west longitude."

"You must be a teacher," said the balloonist.

"I am," replied the woman, "How did you know?"

"Well," answered the balloonist, "everything you told me is technically correct, but I have no idea what to make of your information, and the fact is I am still lost. Frankly, you've not been much help so far."

The woman below responded, "You must be an administrator."

"I am," replied the balloonist, "but how did you know?"

"Well," said the woman, "you don't know where you are or where you are going. You have risen to where you are due to a large quantity of hot air. You made a promise that you have no idea how to keep. You expect someone else to solve your problem. And the fact is you are in exactly the same position you were in before we met, but now, somehow, it's my fault."

It is easy to substitute physician, nurse, health claims adjuster, or actuary into this parable. The point of it is that different measurements produce different ways of looking at the same situation. One way to ensure that ACO participants are looking at the same (and the right) measurements is to rework the organizational performance dashboard.

As covered in Chapter 7, the emergence of the new delivery and financing model invites the redesign of the organizational performance dashboard. Recalling one of the oldest management principles, "what gets measured is what gets done," nothing makes change more tangible to those within a system than changing performance measurement. Often, it is only when organizational leaders present the new performance dashboard that employees fully appreciate the organization's new goals and intentions. That's when the goal becomes tangible to them for the first time. Exhibit 9.2 provides a sample dashboard.

One example of how important dashboards are involves a workshop we recently led for a community teaching hospital. We created a new physician productivity dashboard. It was met by fierce resistance by the medical staff. But one month after it was implemented, a remarkable two-thirds of the physicians were meeting the new performance thresholds. The lesson: What gets measured is what gets done.

There's also a real-world example: signs put up by police that show drivers their actual speed. Drivers invariably slow down when they encounter these signs, even if there are no police nearby. Real-time feedback has a profound impact on behavior.

Changing the measurement system involves five integrated steps:

1. *Decide on the definition of "success."* Select what performance outcomes reflect and can be used to track success.
2. *Decide what should be measured.* Select measures that will inform the operating system about how it is performing.
3. *Decide how each measure should be obtained.* Design a system to capture performance data, and convert them into useful information.
4. *Decide how the information should be reported.* Design the reports, and determine to whom they will be distributed.
5. *Decide on the standards.* Create a first pass at the desired (ceiling) or acceptable (floor) performance standard for each measure; decide what's an A-, B-, or C-level performance.

Exhibit 9.2 A Sample Dashboard

Functional Area	Traditional Metrics	Emerging Metrics
1. Revenue Management	• Days in A/R • Collection/denial rate	• Cost to collect (e.g., per case) • Revenue per adjusted available bed day, machine hour, etc. • Contracted rates at percent of market, cost, and Medicare
2. Overhead (Fixed) Costs	• Cost per adjusted discharge	• Fixed and semi-fixed cost drivers by DRG and department
3. Variable Costs	• Inventory turns • Cost per adjusted discharge • Rx or supplies per adjusted discharge • FTEs per AOB • Percent scripts filled • Cost per adjusted discharge	• Variable cost drivers by DRG and department • Labor cost as a percent total versus peer • Cost of avoidable complications • Generic utilization • TAT
4. Operations	• CMI-adjusted ALOS • Capacity utilization • Risk-adjusted mortality • Labor hours/patient day	• Door to floor • On-time starts • Discharges after 1pm • Sepsis, VAPs, CLBSI, LOS • Premium pay hours; semi-fixed versus fixed versus variable
5. Physician Productivity	• RVU percentile	• Revenue and cost per available clinic slot • High utilization or unit reimbursement outlier
6. Access	• Specialists/1000 • PCP/1000	• NPs/1000 • PAs/1000 • Telemedicine visits/1000

Note: AOB = adjusted occupied bed; ALOS = average length of stay; A/R = accounts receivable; CLBSI = catheter-related blood stream infection; CMI = case mix index; DRG = diagnosis-related group; FTE = full-time equivalent; LOS = length of stay; NP = nurse practitioner; PA = physician assistant; PCP = primary care physician; RVU = relative value unit; TAT = turn-around time; VAP = ventilator-associated pneumonia

Source: Data from Navigant, Geisinger Health System.

Outcomes will change as organizational priorities change. Measures will change as new technology enables more refined measurement. Changes in outcomes, priorities, and measures will inform the measurement process, and the reporting will be modified according to internal customer needs. Finally, the standards will necessarily change over time on the basis of external (environmental or competitive) factors, internal drivers of enhanced performance, and advances in science and technology.

Data are simple observations. When analyzed and processed, against themselves or a standard, data become information. Information that is further analyzed becomes knowledge—a useful tool that shows causal relationships. Knowledge can be put to action. When the performance dashboard is properly designed, clinical and business leaders will have the knowledge they need to make crucial decisions at their fingertips. Improperly designed dashboards generate a lot of data but aren't helpful in guiding decision making. For the balloonist in our parable, too much raw data was just disruptive background noise.

Work with Payers Before, During, and After Start-Up

Healthcare providers ready to implement the ACO strategy have already been engaged in high-level discussions with their payers. Together, the providers and payers have looked at ways to move away from the traditional "pay me more" versus "pay you less" rhetoric to "pay me right." They have mutually acknowledged the difficulties each face in sustaining margins in a soft reimbursement and volume environment. They have begun to explore value-based fee schedules as a means to maintain or earn extra income.

Before start-up, there will be a tremendous need to communicate with health plan members (from the payers' perspective) and patients (from the providers' perspective). Both sides should collaborate on a user-education program. Elements can include direct mailings, online tutorials, and an ACO members' handbook or users guide. The goal is to change the patients' way of thinking so that their behavior changes as well. The concept of a medical home, while old hat within the industry, is still vague and somewhat threatening to patients. Make sure they understand the medical home model and how it will work for them. Many patients have not had a consistent point of contact with caregivers; this is the time to ensure they understand how to work with the new system. To add emphasis to this point, in a recent survey within a respected healthcare organization for which we consult, fully 30 percent of the more than 5,000 employees did not have an identified primary care clinician. And these are informed consumers!

Ultimately, patient education is about improving compliance with medication and other treatment regimens. It is a win–win for both payers and providers and may provide a relatively nonthreatening way for the two sides to work together.

Once ACO Version 1.0 is up and running, the job changes to monitoring. Constant monitoring of utilization, unit costs, patient behavior, and compliance with protocols will yield crucial insights into what works and what doesn't work. Planning for Version 2.0 should begin immediately. This is another task for which the payers and providers can cast aside previous differences and roles and work together. Sharing of data will help cement the new partnership.

Culture Assessment: Changing the Rules

The concept of simple rules was introduced in Chapter 5. Simple rules are powerful shapers of organizational design and direction and, therefore, are reasonably accurate predictors of the capacity for organizational performance. By design, the ACO itself will operate as a separate clinical and business entity yet will most often be integrated into organizations that have non-ACO-related business and clinical goals. Therefore, the design and delivery of care and the business functions that support them will almost certainly interface with other clinical and business operations of the organizations that contribute to and operate within the ACO.

Predictably, the simple rules needed to support success within the ACO are likely to be different from, and potentially in conflict with, those that operate within the organizations that make up the ACO. A review of the suggested simple rules for ACO success from Chapter 3 reveals the likelihood of culture clash and conflict between the participating organizations.

When the possibility for culture conflict is high, it is often helpful to confront potential conflict proactively through a process we call "Changing the Rules®." This process exposes the simple rules most influential in an organization at any given point in time and then evaluates those influential rules in light of the organization's strategy moving forward. It concludes with the central question, "Can we reach our intended goals operating according to these rules?"

In the case of the ACO, the central question would be, "Where are our current simple rules likely to conflict with the simple rules necessary for success of our ACO?" Just declaring a set of new rules to govern the ACO is an exercise in futility. However, inviting those within the participating organization to talk openly about how the culture conflict can be managed will often provide a handle that enables thoughtful dialogue and problem solving whenever the tension is getting in the way of ACO progress.

Bring the Technology Online

As anyone who has experienced the installation of a new office phone system or software platform knows, the transition from one technology to another is what creates the greatest risk of discontinuity. For the highly integrated healthcare provider, or the nascent ACO, complete collapse of the electronic health record (EHR) system could prove a disaster. Therefore, it's essential to follow these steps:

- Begin the transition to the new system before the ACO is up and running. Let the bugs appear while there is still time to solve them.
- Maintain a fail-safe legacy pathway to the EHR that can be relied on in case new systems or modules fail.
- Ensure that 24/7 technical support is available during crucial switchovers.
- Coordinate with affiliated providers so that your information technology (IT) failure does not affect their access.

To the extent possible, training in the new EHR system should begin well before the ACO goes live. IT training is an onerous experience for most healthcare providers, whose primary interest is in helping patients. As we note again later, small rewards can go a long way during change processes.

The Little Bang Theory of the ACO

No ribbon cutting, press releases, or grand opening signs will announce the start of ACO operations. There will be no Big Bang heralding the start of a new healthcare universe.

It is also highly unlikely that a provider organization will start delivering fully loaded ACO care. It's far more likely that it will ease into the model over time through enhanced pay-for-performance strategies, payer-sponsored shared-savings programs, focused bundled payments, alternative quality contracts, or a limited number of (attributed) "enrollees," as with the demonstration projects and early pilots. Such an approach will enable both the payer and the provider organizations to experiment and evaluate results. This is the most common way to introduce innovation like this. There will be much uncertainty, no road maps, no guardrails, and no troubleshooting manual. It's very much like a conversation once overheard between a father and his 13-year-old firstborn after a particularly egregious case of adolescent misbehavior: "The problem, of course, is that neither of us knows how to behave here. You've never been a teenager, and I've never been the father of a teenager. We'll just have to learn together."

The components of the ACO that will need to be operational at the outset include the governing body, the executive and senior management teams, whatever integrative clinical councils are being used initially, and whatever business infrastructure councils are being used to support the business operations of the ACO.

Some organizations are initiating this strategy by building integrated clinical service lines and then coalescing the service lines into an integrated delivery system. Rather than creating the system and then building out its components, these organizations are building out the components and aggregating them over time into a delivery system. Systems that use this strategy often are forced to do so because of limited physician leadership. As noted earlier, organizations that plan to use this strategy might want to consider including their anticipated managers in the design process. Conversely, those involved in the design process should be considered for management once the service lines or centers of excellence are up and running.

By using this strategy, the design team, which has begun to knit together during the design phase, transitions naturally and seamlessly into the initial governance, management, and clinical operations teams. With that in mind, it is often a good idea to have the design teams participate in telling the (organization's) story, as discussed earlier. This will help physicians and frontline staff build trust in their leaders and witness the trust and comfort developing among physician leaders and system professional managers.

There are four distinct phases to the transition from current to future state, though as implied by Exhibit 9.3, the distinctions between each phase are not entirely clear.

The Design Phase

The design phase has already been described and should "end" with a clear communication strategy customized to the needs of each audience (see the "telling the story" discussion). From a practical point of view, the design phase never really ends, as initial designs will need refinement and potentially even redesign throughout the process.

The Transition Phase

During the transition phase, new systems are introduced into an organization that is currently operating in a distinctly different and potentially contradictory manner. It is in this phase that enhanced care coordination programs are introduced; patient registries are initiated; care pathways are introduced; new committees or councils begin to operate; advances to the medical home are begun; new or enhanced EHR systems are implemented; and new cost, quality, and utilization reporting is integrated into day-to-day activities. Much like the adolescent parenting situation noted earlier, the organization is transitioning from one way of being to another during the transition phase.

Exhibit 9.3 The Four Phases of Transition to Future State

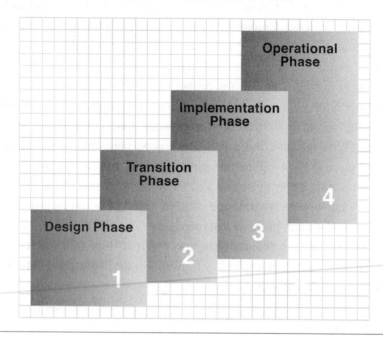

We can expect this phase to be a time of maximum upheaval, chaos, and uncomfortable paradox as the organization is operating within one model while still measuring performance through the lenses of a contradictory model. Highly experienced mid-career professionals will be asked to adopt new systems and tools that will challenge their competencies. For many, this will prove highly unsettling. As is obvious, it is here that the workforce will require the greatest amount of technical and emotional support. This phase can be thought of as the dress-rehearsal phase, as organizations will often create shadow dashboards to track performance within the new model while "officially" measuring results using the old model.

The Implementation Phase

The implementation phase is a bit of a misnomer. Many of the systems for the new model of care delivery will have already been introduced during the transition phase. While the transition phase introduces many pilot activities, the implementation phase introduces larger-scale system changes, such as clinical pathways, disease management programs, new models of care delivery, and new measurement and payment systems. The implementation phase, then, is a period of accelerating change in which major systems are introduced and the delivery system begins to operate differently. This is the period in which participants' behavior has real and measurable consequences. Any healthcare system that has implemented a new EHR can appreciate that this is an unsettling period often filled with anxiety when individuals and work groups suboptimize performance and need significant coaching, support, and assistance.

This is also the period in which the participants need the maximum amount of performance feedback. Leadership will derive great value from catching individuals and work groups "getting it right" rather than focusing on providing critical feedback that exposes those who have "gotten it wrong." Leadership should be highly visible during this period and seek every opportunity to provide affirming feedback to those who operate as desired in the new system. The value of the feedback can be significantly enhanced through small rewards. As noted earlier, leaders always seem surprised by the benefit of a gift certificate for a cup of coffee, a modest lunch, or another small token of appreciation. In change management, a little reward can go a long way.

A technique that can be useful here is focused real-time feedback. Often, a single question on an index card to patients regarding some piloted change program can provide immediate feedback about whether the change, once refined, is likely to produce the desired results. Simply providing an index card to patients at the end of an encounter and tallying the collective responses at the end of the day will provide all the feedback necessary to reinforce or modify a newly introduced system or process. One clever example of how real-time feedback can be used to improve performance took place in a large, multispecialty medical group practice.

The Power of the Marbles

Each improvement effort at this multispecialty medical group practice was accompanied by a process in which patients were asked a single question to which they could respond favorably or unfavorably. For instance, patients were asked at the end of their visit whether they clearly understood the next step in their care process. To register their answers, they were asked to choose an orange marble to indicate full understanding or a white marble to indicate lack of complete understanding.

The patients chose the marbles from a basket that contained both colors and dropped the selected marbles into a cardboard box that had a small hole at the top. At the end of the day, all those in the practice assembled in one room, and the box was opened. The physicians anticipated that most or all of their patients would select orange balls, believing strongly that they were already doing an excellent job communicating care instructions to their patients. To their surprise and chagrin, when the box was opened the first time more than half the balls were white. But within one week, the marbles were virtually all orange.

This is a testament to the power of feedback loops. Without immediate feedback, the physicians and staff all lived with the assumption that they were doing the right thing. With the immediate feedback, they were able to quickly modify their behavior and see the immediate effects of the change. This powerful process was repeated each week with a different question for patients.

The initiation of operations as an ACO, no matter how limited the initial focus, affords payer and provider an opportunity to "run the program" and see how the design, implementation, and measurement cycle combine to improve care delivery and cost. The Centers for Medicare & Medicaid Services and other payers, meanwhile, may enjoy the most valuable by-product—a cadre of learning organizations, all of which possess some elements of a common DNA and are committed to improved care integration and cost management. Over time, common elements associated with success can be identified and shared across participating organizations.

The Operational Phase

The operational phase refers to that period when the systems are fully up and running and the new system is being managed in a relatively steady state. Anxiety is reduced, and new habits are taking hold, although those involved in implementing the changes are, not surprisingly, worn out. This is often an excellent time to promote new managers to maintain momentum, attention, focus, and energy on the newly implemented system. After the period of relative quiescence, the initial wave of *outcome* performance results (as opposed to the initial *process* performance results) will be generated. They will provide the next infusion of energy for analysis and potential systems refinement. It is during this phase that the organization develops the most important habit of all: becoming a learning organization. It is in this phase that organizational leaders must create and reinforce an environment of objective learning and continuous transformation of the learning into action.

Successful operation as an ACO cannot, of course, be guaranteed. The likelihood of successful introduction of large-scale organizational change can be enhanced by adhering closely to the organizational learning cycles of planning, doing, observing, and acting. Leaders are also well advised to be guided in further understanding the "observing" portion of the cycle. If that element has its own cycle of generating data, interpreting the data to produce information, analyzing the information to produce knowledge, and turning the knowledge into action, they will significantly increase their chances of success.

Roll the Cameras

Everyone who has participated in large-scale organizational change appreciates that no matter how much design and planning are used in the change process, unanticipated issues and unpredicted challenges arise. While each situation cannot be anticipated, each class of situations should be anticipated. A solid set of guiding principles developed by the Continental Congress will generally provide the necessary guidelines to create a thoughtful, responsible, and compatible response. Each response becomes incorporated into "case law," which represents the experience-based solutions that appear to have worked well for the organization. The US Constitution shows that it is far more useful to have a strong and enduring set of guiding principles than a detailed and complete set of rules. Rules-based decisions, generally, are not accompanied by individual or collective learning. It is far better to be guided by strong principles than by detailed rules.

This phenomenon can be illustrated by drivers who rely on a GPS in an unfamiliar city. The value of the GPS is appreciated immediately. The limitations of GPS use, however, are that people become reliant on them and never internalize the landmarks, spatial relationships, directions, and so forth. In brief, many people who use GPS acknowledge that while their GPS is helpful in the short term, the unintended consequence is that it often prevents integration and learning. Some users completely forget how to read maps.

When a complex adaptive work environment becomes too reliant on explicit rules, integration and learning can be limited. When confronted by unanticipated issues, those in governance and management/leadership positions need to feel comfortable acknowledging the absence of a rule to guide resolution and instead use the unanticipated opportunity to craft a solution based on one or more operating principles. Keep in mind that the identified solution will often establish a precedent and, if successful, will become incorporated into "case law" so that when a similar situation arises, those in leadership positions can remain consistent and be guided by the earlier solution. Just as every physician essentially learns the trade through on-the-job training, organizations evolve through trial-and-error problem solving and incorporation into enduring case law. Over time, successful solutions either become codified in bylaws or operating procedures, or they simply become accepted as standard operating procedure.

What this means, of course, is that the organization only becomes refined into its final form once it is operational. Striking a balance between planning, design, and implementation activities and the desire to just "get on with it" is always the challenge with respect to the initiation of large-scale change. As a general rule, the stronger the internal commitment to change, the sooner implementation can be initiated. When resistance is high and engagement is low, more time must be spent crafting the rules of the road so that the unexpected does not engender distrust or diminish confidence in leadership.

Organizational Questions

The organizational questions raised in this chapter include the following:

- What other community healthcare providers should we be talking with?
- What clinical area or disease process could we use as a redesign pilot?
- Who should be included in our ACO steering committee?
- Who should we include in our "Continental Congress"?
- What design teams do we want to designate, and who should be included?

Category of Readers	Key Concepts	Actions to Consider
Category A (interested)	• Learn with others	• Initiate conversations with other provider organizations
	• Change cycle management	• Introduce a change and observe the responses in the change cycle
	• Impact of communication	• Tell the story of the changing environment using "storytelling"
Category B (engaged)	• Storytelling	• Tell the story of your organization's ACO intentions
	• Pilot program	• Introduce a pilot program as a "fishbowl" ACO development
	• Steering committee	• Form a steering committee to identify ACO funding sources
Category C (committed)	• Steering committee	• Form steering committee
	• Continental Congress	• Select organizational structure and initiate "fast lane" funding
	• Design committees	• Focus on refinement of the physician organization

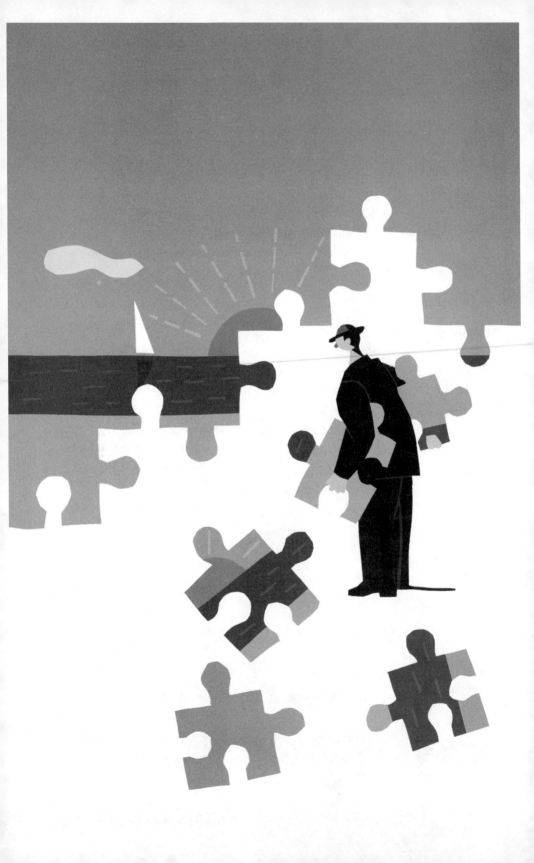

10

Game Time

The ACO is our opportunity to deliver a rational system of healthcare.

—Dennis Keefe
Chief Executive Officer
Cambridge Health Alliance

We introduced Chapter 2 by noting that despite the universal interest and energy in accountable care organizations (ACOs), only four pages of the Patient Protection and Affordable Care Act (PPACA) are devoted to the establishment of ACOs. Among provider organizations, it is the most often referenced section of the PPACA. What is most remarkable is not how many organizations are preparing themselves to participate in this strategy—there are scores if not hundreds—but rather the unprecedented energy and excitement (and it is high) with which many are approaching the challenge. Organizations that prepared for the wave of capitation that never arrived in the early 1990s did so with trepidation and fear. Organizations that braced themselves for consolidation in the late 1990s did so with angst and apprehension. Organizations that readied themselves for safety initiatives shortly after the turn of the century did so with reticence and reserve. Yet today, amid all the uncertainty and ambiguity associated with healthcare reform, many organizations that approach ACO readiness seem to be doing so with optimism and energy. What accounts for the differences?

It is now clear that accountable care has struck a national nerve. Investment income losses, declines in elective surgery, falling reimbursement, decreasing payments, increases in uninsured populations, unfunded pension liabilities, and decreases in charitable contributions have all conspired to place many healthcare organizations in financial jeopardy. At the same time, many healthcare providers are finding their balance sheets pinched by limited access to tax-exempt capital markets and changing debt terms. These factors have limited most healthcare organizations' ability to raise needed investment capital for plant improvements, contemporary updates, acquisition of information, service and care delivery technology, recruitment, pension contributions, and coverage and clinical continuity.

Meantime, increasing demands for better performance from payers, employers, government, and patients; new payer strategies such as pay for performance; and bundling require even more tightly coupled partnerships between physicians and delivery systems. Competition for market share is fierce. All of this is taking place in an increasingly complex and confusing compliance environment. Many healthcare providers find themselves in an increasingly untenable position. Given all the excitement it has generated, one has to assume that the ACO strategy is seen by many leaders and their organizations as a potential answer, or at least a rational response, to these challenges.

For many physicians and healthcare leaders, it seems that accountable care represents the hope of a return to some fundamental and deeply held professional aspirations that have long been subordinated to a different healthcare "game." Within America's healthcare ecosystem, success for many has been determined by how well they have been able to play the transactional game rather than by how well they have been able to improve the lives of those they care for. The transactional zero-sum game has bitterly divided professionals for decades and created adversarial relationships where partnerships were needed. And it has been equal opportunity: Everyone has suffered. Purchasers, payers, providers, and patients are all feeling the pain.

Now even the politicians are feeling the pinch. Those who don't seem to like Plan A don't seem to be offering Plan B. Any pundit who claims to be able to predict the overall effects of healthcare reform is simply ignoring the comprehensiveness, and the unfinished specifications, of the legislation. There are too many moving parts to accurately predict the near-term or long-term effects. Those same pundits can manipulate their data analyses to argue about whether today's healthcare environment is sustainable. We will leave that up to those better positioned to answer. From our point of view, even if it is sustainable, the current healthcare situation is neither fair nor responsible nor simply good enough on the basis of the democratic principles of the United States of America.

We must and can do better. The United States simply cannot afford to be a public health laggard, paying more for poorer results than most other developed nations. We owe it to our citizens, and it is crucial if we are to compete in the global economy.

All sailors know that you can't change direction in a boat that isn't moving. For those of us privileged to interact with healthcare systems across America, the PPACA has already achieved a major accomplishment. By putting some air into the sails of healthcare systems, it has fundamentally changed in some systems the topics of conversations—from revenue, market share, and transactions to clinical integration, partnerships, and efficiency. As we have stated several times in the book, a conversation is the right place to start. And including all stakeholders in the conversation seems like a real accomplishment as well. While everyone is talking about what lies ahead for those who provide and receive care, we can all learn a great deal from observing what's already going on. And a lot is.

Many will argue that healthcare reform went too far. Others think that it did not go far enough. Still others say that the law that emerged only represented one side of the political spectrum. But for many professionals, it represents a small glimmer of hope for a return to a deeply eroded set of principles—principles that guided many people's career choices and, for many decades, were the foundation that supported healthcare in America. For that reason alone it is a reasonable next step in the process of creating a system of care to ensure that every American will have access to healthcare as a right of citizenship.

In brief, there seems to be readiness for change. At the same time, most are realistic and appreciate that the ACO is neither a silver bullet nor a one-size-fits-all solution.

But it's clearly a start.

Chapter-by-Chapter Review

Chapter 1 sets the stage for the healthcare reform law. Cambridge Health Alliance (CHA) is pursuing the ACO model because it is a better strategy for supporting the needs of the patients it serves, and it moves the organization away from a transactional, fee-for-service environment that is slowly strangling the institution. Leaders at CHA are currently assessing their internal capabilities and identifying where they need to develop additional strength to ensure success in accountable care. They have strong and committed leadership, and they are confident they can be successful with this model.

Chapter 2 provides the background and rationale for the ACO model, focusing on requirements, goals, capabilities, and competencies necessary for success. Clinical effectiveness and operating efficiency are stressed as the two crosshairs in the eyepiece of accountable care. We compare operating as an ACO, at least initially, to Michael Crichton's "edge of chaos": a zone of conflict where the forces of change clash with the forces of stability. That clash will be experienced across the American healthcare landscape and within every organization that pursues this strategy. No one feels this tension more keenly today than employed and independent physicians, who will need to partner with one another and with healthcare delivery systems to enable peak performance within the ACO model. The clinical care alignment required for executing this strategy must include many different economic relationships among physicians. Flexibility and generosity of spirit will need to replace rigidity and self-interest in both design and delivery.

While many who think about the ACO strategy erroneously assume there will be a capitated economic model that employs global payments, the initial contracts will involve only shared savings or, at most, asymmetric risk arrangements that provide little or no downside risk and only moderate upside potential. For many, this raises concerns about whether "the juice will be worth the squeeze." Providers may find themselves in a dilemma in which they will have to compare the *certain* benefit associated with an additional transaction against the longer-term *potential* benefit of shared savings associated with forgoing the transaction. Without a strong moral compass and a sturdy clinical quality platform against which all outcomes can be measured, it will be difficult to navigate these choppy waters.

We cannot overstate the importance of effective leadership. As we learned from those involved in the initial pilots, pursuit of this strategy is not for the timid: It represents a total commitment to care process redesign, to new partnerships, and to new ways of thinking. We also predicted that the transition to this delivery model will likely be gradual and initially compartmentalized. Therefore, healthcare professionals will need to live simultaneously in two opposite universes, and leaders will need to feel comfortable managing the paradox created by the juxtaposition of the old and the new.

Chapter 3 explores the anatomy of organizations that pursue the ACO strategy. What becomes clear is that organizations that choose to operate in a fundamentally different way will need to be designed and organized in a fundamentally different way. Their existing systems were designed to produce a totally different outcome—one that is no longer desirable within the ACO strategy. Most systems today were organized within a transactional framework that is not tightly coupled enough to achieve the outcomes required for success within an ACO.

Hospitals will need to redefine themselves as healthcare delivery systems and physicians will need to reorganize themselves as group practices. Both will have to operate as effective partners within those delivery systems. While the attorneys can help create the structural options, it is up to the partners themselves to redefine the nature of their relationships. Once defined, they will need to craft a governance model and management system to build and support the relationship and the outcomes they desire. The best option always lives at the intersection of "this can work" and "this is preferred by those who must make it work." Whatever model is selected will evolve over time, so the best advice is to begin with something flexible and reasonably simple and allow it to evolve organically. While much attention will be paid to organizational structure, it is best to think of the structure like a sports arena: It's the venue, not the game. Organizational structures do not ensure success, though an ineffective structure can make success much more difficult to achieve.

Chapter 4 focuses on the physiology of the ACO. One innovative model for the organization of care delivery is offered to support integration at every patient–system interface. It is not suggested because we feel that it is the best or ideal model. Rather, it is presented as an example of how future leaders will need to envision organizational design and delivery. There are many alternative models that can be used, but the important point, of course, is that all systems need to be operating out of a well-designed and well-executed care delivery model if they are to optimize clinical outcomes, operating efficiencies, patient satisfaction, and appropriate risk management. The principle of "physician led, professionally managed" was reinforced throughout this book and is restated here for emphasis. The system simply will not work unless physicians are authentically included at the leadership table. This is not a physician-centric view of the world; it is an informed conclusion based on years of observation. Those systems that operate most efficiently and effectively benefit from physician leadership supported by professional management.

The flywheel that will make the delivery system efficient and effective is a robust and completely integrated care management system. This cannot be superimposed over the delivery system; it must be embedded deeply within it. The most effective models being used today insert care navigation into the patient-centered primary care medical home. By carrying it out in this way, the care coordinators become extensions of primary care and can best serve their care integration role. Like the systems themselves, primary care physicians are going to have to reinvent their own role from transactional care deliverers to designers of a team of care providers who manage the overall health status of a population of patients. For some, this transition will be difficult, but for others it will be the tonic they have long sought to rejuvenate a stressful and tedious practice. But unless the purchasers and payers see value in such a model, that model will not be developed. For some, such a model will represent an attractive professional opportunity within the healthcare delivery system. And for everyone, the new unit of transaction must become communication and teamwork. Everyone within the system will benefit from this new model of care.

Chapter 5 addresses the sociology of the ACO. These are the cultural underpinnings that will ultimately influence success or failure. While culture is often referred to as the "soft" side of healthcare, it is clear that the "hard" outcomes of quality, safety, patient satisfaction, and business performance are dependent on the "soft" elements of organizational culture. Many leaders are quick to discount organizational culture because it is difficult to understand and even more difficult to influence. But culture will ultimately be the difference between success and failure. Chapter 5 identifies a process to help leaders evaluate and modify their organization's culture.

What Chapter 5 does not address are the potentially conflicting cultures that are likely to exist between organizations that partner within the ACO. Building on the model introduced in Chapter 5, the first step in managing potential culture conflict is identifying each organization's culture and addressing potential conflicts before they start. While every conflict cannot be anticipated, the initial conversations will make it far easier to address conflict when it is recognized. We stress the paradoxical observation that while "I am accountable" has been hard-wired into everyone in today's healthcare ecosystem, that mantra is largely the product of a disorganized and fragmented system in which no individual could reasonably rely on a "system" to be accountable. Until "I am accountable" is replaced by "We (all the members of the system) are accountable," healthcare in America will continue to operate as a series of marginally connected silos within the delivery process and will remain, as the sailors are wont to say, "locked in irons." Twenty-three additional "simple rules" of engagement are offered in the chapter to potentially initiate an organizational conversation about the new culture that will be needed for ACO success. Rules cannot be introduced by fiat, but they can be articulated as intentions and integrated into formal goal setting and performance management systems. Through careful reinforcement, the new rules can become, over time, the bedrock of a new organizational culture. In addition, six parables are offered for use as tools in transforming organizational change. We have used each of the parables over the past 15 years, and they have been effective in introducing change. Each one can be helpful to organizations that plan to operate as an ACO. Once an organization has committed to the strategy and has articulated its vision, each parable can have some utility in framing and facilitating a critical conversation within the organization that can prepare employees for change or support them during that change.

Much like structure, a supportive culture does not guarantee success in accountable care. As noted, however, an unsupportive culture will all but guarantee failure because culture will always supersede strategy. A common misconception is that leaders design the culture to support the strategy. In reality, leaders design the strategy and take purposeful action. Through thoughtful reinforcement, leaders shape behavior, which in turn reinforces cultural transformation. In reality, then, strategy is undertaken and leaders reshape culture through reinforcement of desired actions and behavior. Catching someone doing something desired is far more powerful than catching him when he has done something undesired. A supportive culture emphasizes positive reinforcement.

Information technology (IT) in the form of the electronic medical record is already a crucial tool at most high-performing integrated health delivery systems. In Chapter 6, we look at how IT becomes even more central to the mission of delivering high-quality, cost-effective care within the ACO model. To achieve this, health information systems will need to become ubiquitous throughout the organization, capturing every patient interaction and making that information available at all levels within the ACO, including contracted affiliates. Providers must abandon the notion that a single electronic health record (EHR) is appropriate for all practices within the system and instead look to integrate data across many platforms.

A high-functioning EHR becomes a powerful driver of financial performance, helping to eliminate network leakage. It supports the cultural mission of the ACO by breaking down the silos that exist among various clinical specialties and among the practices and partnerships that comprise the organization. But ultimately, as the ACO becomes more adept at processing information, it becomes a tool for driving care decisions from a patient population level. The health IT system will provide real-time detection of patterns, enabling providers to respond more quickly to health trends and to identify the outliers that drive costs. The system also provides a crucial online interface for patients, providing incentives for them to become more involved in their own care.

In Chapter 7, we examine how healthcare providers will need to attend to the financial side of their business as they change the care delivery side. Most providers are facing significant challenges unrelated to the PPACA. Margins are shrinking. Competition is increasing. Future reimbursement increases are flattening. And patients and purchasers are expressing more resistance to the double-digit annual price increases that became the norm in the early 2000s. To address these issues, providers must abandon not only the transactional mind-set but also many of the ways they have traditionally measured performance. As we have noted, what gets measured is what gets done in most organizations. We introduce a new way of looking at payment on the basis of value and combine that with a strategic margin planning methodology to reduce costs substantially and rebuild the margin gap that many providers will be facing.

Perhaps more important, we examine the toxic and mutually self-defeating games that have become standard practice for negotiations between payers and providers. Changing negotiating style and tactics will do as much to restore healthcare finances as any formal methodology will. As both sides look to create value and integrate care, they will be able to create a new sense of partnership in providing and financing healthcare in the United States. As mentioned, a good starting place for both sides is sharing patient and usage data—information that was previously jealously guarded because it had commercial value or could provide an edge at the negotiating table.

Chapter 8 examines two approaches to assessing ACO readiness. Given the uncertainties and ambiguity associated with accountable care, it was strongly recommended that either approach be accompanied by strategic education about the ACO throughout the delivery system. The shallow dive assessment is used for organizations exploring whether the ACO strategy could be beneficial and realistic for them. This approach enables an organization to answer questions such as "Could it be good for us?" "Should we do it?" and "Can we do it?" The deep dive assessment examines each of the core competencies associated with the ACO and the readiness associated with each. The end product of a deep dive is an organizational road map for filling competency gaps with respect to the design and implementation of the ACO.

Using either approach, the assessment process should be used as an intervention rather than merely an opportunity for data collection. Every interview is an opportunity for engagement. Every analysis is an opportunity for insight. And every identified crisis is an opportunity for new action. The level of interest, enthusiasm, and energy displayed by leaders throughout the assessment process will be a strong predictor of ACO success.

Finally, in Chapter 9, we offer what appears to us to be a rational approach to building the necessary ACO capabilities, recognizing that the process is neither linear nor orderly. But to restate our perspective from the Preface, the fact that each element of the ACO has been introduced successfully in delivery systems across America over the past decades gives us optimism and confidence that such an approach will work.

The evolution of the ACO will not be linear and will undoubtedly involve many starts and stops—some on target, and some misdirected. It is an iterative process, much like decorating a home. For many organizations, the ACO process is ongoing and will never be complete. They will start with Version 1.0 and will continue crafting new versions as they see opportunities to improve. The commitment to the ACO begins with and is supported throughout by multiple conversations. Not only do these conversations advance the strategy, but as a much-desired side benefit, they also build comfort, trust, and momentum.

A Final Word About Leadership Communication

Leaders actually have few opportunities to send signals through their organizations. Whom they hire, whom they fire, and whom they promote send powerful signals. They also send strong signals when they speak. For many, however, the signals are poorly understood. Albert Mehrabian's (1971) classic studies on communication in the late 1960s and early 1970s (published in the book *Silent Messages*), noted in Chapter 9, are important to review. Despite leaders' predictions to the contrary, Mehrabian's studies demonstrated that the verbal content of communication only has a 7 percent impact on whether listeners like the speaker. Tone of voice and body language account for 38 percent and 55 percent, respectively, for whether listeners liked the speaker. Yet many leaders acknowledge that when driving to work the day of an important presentation, their focus is on the word content of their message; they are ignorant of the fact that what they chose to wear that day will probably have more impact on the message.

Everyone in an organization is a leader watcher. They are watching for signals. One of the most important signals is whether the leader seems comfortable, at ease with, and fully committed to a direction, strategy, or initiative. If the words are accompanied by a tone of voice and body language that confirm "I really mean this," the message will have impact. If the body language suggests that the leader is merely mouthing the words, nothing will happen. (The reader might want to review the parable "The Voice of the City" in Chapter 5 to reinforce this point.)

Observations from the Bleachers

We would be remiss if we did not offer some early observations from where we sit in the bleachers. Many healthcare organizations already have pockets within which they operate as ACOs. Care is integrated and quality is market leading or even benchmark. Costs are well managed. And patients are very satisfied. In brief, many delivery systems have pockets of "compartmentalized ACOs" already operating within them, albeit without CMS shared-savings contracts as financial incentives. Most often, these small pockets have been developed by committed teams of clinicians and administrators who operate as small pilots within a large system, or they have evolved on their own with no greater ulterior motive than to deliver better care. Unfortunately, many health system leaders point to these microsystems as evidence that they are ready to "bring on" the ACO. They are surprised to learn how difficult it is to export the "skunkworks" operation into another clinical microsystem or to fully scale it up across the entire system of care.

A compartmentalized ACO is certainly proof of the concept that such a model can work within one's healthcare system. But its presence should not falsely reassure leadership that a broader initiative across a population of patients will be easy or will necessarily prove successful. Certainly, many successful enterprises began as skunk works in somebody's garage; most innovative skunk works, however, do not develop into highly successful enterprises.

As noted repeatedly throughout this book, the ACO is not for everyone. Furthermore, each organization's model will be unique to that organization. Delivery systems that try to emulate Kaiser Permanente, Mayo, or Geisinger are almost certainly doomed to fail. Those organizations are highly evolved, reflecting what each has been doing for years. They have developed organically. In addition, virtually all the successful integrated delivery systems in America share a common DNA: They all began as multispecialty group practices. The addition of hospitals (and even health plans) to the system came well into their development. Most of today's emerging integrated systems are being initiated by hospitals or hospital systems attempting to generate group practices in today's competitive, reimbursement, and compliance environment from a patchwork of individual practices. This is a much more formidable task.

Instead, each organization should take stock of its strengths and vulnerabilities and should initiate its model around its strengths. Use the deep dive assessment findings to draw a road map for expanding strengths and overcoming vulnerabilities. Some organizations plan to introduce bundled payment strategies as their first foray into accountable care. Others are planning to expand pay-for-performance reimbursement models before contracting as an ACO. Others are simply trying to eke out better margins by focusing on operational efficiencies and outcomes improvement without any short-term intentions of contracting as ACOs. All are reasonable approaches and are "forward compatible" with an ACO strategy, because all will lead to the acquisition of the five-and-a-half core ACO competencies (see Chapter 2). All are good places to start.

Over the next two years, we intend to chronicle the experience of the ACO innovators and capture the learning from the early adopters. Those will be reported over time. We fully appreciate that by the time this book is available to readers, some policies will have been further clarified, others modified, and still others created or eliminated. During the period of time from inception to publication of this book, much has changed; such is the course of innovation. We regret if any information contained herein has become obsolete simply by the rapid movement within the industry and the government to adopt the ACO strategy.

The ACO is not *the* answer to America's healthcare crisis. But it is a reasonable contribution to a big and complicated set of problems facing our nation. It is a reasonable experiment based on rational objectives, sound principles, and supportable foundations. Those who approach this as an experiment in service delivery and reimbursement will certainly derive some benefit from the model, as will their patients. Innovation, experimentation, and trial and error are, after all, the American way. But over history, most of the innovators have been individuals or small teams of people that have enjoyed the luxury of being able to more or less promote their inventive spirits in isolation from other activities. Healthcare is different. There will be no practices and rehearsals. Providing healthcare is always "show time."

The ACO experiment has had the benefit of some of America's most thoughtful innovators and leaders. This book has been developed on their broad and capable shoulders. Some elements will work; some will fail. Our goal in writing this book was to extract more than 50 years of consulting observations to help organizations succeed well and fail well. There is a lot we will all learn from some noble failures. But as those failures become manifest, what will clearly differentiate the real healthcare reform leaders is their ability to integrate the learning and apply it to the next phase of experimentation. Some of us will join the experiment as clinical providers; others as delivery system managers; others as observers, advisors, and coaches; still others as payer partners; and many as patients. Each of us has a role to play in this drama.

As for us, we are grateful to have had the opportunity to span careers in which we participated in the healthcare experiment of the 1970s called the HMO and are now able to participate in the experiment called the ACO. Both experiments come from the same need, the same desire, and the same spirit.

Fortunately, for CHA, a Temporary Reprieve

In early October 2010 the Obama administration agreed to a plan to infuse $435 million into Massachusetts hospitals (Kowalczyk 2010). Most of that was targeted to the state's two largest safety net hospitals. CHA (discussed in Chapter 1) was slated to receive $163 million in extra federal Medicaid funding. It was a reprieve, but the battle wasn't over.

As part of the agreement with the Obama administration, the hospitals, including CHA, had to begin their transition away from fee for service and toward a new, but undetermined, payment system. "This gives us time," says Dennis Keefe, CHA's chief executive officer. "We can continue what we've been doing, trying to position ourselves for payment reform."

For Keefe, and for the rest of the US healthcare system, this is game time.

References

Chapter 1

Blue Cross Blue Shield of Massachusetts. 2010. "Our History." [Online document; retrieved 8/19/10.] www.bluecrossma.com/visitor/about-us/our-history.html.

Commonwealth Fund. 2010a. "2007 Commonwealth Fund Biennial Health Insurance Survey." [Online information; retrieved 7/27/10.] www.commonwealthfund.org/Content/Surveys/2007/2007-Commonwealth-Fund-Biennial-Health-Insurance-Survey.aspx.

———. 2010b. "2009 Commonwealth Fund International Health Policy Survey." [Online information; retrieved 7/15/10.] www.commonwealthfund.org/Content/Surveys/2009/Nov/2009-Commonwealth-Fund-International-Health-Policy-Survey.aspx008.

Gawande, A. 2009. "The Cost Conundrum." *The New Yorker*, June 1.

Harry S. Truman Presidential Library. n.d. "President Truman's Proposed Health Plan." [Online article; retrieved 8/11/10.] www.trumanlibrary.org/anniversaries/healthprogram.htm.

Krugman, P., and R. Wells. 2006. "The Health Care Crisis and What to Do About It." *New York Review of Books*, March 23.

Lagoe, R., D. L. Aspling, and G. P. Westert. 2005. "Current and Future Developments in Managed Care in the United States and Implications for Europe." *Health Research Policy and Systems* 3 (1): 4.

Oberlander, J., and T. R. Marmor. 2010. "The Health Bill Explained at Last." *New York Review of Books*, August 19.

Organisation for Economic Co-operation and Development (OECD). 2010. "OECD Health Data 2010: Statistics and Indicators." [Online information; retrieved 6/1/10.] www.oecd.org/document/30/0,3343,en_2649_37407_12968734_1_1_1_37407,00. html.

US Census Bureau, 2010. "Income, Poverty and Health Insurance coverage in the United States: 2009." [Online document; retrieved 9/29/10] www.census.gov/ newsroom/releases/archives/income_wealth/cb10-144.html.

Chapter 2

Anderson, G., P. Hussey, B. Frogner, and H. Waters. 2005. "Health Spending in the United States and the Rest of the Industrialized World." *Health Affairs*, 24 (4): 903–14.

Berwick, D. 2010. "Workshop Regarding Accountable Care Organizations, and Implications Regarding Antitrust, Physician Self-Referral, Anti-Kickback, and Civil Monetary Penalty Laws." Transcript of meeting sponsored by the Office of Inspector General, Department of Health and Human Services, 10/5/10. [Online information; retrieved 12/28/10.] http://oig.hhs.gov/fraud/docs/workshop/10-5-10 ACO-WorkshopAMSessionTranscript.pdf.

Crichton, M. 1995. *The Lost World*. New York: Alfred A. Knopf.

Gawande, A. 2009. "Getting There from Here." *The New Yorker*, January 26.

———. 2007. "The Checklist." *The New Yorker*, December 10.

Hanna, D. P. 1988. *Designing Organizations for High Performance*. Upper Saddle River, NJ: FT Press.

Institute of Medicine. 2001. *Crossing the Quality Chasm: A New Health System for the 21st Century*. Washington, DC: National Academies Press.

McClellan, M., A. McKethan, J. Lewis, J. Roski, and E. Fisher. 2010. "A National Strategy to Put Accountable Care into Practice." *Health Affairs* 29 (5); 982–90.

Organisation for Economic Co-operation and Development (OECD). 2010. "OECD Health Data 2010: Statistics and Indicators." [Online information; retrieved 6/1/10.] www.oecd.org/document/30/0,3343,en_2649_37407_12968734_1_1_1_37407,00. html.

Patient Protection and Affordable Care Act of 2010. [Online information; retrieved 8/1/10.] http://democrats.senate.gov/reform/.

Reid, T. R. 2009. *The Healing of America: A Global Quest for Better, Cheaper, and Fairer Health Care*, 1st ed. New York: Penguin Press.

Rich, J. 2010. Personal e-mail with the author. October 3.

Rittenhouse, D. R., S. M. Shortell, and E. S. Fisher. 2009. "Primary Care and Accountable Care: Two Essential Elements of Delivery-System Reform." *New England Journal of Medicine*, October 28 (published online).

Skinner, J., and E. Fisher. 2010. "Reflections on Geographic Variations in U.S. Health Care." The Dartmouth Institute for Health Policy & Clinical Practice. [Online information; retrieved 12/28/10.] www.dartmouthatlas.org/downloads/press/ Skinner_Fisher_DA_05_10.pdf.

Chapter 3

Detroit Medical Center (DMC) Board of Managers. 2010. Memo to DMC physicians titled "An Update for DMC Physicians." September 7.

Chapter 4

Bard, M. 1990. Personal conversation with urologist at Denver conference.

Newton, D. A., and M. S. Grayson. 2003. "Trends in Career Choice by US Medical School Graduates." *JAMA* 290 (9): 1179–82.

Chapter 5

Berwick, D. 2010. "Workshop Regarding Accountable Care Organizations, and Implications Regarding Antitrust, Physician Self-Referral, Anti-Kickback, and Civil Monetary Penalty Laws." Transcript of meeting sponsored by the Office of Inspector General, Department of Health and Human Services, 10/5/10. [Online information; retrieved 12/28/10.] http://oig.hhs.gov/fraud/docs/workshop/10-5-10 ACO-WorkshopAMSessionTranscript.pdf.

Hanna, D. P. 1988. *Designing Organizations for High Performance*. Upper Saddle River, NJ: FT Press.

Reid, T. R. 2009. *The Healing of America: A Global Quest for Better, Cheaper, and Fairer Health Care*. New York: Penguin Press.

Chapter 6

Barrette, K. 2010. Interview with the author.

Centers for Disease Control and Prevention (CDC). 2010. "Electronic Medical Record/Electronic Health Record Systems of Office-Based Physicians: United States, 2009 and Preliminary 2010 State Estimates." [Online document, retrieved 2/4/11.] www.cdc.gov/nchs/data/hestat/emr_ehr_09/emr_ehr_09.htm.

Centers for Medicaid & Medicare Services (CMS). 2010. "Medicare & Medicaid EHR Incentive Program. Meaningful Use Stage 1 Requirements Overview." [Online document; retrieved 10/15/10.] www.cms.gov/EHRIncentivePrograms/30_Meaningful_Use.asp#TopOfPage.

Harris, C. M. 2010. Interview with the author. November 2.

Healthcare Finance News. 2010. "Summit: ACO Success Tied to EHR, HIE Capabilities." [Online article; retrieved 10/21/10.] www.healthcarefinancenews.com/news/summit-aco-success-tied-ehr-hie-capabilities.

Healthcare Financial Management Association (HFMA). n.d. "Healthcare Financial Pulse: Improving Performance, Leading Change." [Online information; retrieved 10/21/10.] www.hfma.org/pulse.

Healthcare Information and Management Systems Society. 2003. "Electronic Health Record Definitional Model Version 1.0." [Online information; retrieved 10/16/10.] www.himss.org/content/files/ehrattributes070703.pdf.

Hedges, D. 2010. Interview with the author.

Hsiao, C. J., P. C. Beatty, E. S. Hing, D. A. Woodwell, E. A. Rechsteiner, and J. E. Sisk. 2008. "Electronic Medical Record/Electronic Health Record Use by Office-based Physicians: United States, 2008 and Preliminary 2009." [Online information; retrieved 10/18/10.] www.cdc.gov/nchs/data/hestat/emr_ehr/emr_ehr.htm.

National Committee for Quality Assurance. 2010. "NCQA 2011 ACO Criteria." [Online article; retrieved 10/21/10/.] www.ncqa.org/tabid/1266/Default.aspx.

Rothenhaus, T. 2010. Interview with author.

Tripathi, M. 2010. Interview with author.

Chapter 7

Aon. 2010. "U.S. Health Care Increases Reach Highest Levels in Five Years, According to New Data from Hewitt Associates." [Online information; retrieved 2/9/11.] http://aon.mediaroom.com/index.php?s=114&item=89.

Bazzoli, G. J., R. C. Lindrooth, R. Hasnain-Wynia, and J. Needleman. 2004. "The Balanced Budget Act of 1997 and U.S. Hospital Operations." *Inquiry* 41 (4): 401–17.

Carlson, J. 2010. "Booster Shot: Despite a Shortfall in Patient-Care Revenue for the Past 25 Years, Hospitals Turned a Profit Thanks to Investments and Other Revenue." *Modern Healthcare.* August 2.

Feldstein, P. J. 1988. *Health Care Economics*, 3rd ed., 252–97. Hoboken, NJ: John Wiley & Sons.

Healthcare Financial Management Association (HFMA). n.d. "Healthcare Financial Pulse: Improving Performance, Leading Change." [Online information; retrieved 2/10/11.] www.hfma.org/pulse.

Kaiser Family Foundation. 2010. "Employer Health Benefits 2010 Annual Survey." [Online information; retrieved 2/10/11.] http://ehbs.kff.org/?page=charts&id=1&sn =13&ch=1578.

Nowicki, M. 2007. *The Financial Management of Hospitals and Healthcare Organizations*, 4th ed. Chicago: Health Administration Press.

Nugent, M. 2004. "The Price Is Right." *Healthcare Financial Management Magazine*, December.

US Department of Health and Human Services (USDHHS). 2010. "Expenditures for Purchases of Prescription Drugs by Geographic Division and State and Average Annual Percent Growth." National Center for Health Statistics.

Chapter 8

Rich, J. 2010. Personal e-mail with the author. October 3.

Chapter 9

Harris, G. 2010. "Obama to Bypass Senate to Name Health Official." *The New York Times*, July 8.

Mehrabian, A. 1971. *Silent Messages*, 1st ed. Belmont, CA: Wadsworth.

Chapter 10

Kowalczyk, L. 2010. "US Offers Lifeline to Massachusetts Hospitals." *Boston Globe*, October 2, p. 1.

Mehrabian, A. 1971. *Silent Messages*, 1st ed. Belmont, CA: Wadsworth.

Index

ARRA. *See* American Recovery and
Reinvestment Act
Associative power, 156
Athos, Anthony, 177
Autonomy, 103, 106
Avoidable costs, 59, 61

Balanced Budget Act of 1997, 241
Barrette, Kenneth, 210
Bayer, Allison, 16-17, 26
Baylor University Hospital, 9
Behavioral health, 14
Bending the trend, 47, 48
Berwick, Donald M., 62, 188, 334
Bethune, Gordon, 150
Bigby, Judy Ann, 15
Billings Clinic demonstration project,
45
Blue Cross/Blue Shield, 9, 10
Body language, 367-368
Boehner, John, 3, 22
Boudrow, Gordon, 16
Brookings-Dartmouth ACO Collabora-
tive, 45
Bundled arrangement, 59-61
Business case, 322-323
Business plan, 287-288

Cambridge Health Alliance (CHA)
    ACO model, 26, 160
    cost-cutting measures, 23-26
    financial reprieve, 371
    Medicaid patients, 14
    9C cuts, 15-16
    reimbursement issues, 25
    uncompensated care, 14-17
    uninsured patients, 13-14
Cambridge Hospital, 13

Cambridge Public Health Commission,
    13
Capital budget, 226
Capital planning, 230-231
Capital sources, 255
Capitation
    gaps, 239-240
    revisits, 25
    risk management, 118
    risk tolerance, 60-61
Care coordination, 109-110, 137
Care coordinator
    clinical specialty, 139
    subspecialty, 140-141
    task force role, 149
    tasks, 140
Care delivery
    management of, 118
    physiology, 119-136
    requirement model, 119
    silo model, 119
Care design
    care pathway, 148-152
    by committee, 149
    80/20 rule, 150
    evaluation, 149-150
    exceptions, 150-151
    modeling, 338-342
    patient cohort, 123-126
    standardization,151-152
    task force, 149-150
Care integration
    foundational work, 308-309
    innovation, 31-32
    level 1 readiness, 293
    level 2/3/4 readiness, 298-299
    level 5 readiness, 302-303
    physician alignment, 51
Care management
    system, 216, 363
    tools, 217

Middlesex Health System demonstration project, 45
Minor/major illness cohort, 257
Motivation-hygiene theory, 189
Multispecialty group practice, 95
Multispecialty group practice model, 79
Multispecialty group practice physician organization model, 146, 147
Murray, Therese, 25

National Committee for Quality Assurance (NCQA)
 ACO standards, 209
 quality-measure recommendations, 44-45
Navigator, 138-139
NCQA. *See* National Committee for Quality Assurance
Network Health, 26
Nixon, Richard, 20
Non-self-limited illness, 122

Obama, Barack, 20, 22
Oberlander, Jonathan, 22
Observations, 368-370
OECD. *See* Organization for Economic Co-operation and Development
Operating budget, 102, 226
Operating division model, 86-88, 90
Operational excellence
 core competency, 50
 foundational work, 302-303
 level 1 readiness, 293
 level 2/3/4 readiness, 296-298
 level 5 readiness, 302
Operational phase, 352-353
Operations
 clinical structure, 112-113

integrated councils, 112-113
organization of, 112-114
Organization for Economic Co-operation and Development (OECD), 21-22
Organizational activities, 279-280
Organizational behavior, 48-49
Organizational culture, 156
Organizational design, 134-135
Organizational stress test, 323-325
Organizational structure, 361-362
Organizational transparency, 187
Overutilization, 8, 47

P4P. *See* Pay-for-performance
Paired management teams, 128-129
Parent corporation model, 84-85, 90
Park Nicollet Health Network demonstration project, 45
Path dependence, 34
Patient
 cost shifting, 228
 education, 346
 health management tools, 217
 information portals, 217
Patient cohort
 array of, 256-257
 care design, 123-126
 categorization, 121-123
 transition, 124
 registries, 54
 retention, 54-56
Patient Protection and Affordable Care Act (PPACA)
 accomplishment, 359
 ACO under, 29, 36-40, 225-226, 357
 contracting provisions, 227
 implementation, 22, 23
 Medicare ACO, 72
 multiple ACO affiliation, 143

Well-patient cohort, 256-257

Wells, Robin, 18

Whidden Memorial Hospi9tal, 13

Wisdom of the River parable, 178-180

Work groups

  decision making, 135-136

  function of, 135-136

  purpose of, 135

Wright, Will, 167

Acknowledgments

This book was made possible by the generosity of Navigant Consulting and in particular by the insight and wisdom of David Zito, Navigant's healthcare practice leader, who supported the value of this effort and showed confidence in the authors. Erin Bowler has offered tireless assistance and support throughout this endeavor. Jeffrey Krasner has been an invaluable resource, partner, confidant, and friend throughout and the authors owe an enormous debt of gratitude for his expertise, good humor, patience, and support.

On a more personal note, I would like to acknowledge a number of people upon whose shoulders this book has been created. In chronological order, I want to acknowledge the late "Uncle" Cliff Barger, my medical school advisor, coach, surrogate parent, and strongest advocate. Second is Ronald Arky, MD, forever my Chief, who supported the unconventional and provided me with my start. James Sabin, MD, believed in me and supported me in the best job I will ever have. My outstanding professional colleagues at Harvard Community Health Plan (particularly my Wellesley partners) taught me what accountability, teamwork, and organization really mean in practice. The late Anthony Athos of Harvard Business School mentored this young physician when I desperately sought insights into leadership. I found them in Tony. Howard Anderson suggested I become a consultant and changed my life, after which Ted Scott taught me how to be a consultant. Thirty years of supportive clients have given me opportunity and experience: I am grateful to every client who showed the confidence to allow me to enter his or her organization. And of course I extend continued appreciation to my clinical and consulting partner, Andy Epstein, who has been by my side for the past 30 years, along with my alter ego Kristen Jacob, without whom I would be figuratively and quite literally lost.

But of course the real gratitude goes to my bride, Carol, who has both created and supported my passions for over 40 years, and to my children Lisa and Wilton, and Jaime and Jon, who have endured my shortcomings and my long-goings and taught me so much about myself. I am indebted to my furry running partner Jake for whom I always aspire to be the person he thinks I am. And, of course, I give thanks for our dear grandchildren Joshua and Benjamin, who have brought us spirit and hope for the future. Finally, let me express deep gratitude to my recently departed parents, Lillian and Bernard Bard, whose inspiration and imprint are evidenced throughout this book.

Marc Bard
Squam Lake
New Hampshire

I wish to thank several colleagues for their mentorship over the years, including Marc Bard, David Burik, Marty Finkler, Cliff Frank, Dieter Hausmann, Donna Kinzer, Casey Nolan, and MarieAnn North, to name a few—not to mention the hard work and dedication of our broader Payment Transformation team. I also wish to thank our clients for letting our team be a part of their daily pursuit of a higher-quality, lower-cost healthcare system. My biggest thank-you goes to Judy, Ryan, and Katie for their support, inspiration, and sacrifices. Together, we're making a positive difference on Main Street America.

Mike Nugent

About the Contributor

Charles R. Buck is a partner in the law firm of McDermott Will & Emery LLP and is based in the firm's Boston office. He is a member of the health practice group and focuses his practice on complex transactions and regulatory compliance. Mr. Buck represents a wide range of clients, including proprietary and tax-exempt hospital systems, academic medical centers and faculty practice groups, pharmaceutical companies, and HMOs and other health insurers. He routinely provides regulatory and transactional representation to such clients in connection with acquisitions, joint ventures, strategic affiliations, conversions to tax-exempt status, and other transactional matters. He is a graduate of Stanford Law School.

About the Authors

Dr. Marc Bard

Dr. Marc Bard, chief innovation officer in Navigant's Healthcare practice, is a nationally regarded expert on physician leadership effectiveness, change management, and organizational design. Dr. Bard is a board-certified internist who now serves as a strategy and leadership consultant. He consults with leading academic medical centers, faculty practices, medical groups, community hospitals, and individual healthcare executives, focusing on physician integration and clinical program strategies as well as performance improvement.

Dr. Bard practiced internal medicine for 18 years at Harvard Community Health Plan (HCHP)—one of the first staff-model HMOs—and served as that organization's chief of internal medicine and director of medical staff development. Dr. Bard oversaw HCHP through mergers with MultiGroup and Pilgrim Health Care, which eventually transformed it into Harvard Pilgrim Health Care. His role in integrating HCHP's employed-physician model with MultiGroup's and Pilgrim's disparate structures gave Dr. Bard unique insight into the relationships between physicians and organizations. In 1997, he founded The Bard Group, LLC, which consults with hospitals, health systems, medical practice groups, and academic health centers to implement organizational change-creating new physician organizations and relationships that promote operational, clinical, and financial improvement.

Michael Nugent

Michael Nugent is managing director and leader of Navigant's Payment Transformation, Managed Care & Pricing Team. With nearly 20 years in the healthcare payer and provider industry, Mr. Nugent is an expert and a nationally recognized writer, speaker, and advisor in the area of pricing, managed care contracting strategy, negotiations, and front-end revenue cycle innovations.

Mr. Nugent has advised a wide range of healthcare payers, providers, and manufacturers on corporate strategy, reimbursement, product, and operational matters. Mr. Nugent and his team have repriced over $40 billion in hospital charges and have designed and implemented myriad shared-risk programs, tiered networks, pay-for-performance programs, and money-back guarantees for some of the nation's top payers, providers, and manufacturers. Mr. Nugent is one of the lead architects of Navigant Consulting's *NextGeneration* Pricing and Managed Care Toolkit, which is used by payers and providers to benchmark and establish rates in partnership with one another. He has undergraduate degrees in mathematics and economics and an MBA from Northwestern University Kellogg School of Management.